Prosthodontics at a Glance

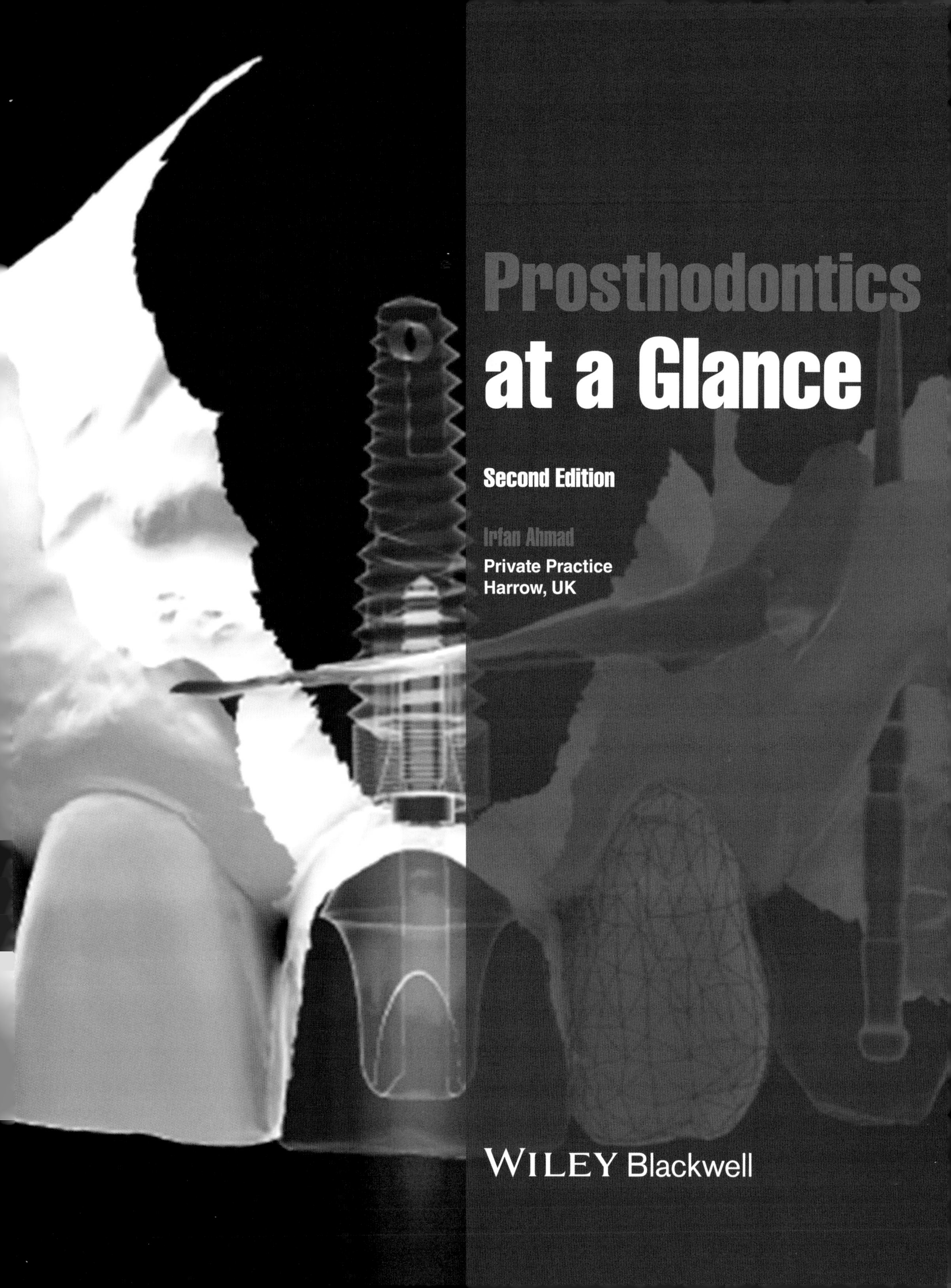

Prosthodontics at a Glance

Second Edition

Irfan Ahmad
Private Practice
Harrow, UK

WILEY Blackwell

This edition first published 2022

Edition History
Blackwell Publishing Ltd. (1e, 2012)

Registered Offices
John Wiley & Sons, Inc., 111 River Street, Hoboken, NJ 07030, USA
John Wiley & Sons Ltd, The Atrium, Southern Gate, Chichester, West Sussex, PO19 8SQ, UK

Editorial Office
9600 Garsington Road, Oxford, OX4 2DQ, UK

For details of our global editorial offices, customer services, and more information about Wiley products visit us at www.wiley.com.
Wiley also publishes its books in a variety of electronic formats and by print-on-demand. Some content that appears in standard print versions of this book may not be available in other formats.

Library of Congress Cataloging-in-Publication Data

Names: Ahmad, Irfan, BDS, author.
Title: Prosthodontics at a glance / Irfan Ahmad.
Other titles: At a glance series (Oxford, England)
Description: Second edition. | Hoboken : Wiley, 2022. | Series: At a glance | Includes index.
Identifiers: LCCN 2021027289 (print) | LCCN 2021027290 (ebook) | ISBN 9781119749721 (paperback) | ISBN 9781119749752 (adobe pdf) | ISBN 9781119749745 (epub)
Subjects: MESH: Prosthodontics–methods | Oral Surgical Procedures, Preprosthetic
Classification: LCC RK651 (print) | LCC RK651 (ebook) | NLM WU 500 | DDC 617.6/9–dc23
LC record available at https://lccn.loc.gov/2021027289
LC ebook record available at https://lccn.loc.gov/2021027290

Cover Design: Wiley
Cover Image: Courtesy of Irfan Ahmad

Set in 9.5/11.5pt Minion by Straive, Pondicherry, India

Printed in Singapore
M112690_011121

'There are no facts, only interpretations' (Nietzsche)

To my children Zayan and Zaina

Contents

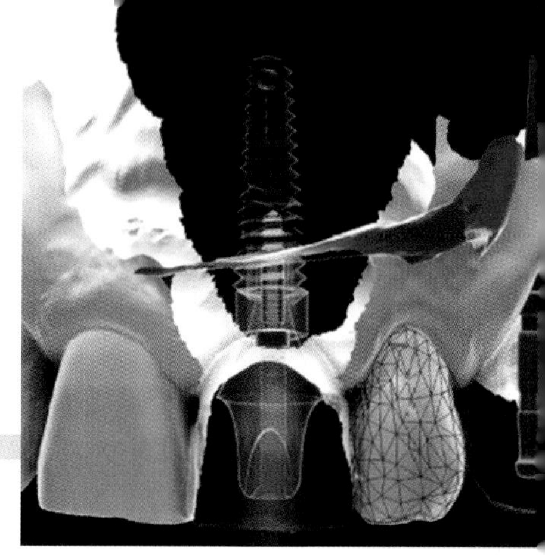

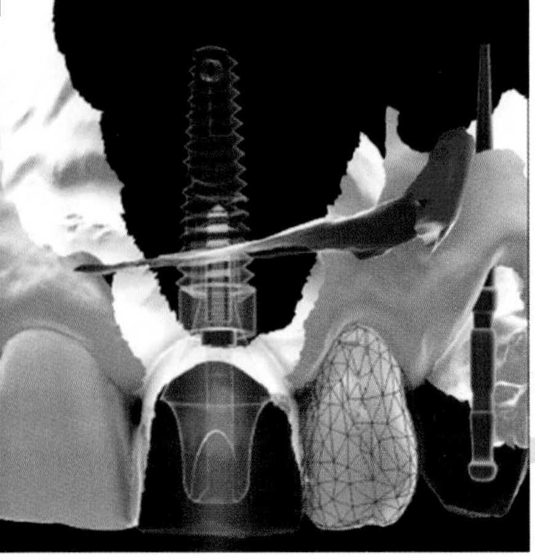

Foreword

'*There is nothing new in art except talent*' (Chekhov).

There is nothing new in dentistry except talent and technique.

Technique is a sign of progress and anyone can learn it, but it is fleeting and constantly evolving. Talent . . . you have it or you don't and it only reveals itself through the grace of technique.

The most perfect techniques are the ones you don't notice. They integrate biologically, functionally, and æsthetically into their environment. This book will guide you through continuous learning of the techniques necessary for successful dental rehabilitations at each step of the way.

With concise text, openness to the future, and beautiful presentation, this book will charm you and be your guide on the path to excellence. Talent is also mastery of technique and accumulation of knowledge.

Without it, nothing remains.

Dr. Claude R. Rufenacht

Preface to the second edition

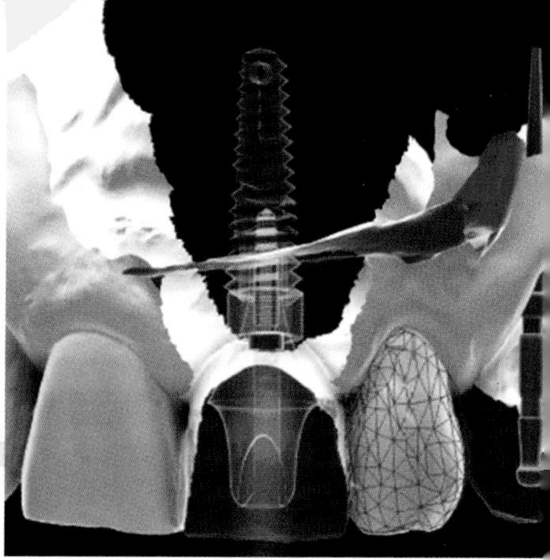

Progress is innovation shaped by intelligence.

There are two aspects that warrant highlighting since the publication of the first edition of *Prosthodontics at a Glance*. First, the ineludible surge in digital dentistry. Few would question that digital procedures are irrevocably redefining the way dentistry is practised, and will be practised in the future. Digital dentistry is the zeitgeist of our times, inexorably rife in nearly every laboratory and clinical protocol. Today, indirect restorations fabricated by CAM/CAM technology are an established protocol, digital impressions are becoming commonplace, and 3D printed surgical guides designed using CBCT and intra-oral scans are the standard of care for placing dental implants. What was once in posse is now in esse. Hence, the digital leitmotif is prevalent throughout this edition.

New technology is either embraced with enthusiasm, viewed with skepticism, or blatantly rejected because of inertia to change from tried and tested methods. Technophiles readily espouse new advances with blind faith, but ignoring the absence of evidence is the basis of true faith.[1] Conversely, technophobes vacillate, awaiting scientific validation or are reluctant to upset the status quo. Besides dedicating time to learn 'new tricks', digital protocols require a new vocabulary, much of which seems arcane and perplexing, and therefore, prolongs dismissal. Moreover, there is nothing more taxing than to unlearn what has always been taken for granted, '*You must empty your cup before it can accept anything new*' (Zen Proverb).

Irrespective of whether or not one is a votary of digital dentistry, there is considerable verisimilitude that digital applications can, and do, eliminate quotidian tasks. For example, laboratory processes of pouring impressions, trimming dies, waxing, investing, and casting are replaced entirely by digital workflows. And in the clinic, who wouldn't trade the oral claustrophobia of tray impressions for the comfort and sophistication of digital impressions? Technology offers efficiency, expediency, job satisfaction, patient friendliness, and improves the delivery of healthcare. But at what price? Of course in the short-term everything is hunky dory, but many dental materials and devices have come and gone, and their demise is usually attributed to mid or long-term failure. Is digital dentistry another fly-by-night phenomenon? Only time will tell. However, judging by the pace at which technology is overwhelming our lives from multitasking mobile phones to auto-driving cars, the answer is possibly just around the corner. In the meantime, digital dentistry is currently a pluralism, commingling with, and complementing conventional analogue procedures.

The second aspect to emphasise is that prosthodontics is not an island speciality. It relies heavily, as do other multifarious disciplines, on a collaborative approach. A truism often overlooked. Dental specialities are categorised according to specific disciplines, and the greater the specialisation, the narrower the scope of application. Unfortunately, a deeper knowledge about a particular subject can sometimes obscure the bigger picture, i.e. the patient, who after all is the ultimate beneficiary of research and translational medicine. Therefore, several chapters of this edition are devoted to satellite topics that transgress the prosthodontic envelope in order to offer a multifaceted understanding, which is essential to build the bigger picture.

Every chapter of the first edition has been redesigned, and where necessary, the accompanying illustrations and text updated to reflect current scientific and clinical advances. Furthermore, the additional 25 chapters deliver a more comprehensive manuscript, for example, the Ethics chapter reconsiders the apocryphal belief that cosmetic dentistry enhances the quality of life, as well as emerging fields permeating dentistry such as artificial intelligence (AI), 3D printing, and the apogee of regenerative medicine represented by tissue engineering and stem cells. These topics contain pertinent material for both the seasoned and neophyte prosthodontist to expand knowledge base, keep abreast of salient breakthroughs, refine clinical techniques or simply stimulate discussion. In spite of the voluminous upgrade, the reductionistic ethos of the '*at a Glance*' series remains the same, represented by succinct and readily digestible bitesize information.

Similar to its predecessor, this second edition endeavours to spark both active and passive learning as part of a poly-didactic eduction that incorporates autodidacticism or self-learning, combined with formal didactic education and hand-on courses. Hence, the keywords and concepts presented in each chapter act as springboards for further learning, or exploring specific topics using a variety of media, including the omniscient, omnipresent (and perhaps omnipotent) 'University of Google'. However, it is worth remembering that clinical techniques need to be acquired by experience rather than merely derived from principle.

It goes without saying that no one can prefigure what lies ahead for dentistry in the coming years, but the recent pandemic has taught us it will be neoteric to what we have been practising in the past: renascent dental care.

Irfan Ahmad
21 February 2021

Note

1. Vidal G. Pink triangle and yellow star. Essays 1952-1992. Random House: New York, 1993.

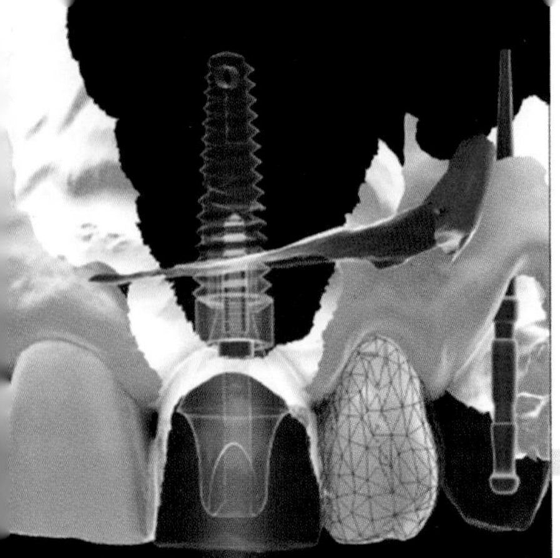

Preface to the first edition

In a Utopian context, a tooth should survive throughout life, unscathed by disease or trauma. However, in the real world, a tooth endures vicissitudes, often necessitating clinical intervention for ensuring its viability. Assuming a pessimistic stance, from nascence to its final demise, a tooth may undergo the following pathological sequelae: incipient fissure or proximal caries, intracoronal decay, pronounced multi-surface caries, endodontic involvement, extracoronal restoration, intra- and periradicular compromises with or without periodontal involvement leading to extraction, and eventual replacement by either a denture (removable or fixed) or dental implants. On an optimistic note, it is not a fait accompli that these events are inevitable; clinical intervention at any stage can prevent progression to the next, more destructive, eventuality. All these aforementioned stages require some form of clinical intervention for salvaging or replacing lost teeth. This is the basic premise of prosthodontics.

Prosthodontics is defined as restoring and/or replacing missing teeth. At times, the line dividing restorative dentistry and prosthodontics can be vague. As a generality, restorative dentistry is concerned with restoring teeth directly, involving a single visit, while prosthodontics is restoring or replacing teeth indirectly, invariably involving multiple visits, usually with impression and employing a dental laboratory. Furthermore, prosthodontics is a multidisciplinary subject, involving specialties such as periodontics, endodontics, orthodontics, implantology and oral surgery.

Besides resolving pathology, another factor requiring consideration is vanity. In an ever-increasing appearance-conscious society, elective cosmetic dental treatment is burgeoning. Although, at times, this type of treatment may be questionable, the communication revolution has created immense patient awareness leading to an escalating demand for patient-driven treatment planning. Hence, cosmetic or aesthetic treatment is now a major part of prosthodontics.

The purpose of this book is to describe the main concepts of prosthodontics. Its aim is to act as a platform for further reading on a chosen aspect of prosthodontics. The ordered format of the 'At a Glance' series accelerates learning, ensures relevance to daily clinical practice, and avoids the tedium and frustration of a verbose text.

Irfan Ahmad

Acknowledgements

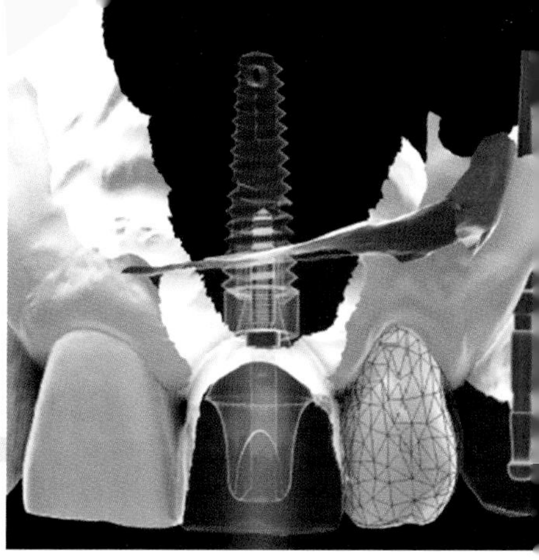

I would like to thank my dear friends Claude Rufenacht et Madame for their continuing support and encouragement, which is an imperishable source of strength and affirmation. A special thanks to Nik Bärtsch for his hypnotic and transcendental music that not only elevates the soul, but actuates creativity and inspiration. And my fidus Achates Manuela Brusoni for always being there – Ciao Manuela!

Finally, a big thank you to the team at Wiley-Blackwell for making this project a reality.

Overview of prosthodontics

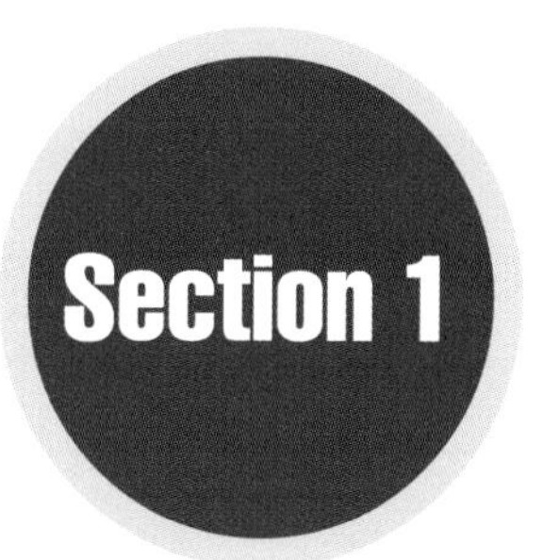

Chapters

1 Overview: rehabilitation of natural teeth

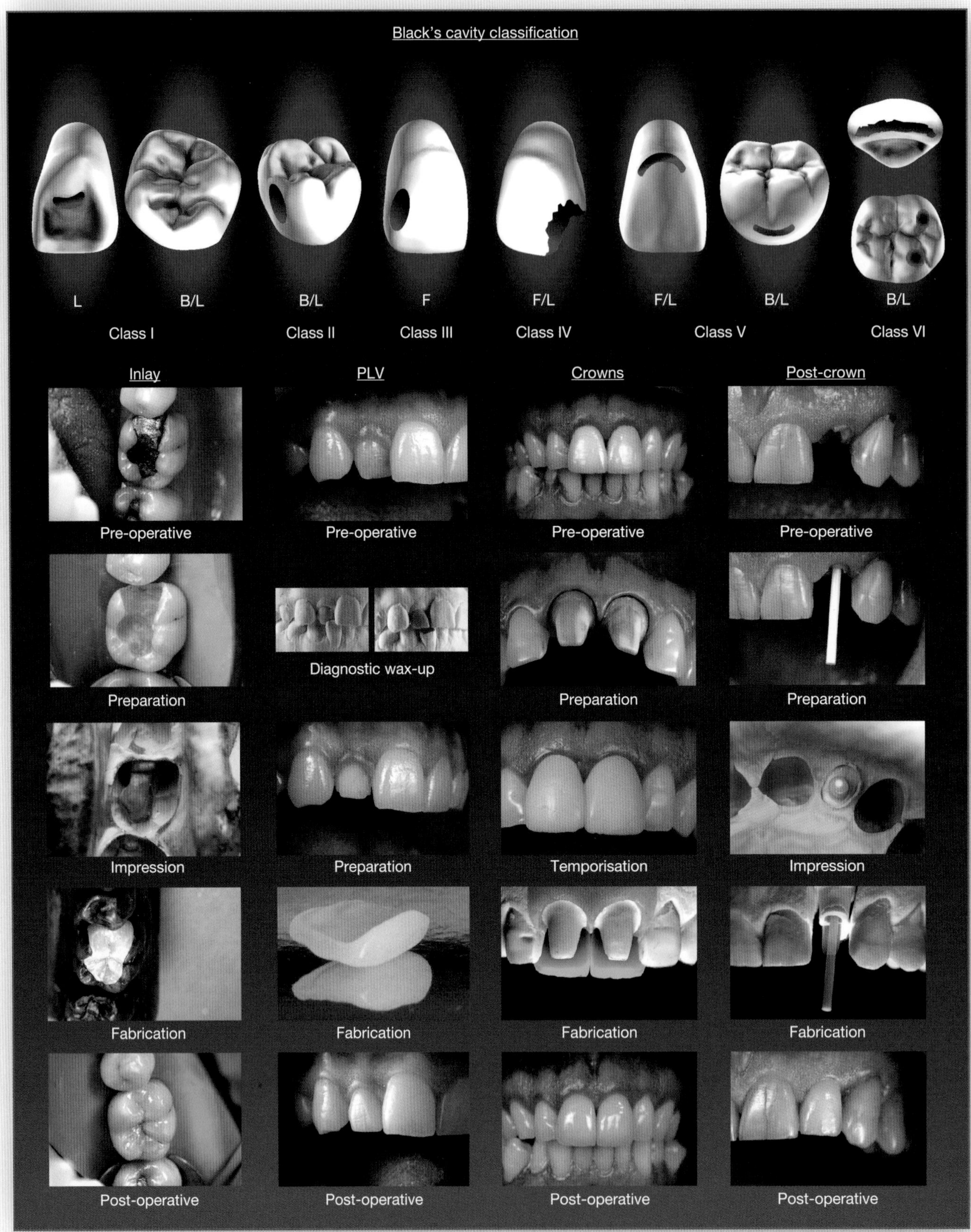

Black's cavity classification

L | B/L — Class I

B/L — Class II

F — Class III

F/L — Class IV

F/L | B/L — Class V

B/L — Class VI

Inlay: Pre-operative, Preparation, Impression, Fabrication, Post-operative

PLV: Pre-operative, Diagnostic wax-up, Preparation, Fabrication, Post-operative

Crowns: Pre-operative, Preparation, Temporisation, Fabrication, Post-operative

Post-crown: Pre-operative, Preparation, Impression, Fabrication, Post-operative

An **indirect restoration** requires taking an impression and employing a dental laboratory to fabricate the prosthesis. Conversely, a **direct restoration** is carried out chairside, usually in a single visit, without using a dental laboratory. Indirect dental prostheses can either be **intracoronal** or **extracoronal**.

Indirect intracoronal prostheses

Intracoronal prostheses are defined as those **surrounded** by one or more natural tooth surface(s). This categorisation is broadly based on **Black's cavity classification**:

- **Class I**: lesions of pits and fissures of all teeth, predominantly in premolars and molars
- **Class II**: lesions on the proximal (mesial or distal) surfaces of posterior teeth, and the restorative cavities are referred to as MO (mesial-occlusal), DO (disto-occlusal) and MOD (mesial-occlusal-distal)
- **Class III**: lesion in the anterior teeth, similar to a class II lesion, the class III lesion typically appears at the contact areas
- **Class IV:** the class IV lesion is a class III lesion, including the incisal corner of an anterior tooth
- **Class V**: typically occurs at the cervical margins on the buccal or lingual aspect of any tooth
- **Class VI**: not originally in Black's classification, but has become accepted as an additional lesion that occurs on the tips and cusps of posterior teeth, or along the biting surfaces of the incisors due to wear (tooth surface loss –TSL)

Three developments have made Black's cavity classification redundant. First, research has elucidated biological mechanisms such as **demineralisation/remineralisation** and the role of fluoride ion, and therefore, removal of infected and affected dentine is no longer a prerequisite. Second, new restorative materials such as **resin-based adhesives and filling materials**, and therapeutic filling materials, which are both bacteriostatic and bactericidal, avoid removing vast amounts of tooth. Third, improved and sophisticated techniques such as **adhesive protocols** allow restorations of small lesions, preventing progression to larger cavities. These advances preserve more of the natural tooth, and the current use of Black's classification is a notation, rather than as a basis for restoring decay. Whereas, in the past, **cavity design** was **geometric** (dictated by the restorative material), it is now **amorphous** (dictated by the extent of disease).

Smaller lesions are restored by a direct approach, while larger Class II or Class IV may also be restored indirectly with inlays or onlays (extracoronal), when a direct approach is judged as mechanically or aesthetically inferior. Inlays and onlays are fabricated in a dental laboratory using a variety of materials including composite resins, ceramics and cast gold alloys.

Indirect extracoronal prostheses

Extracoronal prostheses are defined as those **surrounding** one or more natural tooth surface(s). The indications for extracoronal restorations are:

- Restoring **structurally compromised** teeth
- **Improving function** (e.g. altering vertical dimension of occlusion – VDO or occlusal vertical dimension – OVD)
- **Improving aesthetics** (e.g. anterior maxillary and mandibular sextant)
- **Abutments** for a fixed-partial denture (FPD)

Extracoronal prostheses are categorised as:

- **Inlays and onlays** – the difference between an inlay and an onlay is the extent of tooth loss requiring replacement. Broadly speaking, an inlay **'fits into' the tooth**, while an onlay incorporates cuspal coverage and **'fits onto' the tooth**
- **Porcelain laminate veneers (PLV)** – the principal use of PLVs is improving anterior aesthetics by altering tooth morphology and colour. PLVs are the least invasive of extracoronal restorations, usually involving the buccal surfaces of anterior teeth. If the underlying tooth colour is acceptable, only minimal tooth reduction is necessary (0.3–0.8 mm) for improving contours and colour with a thin porcelain laminate fabricated in a dental laboratory. PLVs are the most prescribed type of restoration for purely cosmetic reasons. However, it should be remembered that preparing vital healthy teeth for PLVs with little aesthetic improvement is contentious, especially if similar results are achievable with less invasive protocols such as **bleaching** or **resin-based composite (RBC)** fillings
- **Partial coverage crowns** – partial coverage crowns are an extension of PLVs. They occupy a midpoint between full coverage and the minimally invasive PLV. Many configurations are possible, e.g. ½, ¾, ⅞, etc. The rationale for partial coverage is retaining as much natural tooth substrate as possible, and hence preserving pulpal and structural integrity
- **Full coverage crowns** and **fixed partial dentures (FPD)** or bridges – a full coverage, 360° crown is indicated for severely broken-down teeth, abutments for FPDs or rarely for elective aesthetic treatment. Various materials are used for fabricating crowns depending on the clinical scenario, e.g. cast metal, metal-ceramic, all-ceramic, composite and acrylic. For vital teeth, a crown can be supported either by coronal dentine or a core build-up. For endodontically treated teeth, a **post and core complex** may be necessary. **Intraradicular posts** are available in many materials, designs, configurations and sizes. A core can be fabricated directly using amalgam or composite, or indirectly using cast metals or ceramics. The sole purpose of a post-and-core complex is supporting the eventual extracoronal crown. **Posts and cores do not reinforce or strengthen teeth**, but weaken an already compromised root and the remaining coronal dentine. A **ferrule effect** is highly desirable for cores, either with or without posts
- **Combination prostheses** – depending on the extent of the clinical requirements, any intracoronal and extracoronal restoration can be combined into a single entity, e.g. inlay + onlay or PLV + inlay (veneerlay).

Key points

- A direct restoration is carried out chairside, while an indirect restoration requires using a dental laboratory.
- Black's classification is useful for describing the site of a lesion.
- Intracoronal restorations are surrounded by tooth surface(s).
- Extracoronal restorations surround tooth surface(s).
- Inlays are examples of intracoronal prostheses.
- Onlays, PLVs and crowns are examples of extracoronal prostheses

2 Overview: rehabilitation by artificial teeth

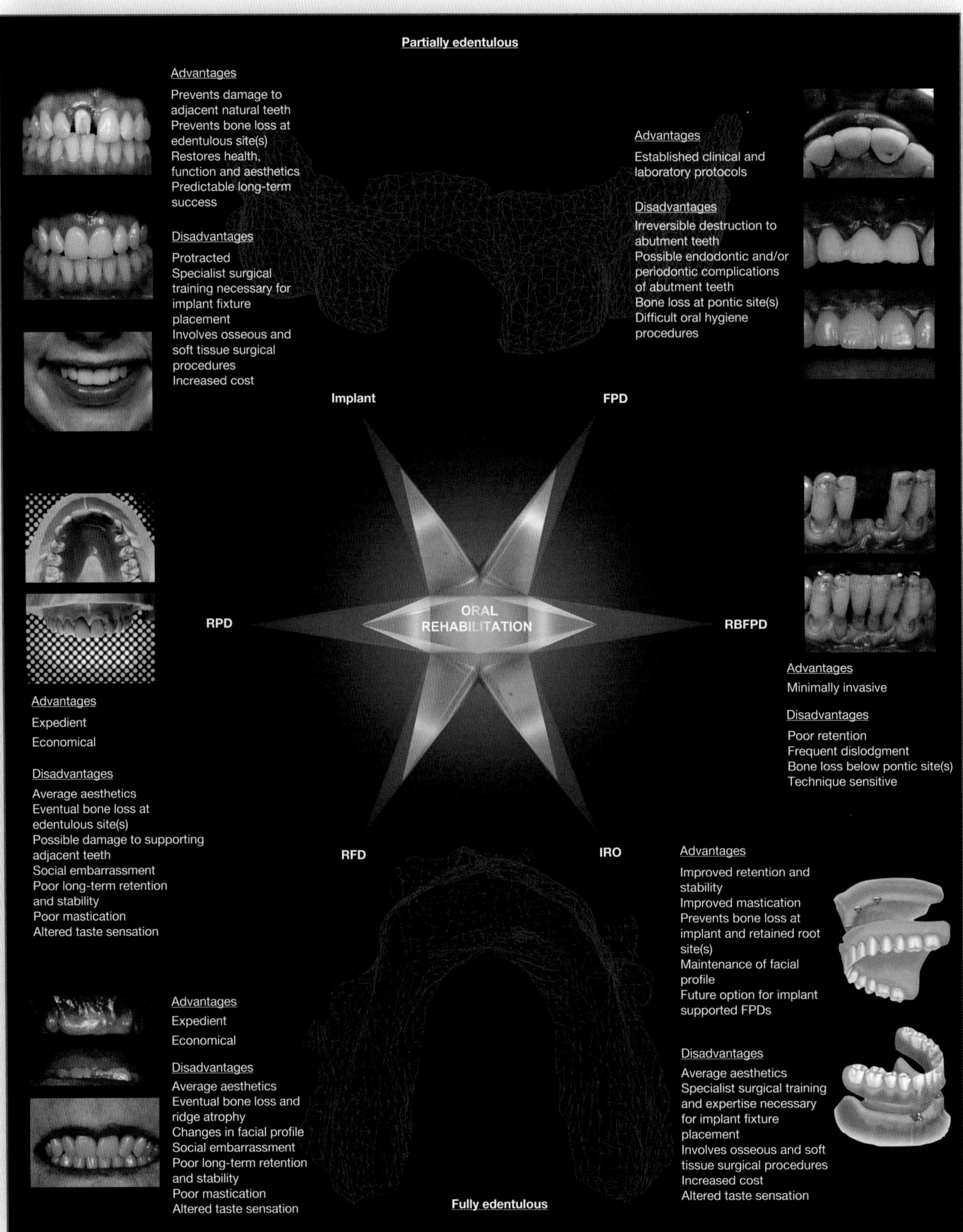

Prosthodontics at a Glance, Second Edition. Irfan Ahmad.

Oral rehabilitation of missing teeth is achieved with **removable** or **fixed** prostheses. The distinction between the two is that removable prostheses are supported by both soft tissues and teeth and/or implants, whereas fixed prostheses are exclusively supported by teeth and/or implants. Before deciding to replace missing teeth, the **shortened dental arch (SDA)** concept should be considered.

Removable full dentures (RFD)

Edentulous rehabilitation is either by full/full dentures totally supported by the alveolar ridges, overdentures retained by natural tooth roots for additional stability, or **implant-retained overdentures (IRO)** supported by strategically placed implants.

Removable partial dentures (RPD)

An **RPD** relies on support from both soft tissues and adjacent or surrounding natural teeth or implants. These dentures can be fabricated entirely from acrylic resins, or in combination with cast metal **frameworks**. **Clasps**, **rests** and **precision attachments** are often incorporated into the denture design for additional retention and stability. A variation of RPDs are **overdentures**, retained by tooth roots or **mini-implants (IRO)**.

Fixed partial dentures (FPD)

Before dental implants, **fixed partial dentures (FPD)** were the state-of-the-art prostheses for replacing missing teeth, but involve gross tooth preparation of supporting abutments. More conservative resin-**bonded fixed partial dentures (RBFPD)**, with minimal or no preparation, include Maryland, Rochette or composite fibre-reinforced bridges. While the advantages of minimal preparation are obvious, these types of bridge are less retentive, requiring frequent recementing and are often used as **transitional protheses**, e.g. during the surgical healing phase following bone grafting or implant placement. Other uses include **splinting** periodontally compromised mobile teeth, or as an interim restoration while awaiting a more permanent restoration.

Conventional FPDs require preparation of abutment teeth for supporting the final prosthesis incorporating **pontic**(s) for replacing a missing tooth or teeth. Numerous FPD configurations are possible, e.g. **fixed–fixed**, **cantilever** and **telescopic**, with or without precision attachments for stress relief for long spans. FPDs have a **cast metal** substructure, which is subsequently veneered with porcelain. Newer **all-ceramic** FPDs use dense ceramic frameworks, e.g. of zirconia or alumina, for supporting the **veneering porcelain**. Although conventional FPDs using natural teeth as abutments are destructive, they still have a place in prosthodontics where medical history or local anatomy contraindicates surgery or implant placement. Besides natural tooth abutments, **implants can also act as abutments for FPDs**.

Dental implants

Dental implants are **titanium root forms** placed into alveolar bone. Following **osseointegration**, the implants are prosthetically restored with a variety of artificial prostheses including implant-retained overdentures or IRO (RFD, RPD) and FPDs. Implants are extremely versatile and used for replacing a single missing tooth, or as abutments for FPDs for replacing several missing units. In addition, implants offer many advantages compared to conventional prostheses including:

- **Improved stability** for IROs
- **Preventing mechanical, periodontal and endodontic insult** of supporting teeth associated with RPDs (e.g. by clasps or occlusal rests)
- **Occlusal rehabilitation** of edentulous areas
- Greater bite force compared to exclusively tissue-borne prostheses, improving masticatory performance and therefore allowing a greater choice of foods
- **Avoiding tooth preparation of natural teeth** bounding missing spaces, e.g. for conventional FPDs, reducing possibilities of endodontic and periodontal complications
- **Preventing further bone loss** (due to bone stimulation by the implants in edentulous areas)
- **Immunity from secondary caries of natural tooth abutments** used for conventional FPD.

Although implants offer numerous advantages compared to conventional treatment modalities, detailed planning, clinical training, experience and meticulous execution are mandatory for avoiding complications and failures. Before deciding whether the patient is a suitable candidate for dental implants, the following requires consideration:

- **MAP** (medical, anatomy and prognosis)

  Medical – age, race, gender, compromised immune system, diabetes, osteoporosis, bisphosphonate therapy, radiotherapy, psychological stress and pregnancy

  Anatomy – soft tissue volume, dental biotype, bone quality and quantity, aesthetics (site: anterior or posterior regions of mouth), reduced vascularity from previous surgical traumas (e.g. apicectomies), proximity to vital structures (nerves, blood vessels, sinuses), occlusal clearance and parafunctional habits (e.g. bruxism)

  Prognosis – not only for an implant, but also for conventional treatment options depending on prevailing clinical situations such as, 'What is the survival rate of a tooth with periodontitis following periodontal surgery?'

  'What is the success of endodontic re-treatment?'

  'What is the longevity of an apicectomised tooth with a post crown?'

A risk assessment is essential before deciding either to pursue conventional treatment options, or to consider implants at the outset. The cost implications of conventional vs implant treatment are also worth consideration. If the prognosis for conventional treatment is poor, it is futile spending time and money which could better be allocated for treatment that has greater long-term predictability. Conversely, implants are not necessary a panacea for replacing every missing tooth or teeth.

Key points

- Missing teeth can be replaced by fixed or removable prostheses.
- Entirely tissue borne removable prostheses, e.g. RFD or RPD, which are economical and have established protocols but are a compromise for long-term oral rehabilitation.
- Conventional FPDs are highly destructive, but obviate the need for bone and soft tissue surgical procedures.
- Implant-supported single or multiple units are the state-of-the-art treatment modality for oral rehabilitation, but require specialist training, experience and meticulous treatment planning for successful outcomes.

3 Ethics

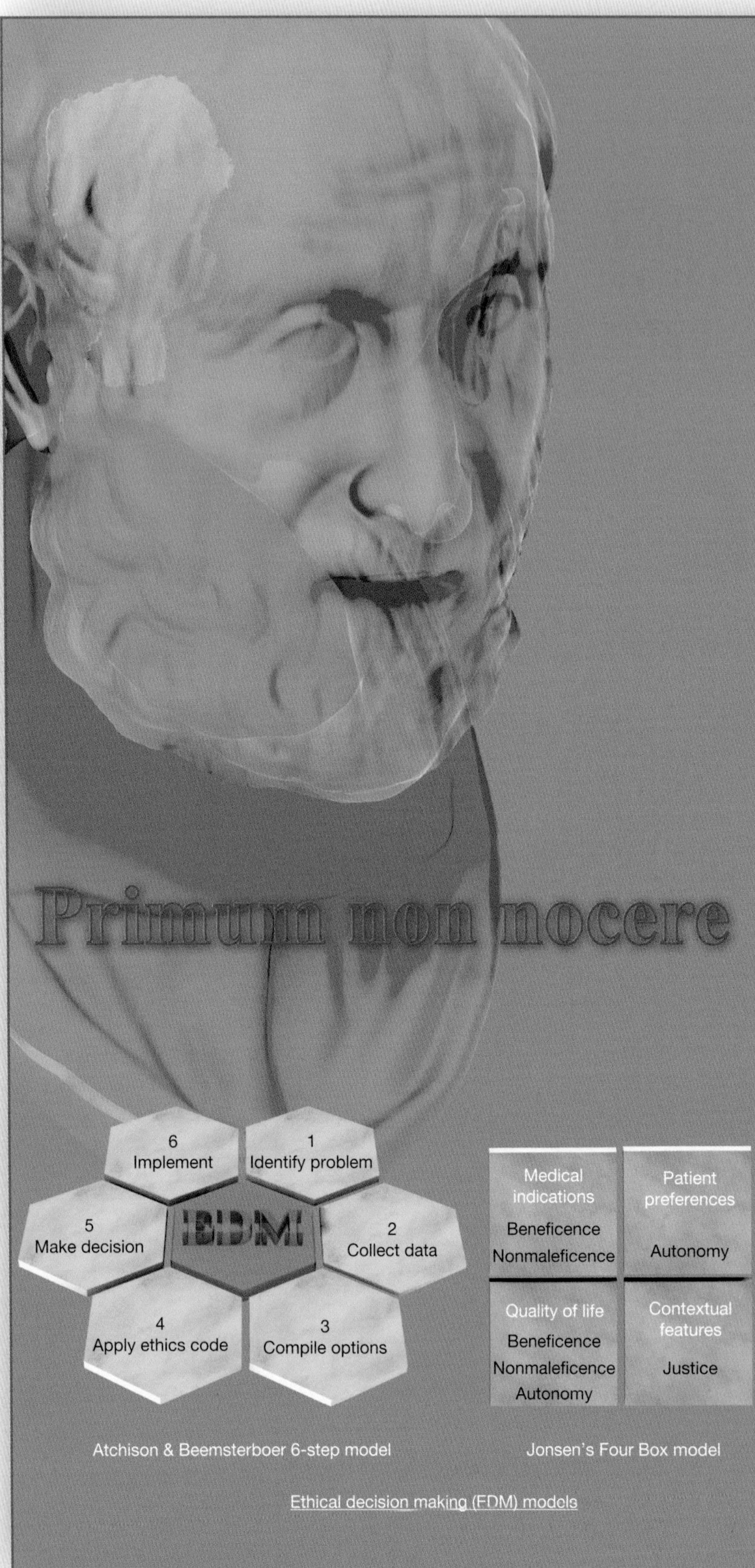

Autonomy

- Patient's right to choose their own destiny
- Maintain confidentiality (except safeguarding public, vulnerable adults & children)
- Involve patients in treatment
- Pros and cons of treatment options to allow patient to give informed consent
- Conflict between patient desires and best interest of patient
- Often antagonistic with cosmetic elective procedures

Nonmaleficence

- First, do no harm
- Clinical self-deprecation
- Continually update knowledge and skills
- Declare personal impairment/infections
- Refer when necessary
- Assess risk/benefit of a modality
- Divulge complications
- Avoid patient abandonment
- Avoid personal relationship with patients

Beneficence

- Remove/prevent harm
- Promote goodness
- Empathise
- Prioritise patient and betterment of society
- Paternalism (parentalism) may conflict with patient autonomy
- Educate patients on importance of oral health
- Preventative measures, healthcare programmes, research
- Prima facia conflict with patient autonomy
- Maintain personal demeanour

Justice

- Egalitarian society
- No discrimination when providing treatment, irrespective of socioeconomic constraints
- In reality, dental care is provided according to resources rather than needs
- Encourage whistleblowing
- Accept constructive or illuminative criticism

Veracity

- Fiduciary in patient–dentist relationship: patient to disclose information, and dentist to offer advice
- Provide treatment options, cost, benefits, disadvantages, longevity (linked with autonomy)
- Keeping promises
- Benevolent deception is questionable
- Avoiding unsubstantiated claims, credentials, misleading advertising
- Disclose conflict of interests
- Resist opportunistic avarice

Prosthodontics at a Glance, Second Edition. Irfan Ahmad.

Ethics in dentistry presents a unique scenario because it encompass several domains: **preventative measures, therapeutic treatment, elective procedures, education, research and academia** (lecturing, publishing, commercial affiliations or sponsorship). Each domain presents specific dilemmas that need to be addressed and solved according to **ethical principles**. Sometimes, an option may violate one principle while favouring another, and deciding which to choose is perplexing, or could border on potential negligence.

The ethics code

The word **ethics** and **morality** are interchangeable and mean the same thing. The **ethics code** is a set of principles of moral conduct derived from **philosophy** and **theology**. However, ethics or morality are independent of faith, and religion not a refuge for unethical behaviour. The **five commandments** or principles of the ethics code, initially proposed in 5 BCE by the Greek physician **Hippocrates** are **autonomy**, **nonmaleficence**, **beneficence**, **justice** and **veracity**. Ethics principles or standards govern the behaviour and judgement of an individual, but are ethics innate or learned? Morality is influenced by education, culture, religion, age, experience and social norms, and is unique to an individual. Ethics are an evolving concept reflecting changes in social, political, cultural and economic climate at a given time; and over the years, the **Hippocratic principles have therefore been revised and modified to have relevance to social norms of contemporary society.** Although every **professional regulatory body** in a country has its own standards, the underlying ethos remains the same.

Professionalism

The distinction between a skilled trader and a professional is that the former has clients, while the latter has patients. If a trader provides poor service, the client seeks **civil litigation**, whereas if dental care is shortcoming, the patient seeks **criminal damages**. A professional abides by ethical obligations, as well as possessing the knowledge and skills to deliver treatment. The first, and foremost ethical obligation is **'primum non nocere'** or **'first, do no harm'**. This is a pivotal ethical obligation, indelibly engraved in stone that cannot be effaced. However, it must be remembered that a bad outcome from treatment does not necessarily indicate unethical behaviour.

The definition of **professionalism** is notoriously ambiguous, but may be stated as **putting the interest of others before one's own**. While professionalism offers status, prestige and benefits, it also carries burdens and responsibilities. In essence, it is a **contract between a professional and society**. The society confers privileges to a professional, and in return the professional is obliged to uphold the ethics code, have integrity and compassion that are universal attributes of any caring society. This task involves, first, maintaining **sagacious minimum standards** to safeguard patients and staff, and second, **maintaining conduct** that is expected of a professional and aspiring to greater heights of excellence. The second aspect is nebulous and relies on '**conscience**', defined as **'whatever it is that makes us behave when nobody is looking'**.

Professionalism starts at the selection process of students wishing to enrol at dental colleges, and is reinforced and maintained throughout a professional career. However, the motivation of some applicants is driven by **financial and status benefits** rather than **altruism**. Hence, screening students presents considerable and perhaps, insurmountable challenge. These include assessment criteria for virtue of character (e.g. recommendations letters), indoctrinating students with the ethics code and managing ethical standards after qualification. Although **DCP (dental care professionals)** are responsible for their own acts and omissions, but on occasion, the dentist's liability and responsibilities may extend to encompass **'repondeat superior'** or **vicarious liability.**

Vocation vs business

With declining caries rate, improved home oral hygiene and increased patient knowledge base, the demand for dental treatment is decreasing. This has resulted in some dentists embracing **plastic aesthetics elective procedures.** While treatment that restores health has a **high benefit/risk ratio**, an enhancement procedure, primarily concerned with beautification, has a **low benefit/risk ratio**. Furthermore, the accompanying backlash is the public's perception of the profession as one that is self-interest orientated. This creates a dichotomy, 'Can a business coexist with the ethics of putting the interest of the patient above profit?' Patients seeking cosmetic or aesthetic treatment fall into two categories, the first who have genuine **tangible reasons** such as decayed, discoloured or misaligned teeth, and the second, for **intangible reasons**, mainly narcissism or psychological or personality complexes, e.g. somatic elusion, transference and body dysmorphic disorder. Although many elective procedures are innocuous (e.g. tooth whitening), but invasive, irreversible modalities place the individual in a vulnerable position, with possible impact on oral health and function at a later date. Ultimately, the **dilemma** is **'What is the right treatment plan for the patient?'** or **'What is the right treatment plan for the business?'**

Ethical decision-making (EDM)

The current trends are practicing defensive dentistry, and abandoning **paternalism** to involve patients in their treatment. To be completely ethical, all five principles of the ethics code should be incorporated in a decision, but a dilemma occurs when one rule conflicts with another and requires making a choice. For example, a conflict may arise when a patient opts for an enhancement procedure (autonomy), that is against the dentist's advice as potentially harmful (nonmaleficence). If the patient decided to proceed, (s)he should forgo the right for compensation if the outcome is not as expected, i.e. **caveat emptor** – **the buyer, not supplier is responsible for purchased commodities or services,** which is particularly relevant for **dental tourism.**

The dentist must juggle between three roles: **clinician**, **professional** and **business(wo)man**, which causes **moral distress** facing a situation where (s)he is impotent. The range of ethical dilemmas are unique to an individual, practice or institutions and can range from **breach of confidentially**, **overtreatment** to blatant **fraud**. An **ethical decision-making (EDM) model** is as systematic reasoning approach used by healthcare professionals to resolve ethical dilemmas, e.g. the six-step Atchison and Beemsterboer approach, or Jonsen's Four Box model. Finally, is feeling healthier becoming less important than looking better? Perhaps the following adages are worth remembering, **'There is nothing permanent in dentistry'**, and **'Why solve a problem that doesn't hurt you?'**

Key points

- The ethics code consists of five principles: autonomy, nonmaleficence, beneficence, justice and veracity.
- Professionalism is maintaining minimum standards and aspiring to greater heights.
- Experience cannot be substituted for chance success.
- Can business values be reconciled with ethical virtues?

Diagnostics

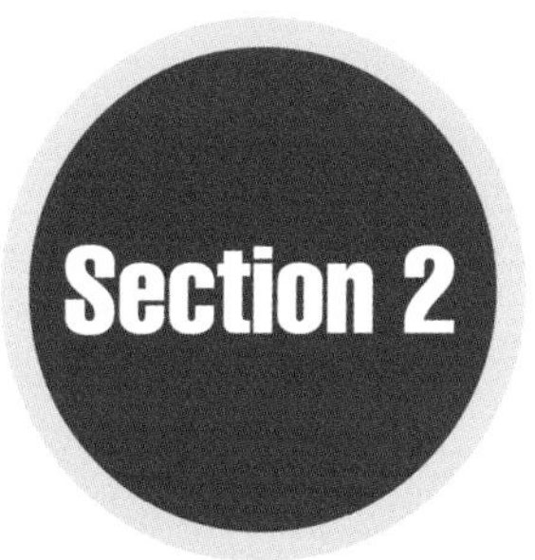

Chapters

4 Diagnostics: history taking

European Medical Risk Related History (EMRRH) questionnaire

1. Do you experience chest pain upon exertion (angina pectoris)? If so, (II),
   Are your activities restricted? (III)
   Have the complaints increased recently? (IV)
   Do you have chest pain at rest? (V)
2. Have you ever had a heart attack? If so, (II)
   Are your activities restricted? (III)
   Have you had a heart attack in the last 6 months? (IV)
3. Do you have a heart murmur, heart valve disease, or an artificial heart valve? (II)
   Have you had heart disease or vascular surgery within the last 6 months? (II)
   Have you ever had rheumatic heart disease? (III)
   Are your activities restricted? (IV)
4. Do you have heart palpitations without exertion? If so, (II)
   Are you short of breath, pale or dizzy at these times? (IV)
5. Do you suffer from heart failure? If so, (II)
   Are you short of breath when lying down? (III)
   Do you need two or more pillows at night due to shortness of breath? (IV)
6. Have you ever had high blood pressure? (II)
7. Do you have a tendency to bleed? If so, (II)
   Do you bleed more than one hour following injury or surgery? (III)
   Do you suffer from spontaneous bruising? (IV)
8. Have you ever suffered a cerebral congestion? If so, (II)
   Have you suffered from one in the last 6 months? (III)
9. Do you have epilepsy? If so, (II)
   Is your condition getting worse? (III)
   Do you continue to have attacks despite medication? (IV)
10. Do you suffer from asthma? If so, (II)
    Do you use any medication and/or inhalers? (III)
    Is your breathing difficult today? (IV)
11. Do you have other lung problems or a persistent cough? If so, (II)
    Are you short of breath after climbing 20 steps? (III)
    Are you short of breath while getting dressed? (IV)
12. Have you ever had an allergic reaction to penicillin, aspirin, latex or anything else? If so, (II)
    Did this require medical or hospital treatment? (III)
    Was it during a dental visit? (IV)
    What are you allergic to?
13. Do you have diabetes? (II)
    Are you on insulin? If so, (III)
    Is your diabetes poorly controlled at present? (IV)
14. Do you suffer from thyroid disease? If so, (II)
    Do you have an under-active thyroid? (III)
    Do you have an overactive thyroid? (IV)
15. Have you now or in the past had liver disease? (II)
16. Do you have a kidney disease? (II)
    Are you undergoing dialysis? (III)
    Have you had a kidney transplant? (IV)
17. Have you ever had cancer or leukemia? (IV)
    Have you received drug therapy or had a bone marrow transplant for this? (III)
    Have you ever had X-ray treatment for a tumor or growth in the head or neck? (IV)
18. Do you suffer from any infections at present? (II)
    If so, which is it?
19. Do you suffer from hyperventilation? (II)
20. Have you ever fainted during dental or medical treatment? (II)
21. Do you have to take antibiotics before dental treatment? (II)
22. Are you on any medication at present? (II)
23. Women only, please: are you pregnant? (II)

The ASA rating is stated in parenthesis, no abnormality is rated as I. The higher the number, the greater the risk of medical complication for dental treatment

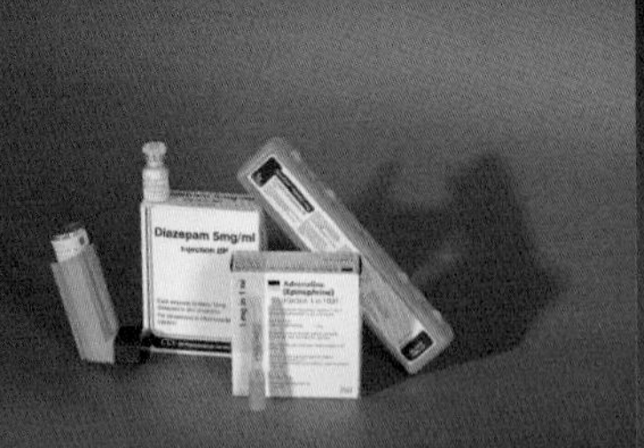

Medical emergency drugs commonly found in a dental practice

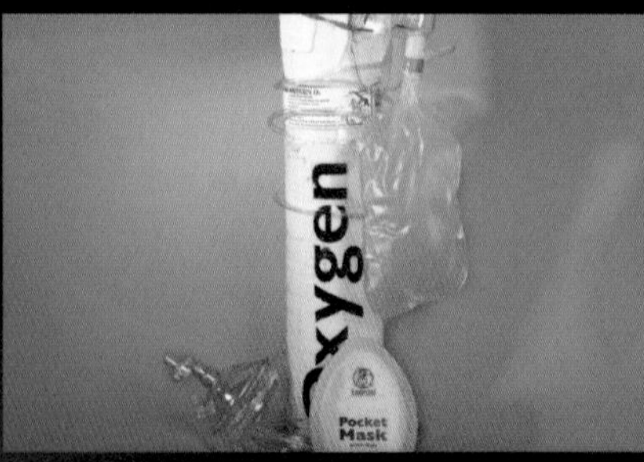

Cardiac problems are the most frequent form of medical complications effecting dental treatment. A knowledge of CRP and readily available oxygen can avert fatal consequences

Prosthodontics at a Glance, Second Edition. Irfan Ahmad.

History taking is the first stage before embarking on dental treatment. Recent medical advances have prolonged life expectancy, and age-related and chronic illness treated with long-term medication influences an individual's **medical status.** Furthermore, the ever-increasing elderly population retain more of their natural teeth, requiring regular dental maintenance. Collating a patient's history is not confined to **medical anamnesis**, but also takes account of **familial medical traits** and **social habits**. All these factors can, and may, affect dental procedures.

Family medical history

There is widespread consensus among physicians that many diseases have a **genetic origin**, and a sibling may harbour genes which may or may not manifest as an eventual ailment. Also, many diseases are **multifactorial**, and even if an individual carries a given gene for a specific disease, it is not a foregone conclusion that disease will follow. For example, having a gene for cardiac problems does not mean that a myocardial infarction is inevitable. If **diet**, **smoking** and **lassitude** are controlled, an individual with a cardiac family history may never suffer a heart attack. The same is applicable with a family **history of chronic periodontitis**.

However, knowing the family medical background helps **risk assessment** and tailoring treatment plans unique for each patient. For example, an individual with a family history of diabetes and periodontitis will require more frequent periodontal maintenance to prevent activation of the offending gene(s) that cause periodontal destruction.

Social history

Many patients are reticent to divulge social practices since they do not perceive that this will influence their dental care. A caring and sympathetic approach, combined with detailed explanations, is necessary to obtain this information. For example, smoking, **drug addiction** or **alcohol abuse** affect many dental procedures and their prognosis. Another increasingly prevalent dental 'disease' is **tooth wear (tooth surface loss – TSL)**, which is non-infectious loss of tooth substrate (erosion, attrition and abrasion) due to **lifestyle choices** such as drinking effervescent acidic beverages or stress-related occlusal grinding.

Gauging the **persona** of a patient is more difficult and takes time, especially when treatment is protracted. A patient's personality, expectations and wishes may be irrelevant for simple procedures or for alleviating pain, but are decisive for certain aesthetic or cosmetic treatment outcomes.

Personal medical history

Medical history taking involves completing a questionnaire, a medico-legal document, which is regularly updated, reflecting the patient's changing health status. Diligent questioning is necessary to establish all **medical history and medication**, especially if the patient does not realise the relevance of divulging this information for dental care. The choice of **medical questionnaire** can be bespoke for a given practice, a proprietary form purchased from dental stationers, the **Medical Risk Related History (MRRH)** or the **European Medical Risk Related History (EMRRH)** form. The bespoke and proprietary are both non-standardised questionnaires and the risk assessment is piecemeal, depending on the prevailing medical conditions. The MRRH and EMRRH forms are an attempt to standardise risk assessment, using the **American Society of Anesthesiologists (ASA)** scale for rating the severity of medical complications for easier assessment of the state of the patient's health.

Medical complications

A significant proportion of the population have medical histories or medication that affects numerous dental procedures. Furthermore, some diseases can place the dental team at risk of contracting illness or exposure to pathogenic organisms. The most significant systemic diseases affecting dentistry are summarised below:

- **Cardiovascular diseases** include hypertension, ischaemic cardiovascular disease (angina), myocardial infarction (heart attack), congestive cardiac insufficiency, valvopathy and cardiac arrhythmias (with or without a pacemaker). A practical knowledge of **cardiopulmonary resuscitation (CPR)** is essential
- **Allergies** can either be constitutional, e.g. asthma, or drug induced. The most common **anaphylactic** reaction is due to penicillin **(Type 1, IgE-mediated and immediate reaction)**, but can also be precipitated by many other drugs (e.g. neuromuscular blocking drugs, aspirin). The symptoms are usually apparent within 15 minutes of taking the offending drug. Other allergies that may complicate dental treatment are natural rubber latex (NRL), allergy from latex gloves, local anaesthesia, mouthwashes (e.g. chlorhexidine), patent blue dye or dental materials (amalgam, acrylic monomer, eugenol) and particularly alloys containing nickel **(Type IV, IgE-mediated and delayed reaction, e.g. contact dermatitis)**
- **Diabetes mellitus** (types 1 and 2) is not only a debilitating systemic disease, but may also increase the severity of periodontal destruction and complicate surgical or implant procedures. Many patients are oblivious to their condition until symptoms appear, and if detailed questioning arouses suspicion, referral to a medical practitioner for further tests is advisable
- **Infectious diseases**, e.g. hepatitis A, B, C, coronaviruses (MERS-CoV responsible for MERS, **SARS-Cov-2 responsible for COVID-19)**, HIV and tuberculosis, do not contraindicate dental care, but stringent cross-infection control and PPE (personal protective equipment) are mandatory
- **Epileptic convulsions** are controllable by medication in the majority of cases, but the dental surgery environment may cause stress and trigger an epileptic attack
- **Tendency to bleed** may be due to haemophilia or anticoagulant therapy. In both situations, a medical consultant's report is essential before embarking on deep scaling or surgical procedures
- **Drug-related complications** are secondary effects that may interfere with certain treatment; for example, antidepressants interacting with local anaesthetics, or bisphosphonate therapy causing osteonecrosis following soft tissue or implant surgery
- **Other conditions** include pregnancy, thyroid disease, radiotherapy, kidney disease, stroke and carcinomas

Key points

- A detailed family, social and personal medical history is essential before starting dental treatment.
- Gauging a patient's persona is helpful for aesthetic treatment outcomes.
- A standardised MRRH or EMRRH questionnaire with an ASA rating is useful for assessing severity of medical complications.
- A working knowledge of dealing with medical emergencies is essential.

Diagnostics: initial consultation

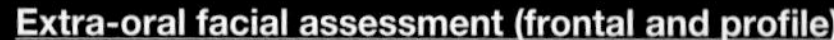

Extra-oral facial assessment (frontal and profile)

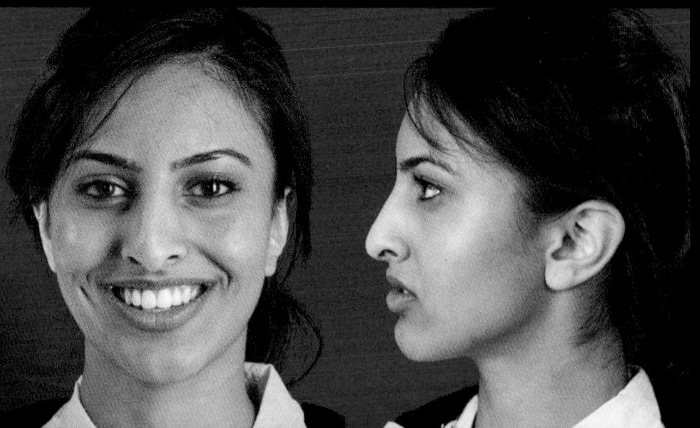

Photographs of the face are an excellent method for studying in detail extra-oral pathology, variations and asymmetries that affect treatment planning. For example, parallelism of the interpupillary line with the incisal plane is essential for aesthetic approval

Intra-oral soft tissue examination chart

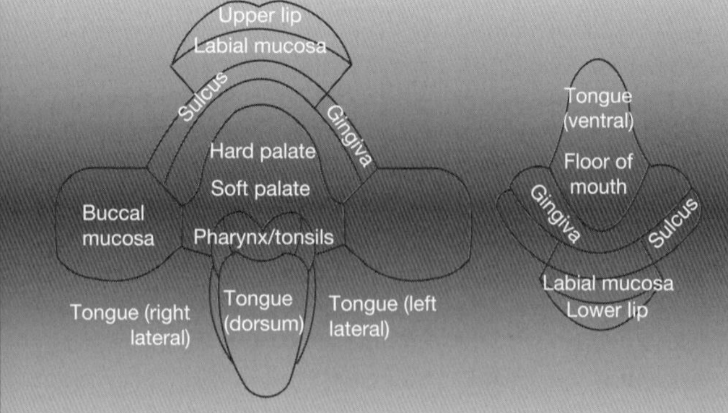

An intra-oral soft tissue examination noting all pathology, which is an essential record of any cancerous or pre-cancerous lesions that require further investigation

BPE sextants

UR7-4	UR3-UL-3	UL4-7
LR7-4	LR3-LL-3	LL4-7

BPE scores

4*	2	3
X	3	4*

*furcation involvement, 'X' edentulous sextant

Computer-generated dental and periodontal charting

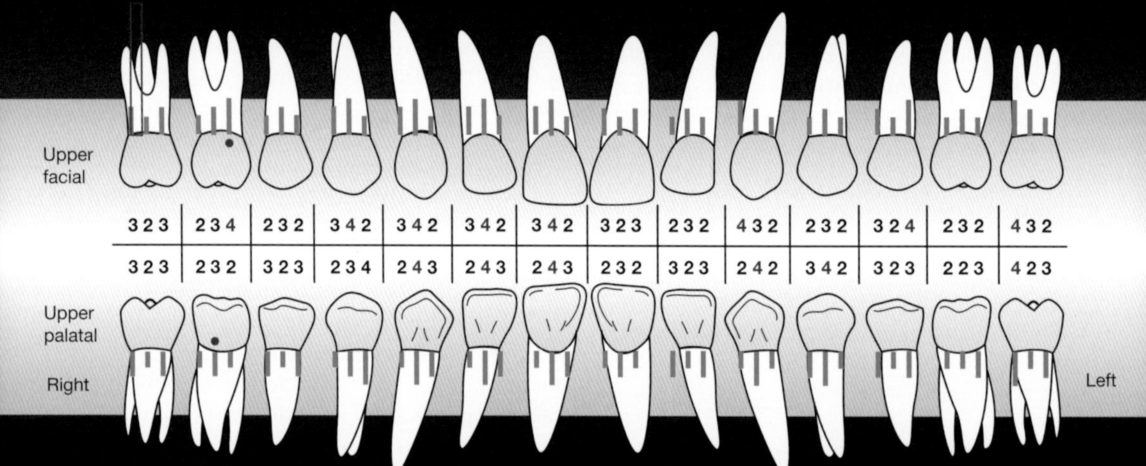

Dental software allows a comprehensive dental and periodontal charting, which can be readily reviewed and modified

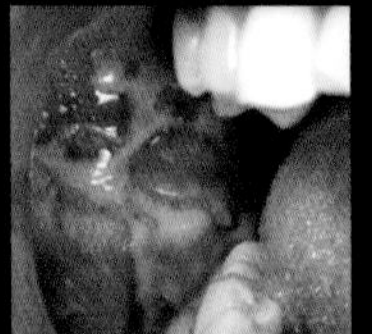

Early detection of cancerous and precancerous lesions are life saving

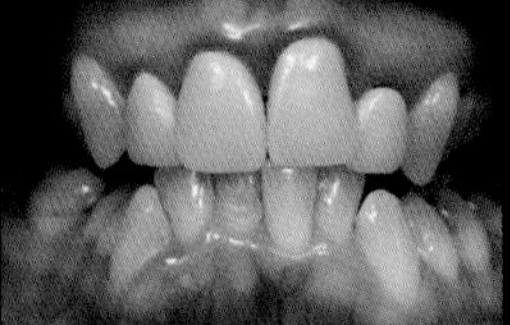

Uneven gingival margins detract from 'pink' aesthetics, especially with a high lip line

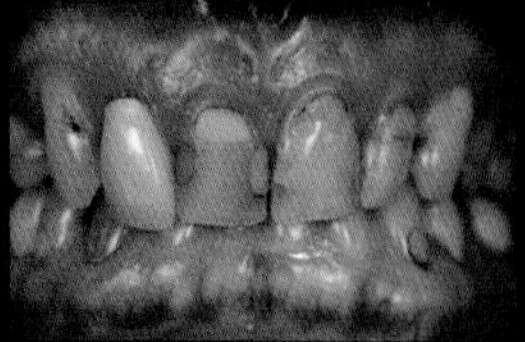

Angle's Class II(ii) anterior relationship is associated with a steep anterior guidance

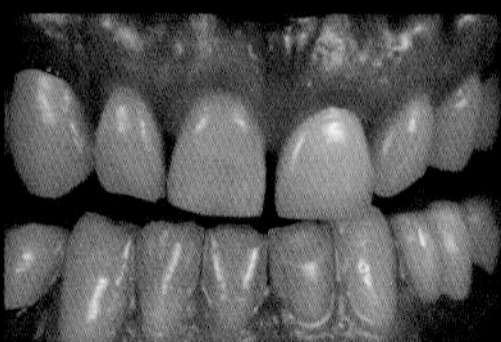

Tooth wear is non- infectious loss of enamel and dentine, e.g., due to attrition

Prosthodontics at a Glance, Second Edition. Irfan Ahmad.

The initial consultation is to assess the patient's current **dental status** and determine which, if any, detailed investigations or referral are necessary before arriving at a diagnosis.

Initial complaint

The first point to ascertain is the **reason for attending,** which can be pain, dissatisfaction with previous dentists, referral, coercion by family, friends and colleagues regarding poor dental health and/or appearance, second opinion or a personal desire to improve dental health and aesthetics.

Dental history

Dental history taking includes the following:

- **Attitude** to oral health
- **Regular or occasional attender**
- **Dental records**, models, photographs and radiographs from previous dentist(s)
- Dental **phobias**
- **Hobbies or habits** that affect the dentition, e.g. playing a wind instrument
- Sports, **occupational hazards** or other risky activities
- **Persona** and expectations about dental treatment
- **Financial** status

Extra-oral examination

The extra-oral examination consists of a **visual** and **tactile** assessment. The skeletal structure, tegumental (skin) structure and the musculature are scrutinised and deviations from the norm or pathological changes are recorded.

- **Skeletal**: facial shape (ovoid, tapering, rectangular or square), facial profile (class I, II or III base), zygomata (prominent, receding), angle of mandible (prominent, receding), **temporomandibular joint [TMJ]** (deviation and/or clicking during movement, hypo- and hyperplasia of condyles) and maxilla (parallelism, prominent, receding and canting).
- **Tegumental**: swellings, lacerations, bruising, scarring (e.g. healing of previous disease or surgery, or result of facial cosmetic procedures), indelible tattoos, suppuration, pathological pigmentation and hirsutism, loss of tonicity, prominent facial grooves and ridges (e.g. nasolabial). Other soft tissues to consider are the shape and size of the nose, lips and chin. Facial asymmetries are assessed during musculature stasis and contraction (e.g. conversing, smiling and laughing).
- **Musculature**: paralysis, hypertrophy and twitching. In addition, palpation of the oral muscles is performed including the temporalis, masseter, medial and lateral pterygoids. During this tactile examination, tenderness or trigger points that elicit pain or spasm are recorded. Lastly, the degree of mouth opening and trismus is noted

Intra-oral examination

As well as a visual and tactile assessment, intra-oral examination is expedited by using **diagnostic adjuncts** to elucidate and confirm clinical findings (see Chapter 6).

Soft tissues

The areas to examine are the **oral mucosa, buccal mucosa, palate, uvula, floor of the mouth, the tongue** (especially the **lateral aspects**, together with tongue thrust) and, in children, habits such as **thumb or dummy sucking**. Any abnormality or findings are recorded, especially pathological, **cancerous** and **precancerous** lesions. Finally, impediment to phonetics is ascertained with sounds such as 'M', 'F', 'V', 'S' and 'TH'.

Dental charting

Nowadays, most dental charting is performed using computer software, which prompts the user with specific items to record, thereby avoiding omissions. The charting should include **DMF** score (decayed, missing and filled teeth), diastemata, **imbrications**, **tooth wear** (erosion, attrition, abrasion and abfraction – Smith and Knight index), **primary caries** (in virgin teeth) and **secondary caries** (around restorations or prostheses), direct restorations (amalgam or composite), indirect prostheses (veneers, crowns, inlays and bridges), **defective margins**, **discolouration** (intrinsic and extrinsic), **fractures** (tooth, restorations or cuspal), **tooth vitality**, **removable prostheses** (acrylic, metal dentures, mouthguards and bleaching trays), **implant-supported prostheses** and fixed or removable **orthodontic** appliances.

Periodontal charting

Periodontal screening is the **basic periodontal examination (BPE)** for all patients, including children. BPE is economical and allows rapid assessment of simple or complex cases, but does not indicate disease activity, distinguish false pocketing and **cannot be used for diagnosis**. BPE divides dental arches into sextants and using either a **WHO-C** (World Health Organisation – Clinical), or **WHO-E** (World Health Organisation – Epidemiological) **probes**, records values from 0 to 4 representing periodontal pocket depths. The highest measurement is noted in each sextant, including those around implants to **detect early peri-implantitis.** A **score of 3 or more** requires further diagnostics such as full periodontal charting and radiographs. **Computer-aided charting** also expedites periodontal charting, to record halitosis, inflammation, suppuration, plaque score, calculus, bleeding on probing, **pocket measurements**, location of the cemento-enamel junction (CEJ), **gingival recession** (Miller's Class I, II, III and IV), **mobility** (Class I, II, III and IV), width of attached gingivae, **altered passive eruption (APE), furcation** involvement (Class I, II and III), pronounced gingival embrasures ('black triangles'), degree of maxillary **gingival exposure** during a relaxed and exaggerated smile (norm is <3 mm) and the **gingival aesthetic line (GAL)** for assessing the maxillary anterior sextant gingival zeniths. A useful online based tool is the **PreViser risk calculator** to measure and communicate patient susceptibility to various oral diseases.

Occlusion

The basic occlusal examination includes **arch shape** (narrow, wide, oval and square), **Angle's classification** (Class I, II(i), II(ii) and III), measurement of overjet and overbite, slide from **centric relation (CR)** to **centric occlusion (CO), lateral contacts** (canine guidance, group function), **anterior guidance** (steep, normal and shallow), **fremitus, occlusal interferences, parafunctional activity** (e.g. bruxism), **temporomandibular disorders (TMD), trauma from occlusion** and loss of **vertical dimension of occlusion (VDO).**

Key points

- After ascertaining the initial complaint, a dental history is recorded.
- Extra-oral examination assesses the facial skeleton, tegument and muscles.
- Intra-oral examination includes soft tissues, dental and periodontal charting and occlusal assessment.
- The initial consultation determines whether to start treatment, carry out further investigations or refer to a specialist for further advice or treatment.

Diagnostic adjuncts 1

As well as choosing the magnification factor, it is important to select the correct working distance of loupes to ensure correct posture, and prevent musculoskeletal strain. A fibreoptic cable can also be attached for shadow-free illumination

Transillumination is useful for detecting cusp and restorative material fractures

Although the learning curve is more challenging than for loupes, an operating microscope offers innumerable benefits such as dual binocular vision for both the clinician and dental assistant, as well as the facility to attach a camera

Using a fluorescent disclosing agent allows visualisation of plaque biofilm with UV illumination

ILLUMINATION

MAGNIFICATION

ORAL CANCER

VITALITY TESTS

OTHER

Leukoplakia

Transient paraesthesia gives a false-negative result when vitality of traumatised teeth is tested using thermal or electrical stimulation

CBCT

Digital smile design

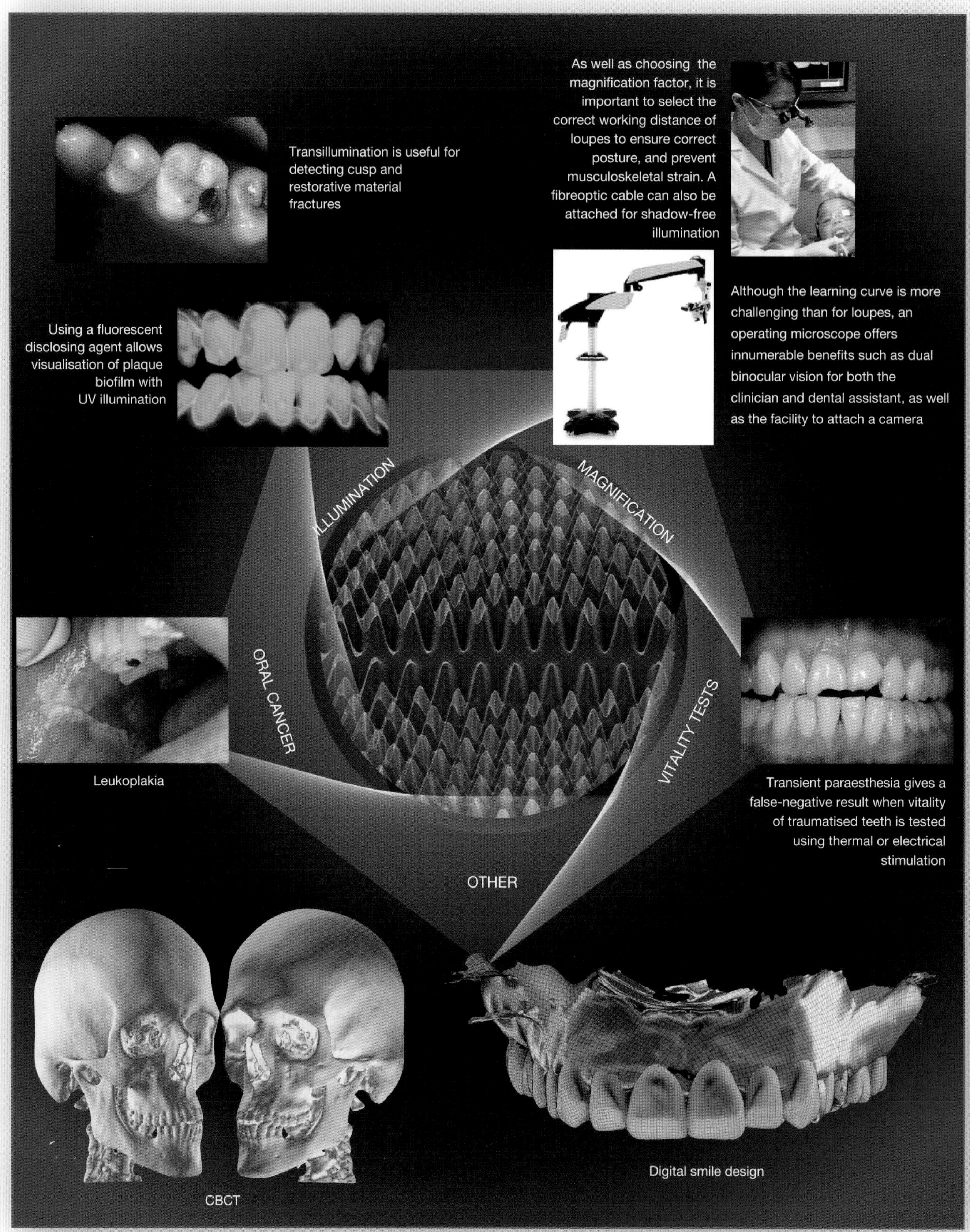

Prosthodontics at a Glance, Second Edition. Irfan Ahmad.

Besides visual and tactile examination, many conditions and lesions require specific tests and adjuncts to elucidate findings and confirm diagnosis.

Illumination

The typical illumination in a dental practice is the **operatory light,** which delivers incident light that is suitable for most examinations. However, other types of illumination allow visualisation of features that may be missed by traditional light sources, e.g. **transillumination** via a fibreoptic cable emphasises fractures (tooth and restorations), defective restorative margins and caries. In addition, **ultraviolet (UV) illumination** is useful for detecting plaque biofilm (with fluorescent disclosing solutions) or porosity in ceramic restorations.

Magnification

Visual enhancement is not limited to specific specialties such as endodontics, but is invaluable in many dental disciplines such as prosthodontics and periodontics, and in detecting lesions that may be 'invisible' to the unaided eye. **Magnification elevates visual acuity** using **loupes**, **intra-oral cameras**, **operating microscopes** and **projection stereomicroscopes** using 3-D video technology. Loupes offer magnification from ×2 to ×5, while microscopes have the capability for ×20 or greater levels of reproduction.

The advantages of magnification are:

- Enhanced visual access to detail
- Improved precision
- Increased efficacy
- Compensate for presbyopia
- Comfortable ergonomics, avoiding musculoskeletal injuries.

The disadvantages of visual aids are:

- Limited field of view (beyond ×2.5)
- Reduced depth of field (with extreme magnifications >×10)
- Cross-infection concerns
- Damage to optics (by dental debris or air abrasion procedures)
- Learning curve (especially with microscopes)

Oral precancer and cancer lesions

Oral (or mouth) and oropharyngeal cancer accounts for 3% of all malignancies, **with a 50% mortality rate for oral cancer.** Early detection and management are therefore essential for increasing survival rates and minimising metastases and recurrence. The aggressiveness of **squamous cell carcinoma** depends on age, sex and its location, which includes **vermilion border of lower lips, ventral surface of the tongue, floor of mouth**, palate, buccal mucosa and oropharynx.

Examples of precancerous lesions are **leukoplakia (dysplasia** ranging from 3% to 18%), **erythroplakia** (high incidence of dysplasia [91%] at clinical detection) and possibly **human papillomaviruses (HPVs)**. The **probability of malignant changes** depends on:

- Site of lesion (e.g. ventral surface of the tongue, floor of mouth)
- Proliferative verrucous appearance
- Erythroplakia within a leukoplakia
- Multiple lesions and
- Surprisingly, in some non-smokers

However, not all dysplasia develops into **carcinoma in situ** or **full-blown carcinoma.** The early stages of cancer are asymptomatic, while the late stages (carcinoma in situ) show ulceration and bleeding accompanied by pain, dysphagia and lymphadenopathy. Visual inspection is insufficient for diagnosis and must be investigated with **active stains** (toluidine blue), **oral cytology** (scraping and brush biopsy) and **scalpel biopsy.** However, staining and scrapings may be inconclusive, and an **USC (urgent suspected cancer) referral** with a brush biopsy is advised for lesions that **do not heal in 10 days. Differential diagnoses** include lichen planus, frictional keratosis, leukoedema, nicotinic stomatitis, white sponge naevus, etc., where a cause cannot be elucidated. The **gold standard for definitive diagnosis** is a scalpel biopsy and **histology examination**.

Vitality testing methods

Methods to determine **pulp vitality** include **thermal**, **electrical**, **drilling** cavities into dentine, **anaesthesia**, **laser Doppler flowmetry, dual wavelength spectrophotometry** and **pulse oximetry**. The most commonly used are **thermal and electrical stimuli that are subjective,** while pulse oximetry is objective. Thermal and electrical tests measure neural responses and are erratic and inconclusive, especially when used in children. **Heat stimuli are less reliable than cold liquids** (e.g. 1,1,1,2- tetrafluoroethane). In addition, a false-negative result is often obtained with traumatised teeth due to transient paraesthesia of nerve fibres. Conversely, a false-positive result is elicited when necrosis of the pulpal vascular tissues has occurred, leaving vital nerve fibres, which are more resilient. Both of these situations delay diagnosis and treatment of the affected tooth, often leading to root absorption. **Pulse oximetry is objective**, measuring the **blood oxygen saturation levels** or circulation within the pulp. The pulse oximeter consists of light-emitting diodes (LED) of two wavelengths (red light, 640 nm and infrared light, 940 nm) and a receptor which records the spectral absorbance of the oxygenated and deoxygenated haemoglobin in the tooth pulp. A computer calculates the percentage of oxygen saturation levels, which are approximately 75–80% for vital teeth, compared to values at the fingers or ear lobes of 98%. The saturation levels of teeth are lower than soft tissues due to the dentine and enamel enclosing the pulp, which scatters the LED light.

Other methods

Other methods used for diagnosis and treatment planning include:

- **Caries detection** and **periodontal assessment** (Chapter 7)
- **Radiography** (Chapter 8)
- **Digital acquisition,** e.g. computed tomography (CT), **cone beam-computed tomography (CBCT)** and **intra-oral scanners (IOS)** (Chapters 9–12)
- **Dental photography** (Chapters 13 and 14)
- **Occlusal analysis** (Chapter 15)
- **Shade analysis** (Chapter 16)
- **Plaster casts/3D printed models** and **simulations** (Chapter 17)
- **Smile design** (Chapter 33)

Key points

- Transillumination is used for detecting caries, fractures and deficient restorative margins.
- Magnification facilitates diagnosis, using loupes or operating microscopes.
- Precancerous lesions such as leukoplakia and erythroplakia that do not heal in 10 days should be biopsied.
- Frequently used tests for tooth vitality include thermal, electrical and pulse oximetry.

7 Diagnostic adjuncts 2

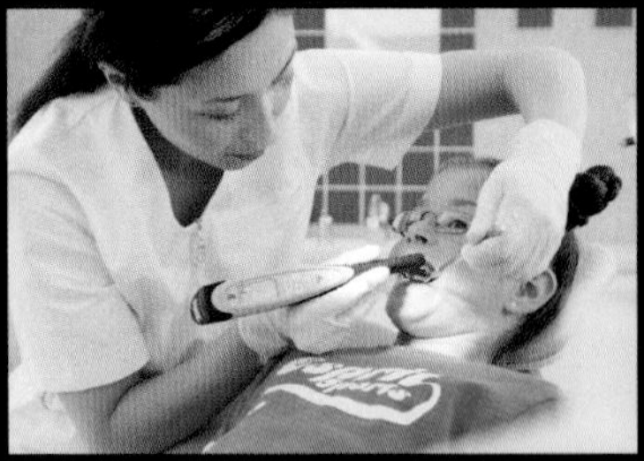

QLF is an objective method for detecting caries

Digital score	Clinical interpretation
0–9	Sound enamel or early enamel lesion
10–17	Enamel caries
18–99	Dentine caries

Quantitative laser fluorescence (QLF) scores

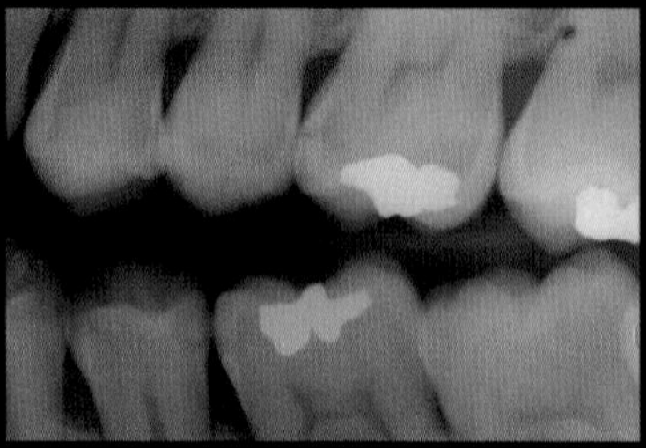

Bitewing radiographs are an excellent method for detecting inter-proximal (smooth) carious lesions

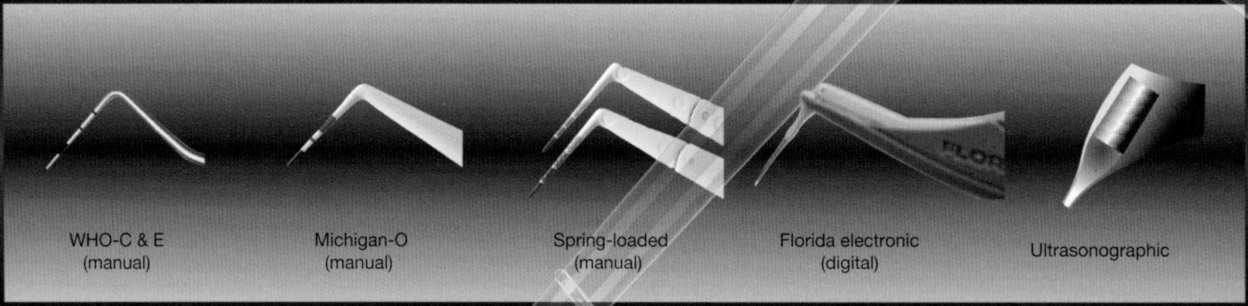

WHO-C & E (manual)

Michigan-O (manual)

Spring-loaded (manual)

Florida electronic (digital)

Ultrasonographic

A section of periodontal probes

Level	Process	Diagnostic tools
Clinical	Attachment and bone loss	Periodontal probing, radiographs
Tissue	Apical migration of epithelial attachment, connective tissue and bone loss	Histomorphometry, immunohistochemistry
Cellular	Presence of inflammatory cells (neutrophils), osteoclast activation	ELISA, immunohistochemistry
Molecular	Activation of receptors for endotoxins: CD-14, toll-like receptors	Polymerase chain reaction, DNA–DNA hybridisation, laser-capture microdissection

Methods of diagnosing periodontal disease

Prosthodontics at a Glance, Second Edition. Irfan Ahmad.

Caries detection

Dental caries is the most prevalent lesion in the oral cavity that is diagnosed and treated in a dental practice. **Caries** describes both the **lesion and disease process**, and its incidence in industrialised countries has decreased over the last four decades. Specifically, interproximal or **smooth surface caries** has shown a greater decline than occlusal lesions. Consequently, **occlusal caries** presents a greater challenge for early detection and treatment to prevent progression into larger cavities. Also, **Caries-risk Assessment Tools (CATs)** are useful for objectively classifying patients into low-, medium- or high-risk categories. Ideally, caries diagnostic tests should fulfil the following criteria:

- **Sensitivity** – ability to truly determine presence of caries
- **Specificity** – ensure that sound tooth is registered as negative
- **Accuracy** – number of positive and negative tests should sum to the total examined tooth surfaces

Methods for caries detection include the following:

- **Histology** – remains the gold standard for evaluating caries, but is obviously impractical, and is predominantly limited to research, especially of the primary dentition following exfoliation or extraction
- **Visual inspection** – most common method for caries diagnosis, e.g. using the **International Caries Detection and Assessment System (ICDAS)**, but is affected by operator experience and subjectivity
- **Enhanced visual inspection** includes:
  - **Magnification** – using loupes or operating microscope
  - **Fibreoptic illumination** – widely used for detecting interproximal caries, but can also be used for occlusal lesions, e.g. FOTI (fibreoptic transillumination) and DIFOTI (digital imaging fibreoptic transillumination). Sound enamel appears translucent, enamel caries appears grey and opaque, and dentine caries casts an orange/ brown or bluish shadow
  - **Enamel porosity** (Ekstrand method) – assesses difference of refractive indices between air, water and enamel
  - Combination of fibreoptics and enamel porosity
- **Electrical conductance measurements (ECM)** – measures electrical resistance of teeth. Intact enamel has greater resistance than carious lesions, which are porous and have a higher water content. Dentine has lower resistance than enamel, and therefore allows differentiation between enamel and dentine lesions
- **Tactile** – explorer probes suffer from subjectivity and clinical experience, and should be used with caution to avoid piercing non-cavitated enamel (possibly reversible) carious lesions
- **Bitewing radiographs** – the most popular method, especially for interproximal lesions. In addition, digital radiography allows image manipulation for highlighting salient lesions
- **Caries detection dyes** – stain carious dentine, especially useful for deep caries excavation and avoiding inadvertent pulpal exposure
- **Tuned aperture computed tomography (TACT)** – reconstruction of anatomical 'slice' images to form a pseudo- or true 3D representation of a tooth, known as a **pseudohologram**.
- **Tooth staining and hydration** – produce erratic values
- **Fluorescence** – either **quantitative laser fluorescence (QLF)** using a diode fluorescence device that illuminates the tooth with a pulse light of wavelength 290–450 nm, or DIAGNOdent that uses infra-red light of wavelength 655 nm. The emitted fluorescence correlates with the extent of enamel and dentine demineralisation, e.g. a digital scale representation from 0 to 99. This is an objective assessment, but intrinsic or superficial tooth stains or hypomineralisation create variable light scattering and therefore unpredictable readings

Periodontal assessment

The crucial factor for periodontal disease is **host genetic susceptibility.** Individuals who are susceptible to severe chronic periodontitis should be screened and identified as **genotype positive**, which helps with treatment planning and monitoring. **Periodontal disease is diagnosed** at the **clinical**, **tissue**, **cellular** and **molecular levels.** The clinical assessment of periodontal disease is the most popular method for ascertaining destruction caused by previous episodes of disease, or the effectiveness of recent periodontal therapy. This includes recording **bleeding on probing (BOP)**, **pocket depth (PD)**, **loss of attachment (LOA)** and **clinical attachment level (CAL)** using periodontal probes. It is advisable to perform prophylaxis, remove plaque retentive factors and oral hygiene counselling before probing to avoid **false pocket** measurements. The types of **periodontal probes** include:

- **Manual**, e.g. WHO BPE probes, Michigan-O, Williams, Colorvue, UNC-15 or Marquis. The degree of reproducibility varies with the type of probe and there are conflicting reports on whether a manual or electronic probe is more reliable. Manual probing is convenient and expedient but measurements may be erratic due to prevailing inflammation, presence of plaque, calculus, overcontoured restorations, tooth location and angulation, patient compliance, probe diameter, angulation and pressure and visual recording errors.
- **Spring loaded**, e.g. Brodontic Probe (Prima, Byfleet, UK) and Click-Probe (KerrHawe SA, Switzerland). Unlike manual probes, these varieties deliver a predefined consistent force (0.2–0.5 N (20–25 g) probe force or 255 N/cm^2 probing pressure)
- **Electronic or computerised pressure-sensitive (digital probes)**, e.g. Florida Probe (Florida Probe Company, Gainesville, FL, USA) and Jonker Probe (Jonkers Data, Staphorst, Netherlands). These probes deliver a constant pressure and electronic recording or displaying data using appropriate software. However, the probing pressure in many probes is less than 250 N/cm^2, which is necessary to enter periodontal pockets deeper than 5 mm
- **Ultrasonographic** periodontal probes are non-invasive, using ultrasound echo waveforms to measure periodontal pocket depth

Radiography is an adjunct tool for detecting and confirming periodontal disease. The various views include panoramic, horizontal and vertical bitewings and periapicals (presence or absence of lamina dura). Bone loss quoted as a **% is more meaningful** than a millimetre measurement. At the tissue, cellular and molecular levels, biomarkers in **gingival crevicular fluid (GCF)** are useful diagnostic indicators for assessing periodontal disease. Biomarkers include microbial factors, host response factors and connective tissue breakdown products, bone resorption factors (e.g. ICTP; type I collagen carboxyterminal telopeptide), and their levels found in plaque biofilm, GCF or saliva are diagnostic markers for periodontal disease activity and its progression. Future developments may allow GCF analysis for biological markers with chairside assay.

Key points

- Although the incidence of dental caries has declined, caries remain the most common disease treated in the oral cavity.
- Subjective caries detection includes visual, tactile and enhanced visual inspection.
- Objective caries detection includes radiography and QLF.
- Periodontal probing remains the most popular and convenient method for detecting, charting and monitoring periodontal disease.

8 Radiography

Digital radiographs can be manipulated to enhance salient features
Digital CCD sensor
ABC
Sally Smith
DENTAL BADGE
luxel
Radiation monitor badge
Digital sensor with paralleling holder
GENDEX
KAVO
FOCUS
Digital intra-oral dental X-ray unit (KavoKerr)
Panoramic dental unit (KavoKerr)
L
Lateral cephalometric radiograph
Panoramic radiograph
Periapical radiograph
Bitewing radiograph

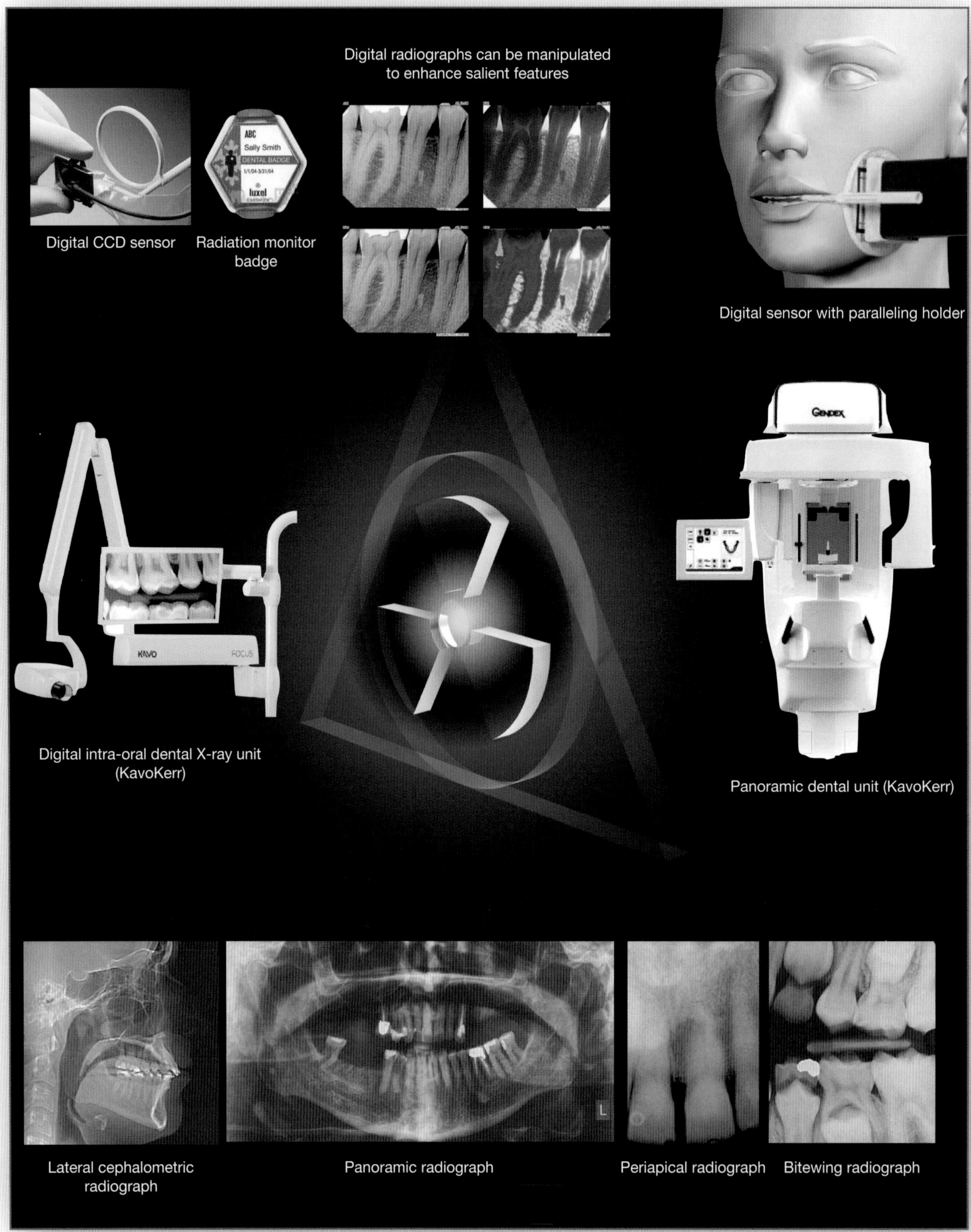

Prosthodontics at a Glance, Second Edition. Irfan Ahmad.

Besides a clinical examination, **projection dental radiography** is the most frequently used diagnostic tool in dentistry. Its uses range from detecting caries to more elaborate findings such as gross pathologies of the jaws. **Cone beam-computed tomography (CBCT),** discussed in Chapter 9, is the latest radiology tool, offering enhanced and sophisticated 3D visualisation of dento-maxillofacial anatomy.

X-ray tube

The production of X-rays has changed very little since they were discovered by **Röntgen in 1895**. X-rays are produced when electrons are accelerated to strike a metal target. A contemporary dental X-ray tube for producing radiation is a **DC (direct current) or Constant Potential** device that reduces soft X-rays, which cause DNA damage. It is housed in a casing and has an appropriate sized **collimator** to restrict the emitted beam and reduce the **Equivalent Dose** by 60%. The typical setting for intra-oral dental radiography is 60 kVp, 7 mA, with varying focus to skin distances of 20–32 cm. The **exposure time (for AC units)** or **kilovoltage (for DC units)** is selected according to tooth, age and the physical build of the individual.

Radiation safety and precautions

X-rays are part of the **electromagnetic spectrum** classified as **ionising radiation,** which are potentially hazardous for living organisms, causing irreversible ailments such as **cancer**, **sterilisation** and **gene mutation.** The aims of radiation safety are:

- **Justification** for its use, i.e. risks vs benefit
- **Optimisation** of protection using the lowest possible dosage, e.g. for a periapical exposure the limit is 2.3 mGy
- **Limitation of exposure** by conforming to recommended limits as specified by law. In the United Kingdom, Ionising Radiation Medical Exposure Regulations (IR(ME)R) 2000/2018 guidelines must be observed for all types of radiographic examination, i.e. **ALARP (as low as reasonably practicable)**. **Radiation protection** is for the operator, patient, ambient environment and third parties (other patients and staff members in the practice). **Precautions** include regular **equipment testing** and maintenance, **thyroid lead aprons, monitoring devices/badges** and **restricted areas of operation**. Finally, **operator training** is essential in the taking and interpreting radiographs, thereby avoiding the need to repeat exposures unnecessarily.

Conventional dental radiography

Film or conventional dental radiography is similar to conventional photography. A cellulose acetate sheet (film) is coated with X-ray sensitive chemicals which react when exposed to radiation. Subsequently, the film is processed with chemicals (developer and fixer) to create a black-and-white indelible image on the cellulose acetate sheet. The processing can be performed manually in tanks of appropriate chemicals, or in an automated processing unit, which also dries the film ready for storage. The films are available in various sizes for taking **intra-oral periapical, bitewing, occlusal,** as well as extra-oral **lateral cephalometric or panoramic views**. In addition, radiation dosages can be reduced using films of varying sensitivities (**high film speeds**, e.g. 'F' speed requires 60% less dosage than 'D' speed films) or rare earth **intensifying screens** in film cassette holders (panoramic and lateral cephalometric). The major advantage of film radiography is familiarity with established protocols. The **drawbacks are a relatively higher radiation dose** (compared to **digital radiography that requires 70% less exposure**), the need for visual magnification for proper analysis, environmentally toxic chemicals and the inability to store and transmit images electronically. However, **scanners** are available to **digitise film radiographs**. The two main methods for intra-oral dental periapical radiographs are the **parallel** and **bisecting angle techniques.**

Digital dental radiography

Similar to digital photography, **digital radiography** has revolutionised dental radiology. The advantages are **instantaneity**, no chemical processing, **reduce radiation dosage**, ability to manipulate and enhance images for improved and **accurate diagnosis, electronic storage** and **transmission via the Internet.** The disadvantages are the initial capital outlay for equipment purchase and training, which are rapidly offset by the innumerable benefits mentioned above.

With digital radiography, the film is substituted with a **sensor**. Currently, three types of sensor are available, **CCD** (charge-coupled device), **CMOS** (complementary metal oxide semiconductor) and **PSP** (Photo-stimulable Storage Phosphor plate). Each type of sensor has advantages and limitations regarding altering the exposure, signal-to-noise ratio or image resolution. For accurate diagnosis, the resultant image resolution is paramount. **Image resolution** is determined by spatial resolution expressed as pixel size, **dots per inch (dpi)** or **line pairs per millimetre (lp mm^{-1})**. For example, a high-resolution CCD sensor is 15–20 lp mm^{-1}, while an SPP system is 8 lp mm^{-1}. The required **resolution depends on the diagnostic requirements**, e.g. medium resolution is sufficient for detecting caries or gross pathology, while high resolution is beneficial for discriminating minute tooth or root fractures and for locating root canal anastomoses during endodontic treatment. However, high resolution images create larger files, requiring increased computer hard drive storage capacity and present a challenge for transmission via email.

The process of digital radiography is as follows. After exposing the sensor (e.g. KaVo IXS) to radiation from an X-ray unit, an **analogue/digital (A–D) converter** converts the analogue signal to digital data that is processed by either a dedicated or generic software for displaying as an image on a computer monitor. The radiograph image can be manipulated by altering **magnification** (best method for enlargement is bicubic convolution), **gamma curve**, **density**, **contrast**, **brightness** or **applying filters (e.g. polarising)** for emphasising or **enhancing pertinent detail**.

Key points

- Projection dental radiography is the commonest diagnostic tool in dentistry.
- A dental X-ray unit produces potentially hazardous ionising radiation.
- An X-ray detector can either be analogue (film) or digital (sensor).
- Radiation safety and appropriate training are paramount for preventing irreversible damage to health.
- Digital radiography offers innumerable advantages compared to X-ray films.

9 Digital acquisition: computed tomography

Volumetric data reconstruction creates axial, sagittal, and coronal orthogonal planes in the *x, y & z* axes

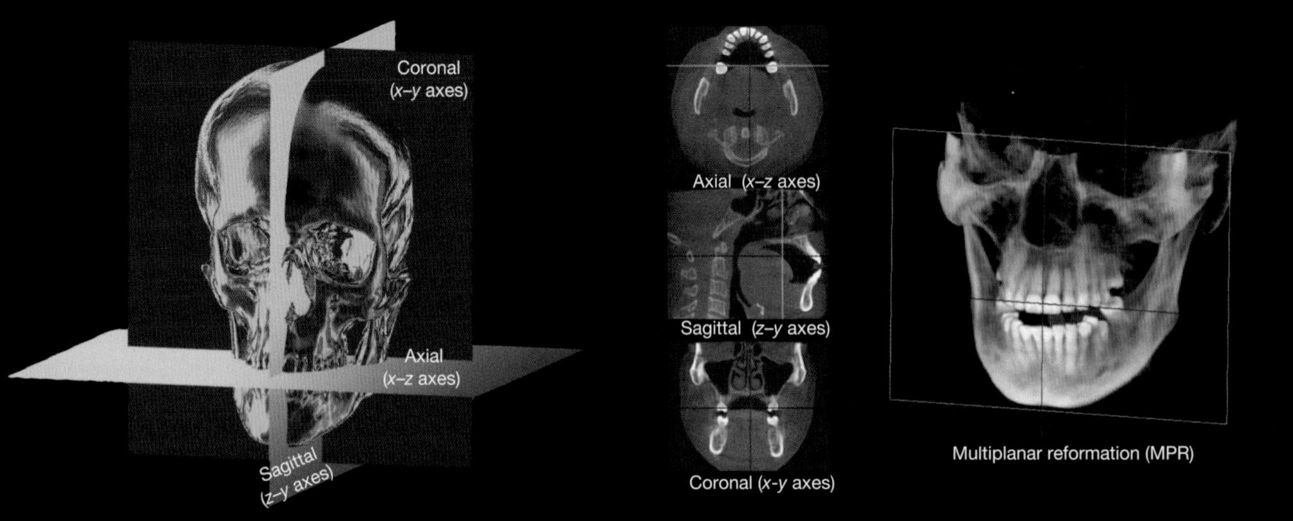

Coronal (*x–y* axes)

Axial (*x–z* axes)

Sagittal (*z–y* axes)

Axial (*x–z* axes)

Sagittal (*z–y* axes)

Coronal (*x-y* axes)

Multiplanar reformation (MPR)

CBCT scan visualised by various rendering methods: MIP, surface & volume modelling and soft tissue overlays

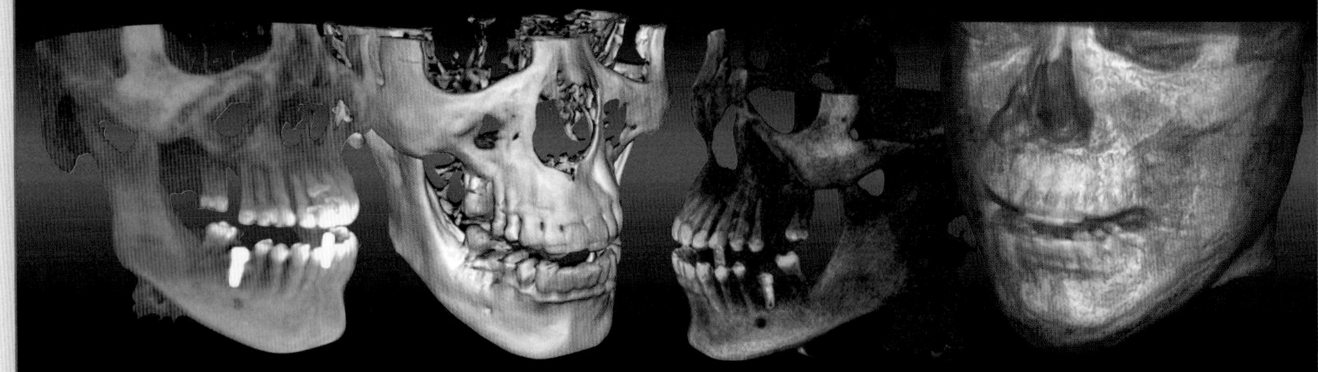

MIP

Surface rendering

Volume rendering

Soft tissue overlay

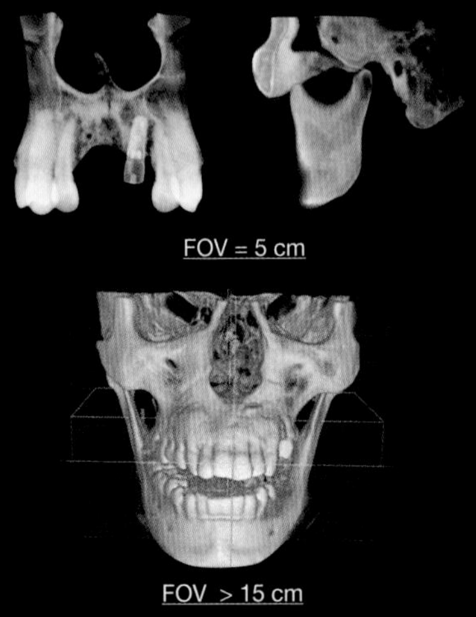

FOV = 5 cm

FOV > 15 cm

Field of View (FOV) & Region of Interest (ROI)

	Radiation dosages (µSv)
Full mouth periapical radiographs	13–150
Panoramic	26
CBCT of jaw	29–477
CAT of jaw	1200–3300
Daily background radiation/year	8–3000

Comparison of radiation dosages

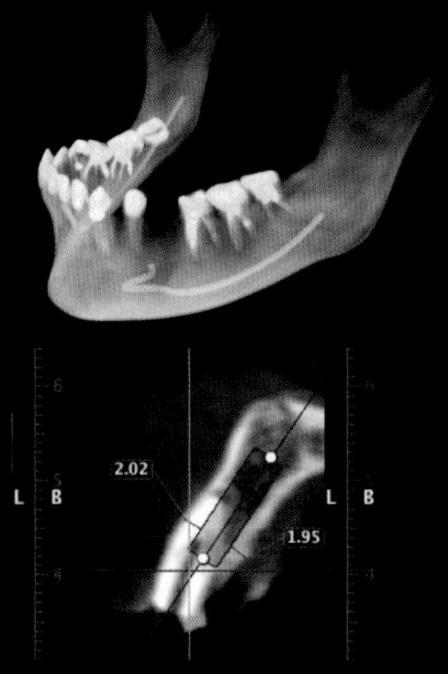

2.02

1.95

L B

L B

Nerve trajectory & implant treatment planning

Prosthodontics at a Glance, Second Edition. Irfan Ahmad.

Computed tomography (CT) is a radiology-based imaging system for evaluating skeletal structures of the body. CT imaging is one method used for scanning the maxillofacial region. However, depending on the symptoms and clinical findings, alternative methods of imaging can be considered including digital radiography, **magnetic resonance imaging (MRI)** and **ultrasonography (ultrasound imaging)**.

CAT (computerised axial tomography)

CAT, synonymous with **conventional CT (cCT)** imaging, uses a rotating helical fan beam X-ray unit and detector to scan the maxillofacial region. The ensuing **digital slice-by-slice images**, usually in the axial plane, are combined to create a 2D representation. The scan can either be a **single-slice** or **multiple detector CT (MDCT),** which substantially reduces the radiation dosage. CT scans are usually limited to hospitals or specialist centres due to their prohibitive cost, large size and the requirements for periodic maintenance, training of operating staff and adherence to strict radiation controls.

CBCT (cone beam computed tomography)

Unlike the layered (or slice) images produced with CAT scans, **cone beam CT (CBCT)** scans are based on **volumetric tomography**. A CBCT apparatus consists of a pulsed or continuous X-ray beam unit with a reciprocating detector to capture multiple basis projections. The CBCT X-ray beam has a **cone beam geometry**, and its **field of view (FOV)** is varied according to the **region of interest (ROI)**, ranging from 5 cm for capturing a specific dentoalveolar areas or TMJ anatomy, to more than 15 cm for recording the entire craniofacial skeleton. A series of raw images are collected at a fraction of a second (around 30 frames/second), referred to as **projection data**. The number of 2D sequential images varies from 150 to 600, according to the desired FOV or ROI. The digital information obtained is in the form of 3D cuboid blocks known as **voxels** or volume pixels (similar to pixels in a digital camera sensor). The next stage is reconstructing the projection data to **volumetric data** by applying **software algorithms** such as Feldcamp, Davis, and Kress (FDK) or algebraic reconstruction technique (ART). The individual projections are reconstructed to form **orthogonal planar images**. This process is termed **multiplanar reformation (MPR)**. As well as images in various planes, other types of possible MPR images include the following:

- **Oblique planar reformation** – 2D non-axial images useful for assessing the temporomandibular joint (TMJ) and impacted molars
- **Curved planar reformation** – similar to panoramic radiographs but without distortion or superimposition of the cervical spine
- **Serial transplanar reformation** – a series of images (1 mm thick, with 1 mm separation) derived from oblique and planar reformations for assessing alveolar bone height and width, relation of nerve canals and sinuses and shape of the condyles for determining TMJ pathologies
- **Multiplanar volume reformation** – formed by increasing the number of voxels of a slice for 'thicker' panoramic (25–30 mm) or cephalometric (130–150 mm) images
- **Maximum intensity projection (MIP)** – isolates the highest value voxels to form a pseudo-3D structure of surface morphology. A true 3D representation is also possible by adding shading effects. Furthermore, user interaction allows the skeletal structures to be visualised in 'real time' in any orientation from limitless angles

The standard files from CBCT scans are **DICOM-3 (Digital Imaging and Communications in Medicine)** with the .dcm file extension. **CBCT is used for many dental disciplines** such as implantology, oral surgery, oral medicine, periodontology, endodontics, prosthodontics, orthodontics, and monitoring pathology and assessing the efficacy of therapy.

Advantages of CBCT

The reduced cost X-ray tubes, development of high-quality digital sensors and the introduction of powerful personal computers have made CBCT equipment more accessible, and within reach of many practitioners. Similar to digital photography and radiography, **image manipulation** is relatively straightforward, e.g. zoom, magnification, isolation, cropping, altering contrast and brightness, adding 'false colours' to visualise specific structures, cursor-driven measurements, image pointers (arrows, lines) and adding descriptive text annotations. Another invaluable advantage is **transmission of CBCT images by the Internet** to specialists for remote diagnosis, and to dental laboratories for prosthetic assessment. Moreover, CBCT imaging offers **numerous benefits** compared to CAT scans or digital radiographs, including:

- **Collimated X-ray beam adjustment** – for altering FOV and concentrating on the ROI, e.g. root canal number and location within an individual tooth
- **Image accuracy** – reduced distortion, no magnification factor
- **Image quality** – superior due to isotropic voxels (76–400 μm), compared to anisotropic voxels of 1–2 mm with CAT
- **Faster scan time** (10–70 seconds, depending on equipment) compared to CAT scans
- **Reduced dosimetry** than CAT
- **Soft tissue rendering** – allows assessment of soft tissues profiles, particularly useful for orthodontic therapy
- **'Stitching' with intra-oral and facial scans** for enhanced 3D analysis of skeletal and soft tissue anatomy
- **Fabrication of surgical guides** – surface rendering allows conversion of **DICOM** files to **.stl** or **.obj** files used for printing 3D biomodels of bone architecture, or for designing surgical guides for implant osteotomies
- **Print 3D models of jaws** (conversion of a DICOM file to .stl files) using 3D printing for **tactile rehearsal treatment planning (TRTP)** to foresee complications before a surgical procedure
- **Reduced image artefacts** using sophisticated software

Disadvantages of CBCT

- **Increased radiation dosage compared to digital radiography**
- **Misuse** by inexperienced operators may cause excess dosage
- **Radiation burden for children**, if used for periodic orthodontic monitoring
- **Irradiation of vital organs** – pituitary gland, salivary glands, eyes, skin, bone marrow, breast, reproductive organs
- **Unreliable caries detection**
- **Scatter from dental materials**, e.g. amalgam, casting alloys or gutta-percha
- **Evolving technology** – obsolescence of equipment and software

Key points

- CAT produces 2D axial images with higher radiation dosage compared to CBCT.
- CBCT is a 3D volumetric representation with several distortion-free views, and is used for many dental disciplines.
- CBCT is a rapidly evolving technology requiring continual capital investment and intensive training.

Digital acquisition: optical scanner technologies

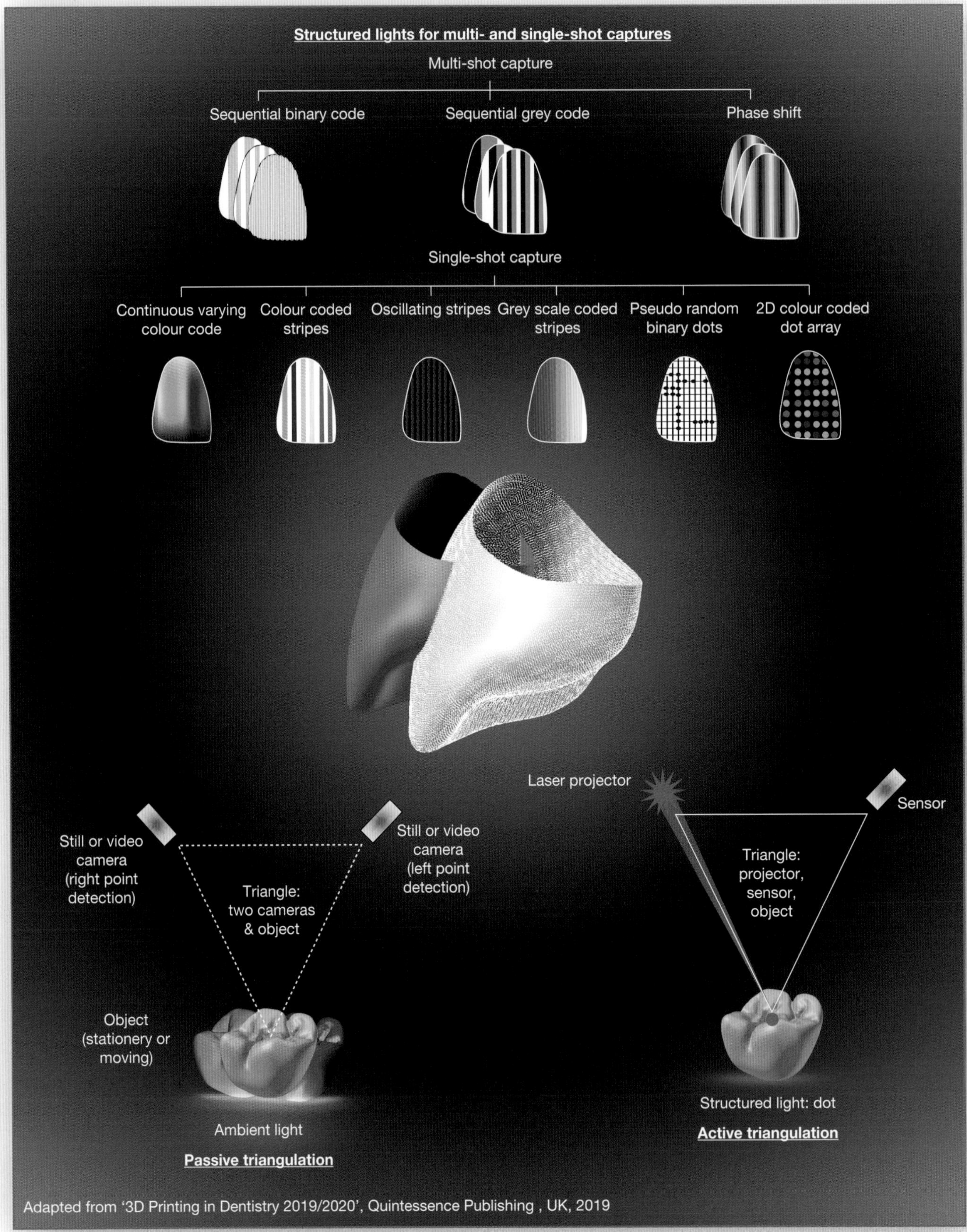

Structured lights for multi- and single-shot captures

Multi-shot capture

Sequential binary code

Sequential grey code

Phase shift

Single-shot capture

Continuous varying colour code

Colour coded stripes

Oscillating stripes

Grey scale coded stripes

Pseudo random binary dots

2D colour coded dot array

Laser projector

Sensor

Still or video camera (right point detection)

Still or video camera (left point detection)

Triangle: two cameras & object

Triangle: projector, sensor, object

Object (stationery or moving)

Ambient light

Passive triangulation

Structured light: dot

Active triangulation

Adapted from '3D Printing in Dentistry 2019/2020', Quintessence Publishing , UK, 2019

Prosthodontics at a Glance, Second Edition. Irfan Ahmad.

3D digital acquisition is accomplished with **intra-oral oral scanners (IOS)**, **extra-oral scanners (EOS)**, **facial scanners** and **CBCT**. Surface scanners map superficial nonplanar topography, while radiographic-based devices capture osseous anatomy below the soft tissues. The technology of **tridimensional surface imaging** is complex and diverse, consisting of **contact** and **non-contact scanning** protocols. The recent trend has shifted to an **optical, non-invasive, non-contact approach** using a variety of scanning technologies. A distinguishing factor of these devices is whether the scanner uses an **active** or **passive** method for acquisition.

Structured light

The difference between **active and passive methods is the type of illumination** used for collecting data regarding the distance of the topography of an object's surface. **Passive** refers to processes that utilise a **non-coherent light source** (usually ambient light), while **active processes** directly or actively illuminate the subject by a **coherent, structured light source**. A structured light (or controlled/contrived lighting) is typically generated by a laser or LEDs (light emitting diodes) that project **stationary or oscillating (time varying or pulse) patterns** known as **codes**. The codes can be a point (dot), multi-points, lines (stripes), meshes or grids, which are projected onto the surface of the object for speeding up the acquisition process. The type of structured light varies depending on whether the image capture is a **single-shot (still)** or **multi-shot (video)**.

3D surface imaging technologies

Optical scanners used several imaging technologies as follows:

- **Passive triangulation**, or time-of-flight, is a method of measuring the distance of objects without physically touching them. Passive triangulation (PT) uses ambient, non-coherent light source to calculate the distance to the target object's nonplanar surface. The configuration of the **emitter(s), object and sensor(s) form a triangle,** and hence the term triangulation. The software algorithms employ the principle based on **Pythagoras theorem of triangles** (law of cosines) to calculate the distance to the object's surface. PT is also used for **stereovision** or **stereophotogrammetry** that involves capturing stereo images that are processed with **photogrammetric** algorithms to produce a 3D still or in-motion video representation. PT provides superior accuracy, but its drawback is precisely matching reference points on the object that are captured from different angles by two separate sensors or cameras. Also, only objects with **distinct features with pronounced outlines** are registered, [illegible] featureless surfaces are poorly recorded, and suffers from **chromatic aberrations** or 'rainbow effect' at the edges of surfaces
- **Active triangulation (AT)** overcomes the deficiencies of PT, by measuring distances using a **structured light source** projected onto the object. Since the distance of the illumination is fixed, only one sensor is required for calculating the distance to the object. The imaging sensor can be either a digital **CCD (charged coupled device)** still/video camera or a **linear array device**. AT is capable of high-speed, non-tactile scanning, which is ideal for delicate, moist and friable oral tissues. However, the drawback is **specular reflections** or scatter off mirror-like shiny surfaces and poor recording of shadow area that result in missed data. Some of these shortcoming can be partially circumvented using higher resolution cameras with large megapixel sensors. Finally, similar to PT, AT image capture can either be stills or videos, and the process is termed **active stereoscopic vision** or **active stereophotogrammetry**.
- **AFI (accordion fringe interferometry)** uses acousto-optics for non-contact 3D imaging by projecting **interference fringes** (e.g. Moiré patterns) onto objects for measuring distances. The advantages of AFI are **infinite depth of field**, **ability to scan shiny surfaces without powder**, unaffected by ambient light and **indifferent to patient or operator induced movements**. Also, AFI produces high-quality images with rapid capture, is portable, which is ideal for hand-held scanners.
- **CLSM (confocal laser scanning microscopy)** – confocal means 'having the same focus' since the process removes all extraneous light from above and below, allowing **only in-focus points of light** to be detected by the sensor by applying spacial filtering. CLSM is an optical imaging technique that traverses point-by-point the topography and texture of the target specimen. A laser point light source in the ***x*, *y* axes builds 2D 'slices'** of the object by optical sectioning. In order to create 3D renditions, either the specimen or sensor moves up or down so that the ***z* axis** can be recorded. The successive 2D image layers (known as *z* stacks), are piled up on top of each other by imaging software to convey depth or a three-dimensional surface profile. Also, since **specular reflections and out-of-focus points are eliminated,** extremely detailed, blur-free, high-quality images are possible. The drawback is that since only a small portion of in-focus light is transmitted, a high intensity laser and highly sensitive **photomultiplier tube (PMT) detectors** are necessary to compensate for the loss of light by the pinhole collimator.
- **AWS (active wavefront sampling)** uses **video non-contact 3D surface technology** for capturing consecutive images (e.g. at 20 fps [frames per second]) to produce tridimensional imagery. The structured light stripes are generated by blue LED and a module with an **off-axis aperture** that rotates around the optical axis of the object. The rotating off-axis aperture can either be located in the illumination path or the imaging path. A single camera with a **lens array** captures the moving points at each position for calculating distance
- **OCT (optical coherence tomography)** is an **interferometric imaging process** that is capable of scanning both **surface and subsurface detail**. This method is similar to ultrasound for mapping internal morphology of biological tissues, but OCT uses a light source instead of sound, and is sometimes referred to as 'optical ultrasound'. For surface analysis, a blue UV (ultra-violet) laser is used to gain profiles of the tomography of the oral tissues, with a resolution of 1–15 μm, which is100 time better than ultrasound scanners. Also, since the light source penetrates about 3 mm below the tissues, OCT is utilised for biopsy of tissues when excision biopsies are contraindicated
- **Ultrasound** or sonography is an established medical imaging technology, which has been adapted for dental IOS. The scanner uses high-frequency ultrasound for capturing challenging areas such as **subgingival crown margins,** and is also capable of **recording the underlying osseous architecture**. The rationale for using ultrasound, rather than light-based systems, is that sound is indifferent to optical distortions caused by saliva, water or blood, and therefore, yields **higher signal-to-noise ratio images**, which require less post-capture processing

Key points

- 3D optical surface imaging technologies allow digitisation of the oral cavity.
- Non-contact, optical scanners use passive or active methods for digital acquisition.
- IOS use several scanning technologies.

Digital acquisition: IOS (intra-oral scanners)

Compassion of technologies & features of IOS

Scanner	Technology (ies)	Powder-free	Scan time (U/L arches)
CEREC AC OmniCam	AT & CLSM	Yes	
CEREC AC BlueCam	AT & CLSM	No	
FastScan	AT & Scheimpflug principle	No	4 min
MIA 3d	AT stereophotogrammetry	Yes	1½ min
DirectScan	AT stereophotogrammetry	?	
BlueScan-I	AT stereophotogrammetry	Yes	
Condor	AT stereophotogrammetry	Yes	
Straumann CARES (Dental Wings)	AT stereophotogrammetry	Yes	2 min
Heron IOS	AT stereophotogrammetry	Yes	
Lythos	AFI	Yes	7 min
ZFX Intrascan	CLSM & AFI	Yes	
iTerio iTerio Element*	CLSM	Yes	10–15 min *(1 min)
3D Progress	CLSM	No	4 min
CS 3500	CLSM	Yes	10 min
Trios	CLSM	Yes	5 min
Lava COS	AWS	No	10 min
True Definition Scanner	AWS	No	5–6 min
Mobile True Definition Scanner	AWS	No	<5 min
PlanScan/Planmeca Emerald	OCT & CLSM	Yes	8–10 min
Aadva IOS (GC)		Yes	
Fona MyCrown		No	
Adin VIZ		No	4 min
Whitesonic IOS	Ultrasound	Yes	

Adapted from '3D Printing in Dentistry 2019/2020', Quintessence Publishing, UK, 2019

Intra-oral image acquisition

2D digital image
IOS image capture
3D digital image

IOS

Confocal laser scanning microscopy (CLSM) IOS

Focus filter
Beam splitter
Sensor
In-focus point
Collimated laser point source

Accuracy

Trueness
Precision

Resolution

High resolution
Low resolution

Prosthodontics at a Glance, Second Edition. Irfan Ahmad.

The concept of an **IOS** is taking a non-contact **digital impression**, using light or other means, for capturing the surface of intra-oral tissues. An **optical scanner** records analogue signals that are translated into electric signals by an **analogue-to-digital converter**, which are subsequently processed by computer software to create 3D digital images.

Principles of IOS

Ideally, a digital impression or scan should faithfully reproduce the teeth and surrounding soft tissues with extreme dimensional accuracy that is comparable, or superior, to a conventional analogue tray/material impression. Current IOS are capable of creating accurate three-dimensional geometric representations that are **clinically acceptable f**or most dental modalities. The physical components of an IOS depend on the type of technology, but usually consists of a **wand**, which houses several items including a **light source emitter**, **lenses**, **beam splitter** and a **still or video camera**. The wand can be either stand-alone, wireless or part of a workstation cart incorporating a **CPU (central processing unit)** and a **touch screen** display monitor. The cart or desktop configuration is an all-in-one unit that can be stored away and accessed whenever necessary without needing an independent computer for operation. The stand-alone IOS offers flexibility and economy, as it can be attached to any laptop via a USB (universal serial bus) cable.

There are **three distinct stages for non-contact, optical recording**; first stage is **projecting light** onto the surface and analysing the deformations of the reflected light for creating 2D images in the **cartesian *x* and *y* coordinates**. The second stage is recording the third cartesian *z coordinate*, in order to create a three-dimensional rendition. This is accomplished either by moving a **hand-held scanner (IOS) over the surface** or **moving the object (extra-oral scanners – EOS)** by servo-motors (turntable) to profile its surface and record successive image layers. In addition, the **zoom factor** of an IOS compensates for variations in **magnification** and **spatial resolution**. The sensor or camera can either record successive still images (single-shot) or continuous video (multi-shot) capture. The last stage is calculating the distance of **points of interest (POI)** on the surface using distance measuring methods such as triangulation or stereophotogrammetry, using **various technologies such as AFI, CLSM, AWS, OCT or ultrasound**. Furthermore, many IOS use a combination of technologies to compensate for the **challenging and unique environment of the oral cavity**, such as confined area of the mouth, simultaneously recording matt and reflective surfaces, subgingival tooth or implant abutment finish lines, wetness and involuntary movements of both the patient and operator. Finally, a **surface reconstruction software** uses the **point cloud** data for recreating the geometry and texture variations, or topography of the surface. A point cloud is a volumetric data set representing the 3D surface of an object in the *x*, *y* and *z* coordinates. It can be considered as a 'RAW' unadulterated capture, equivalent to RAW digital photographic unprocessed images. Although the digital data of a point cloud is extremely accurate, it needs to be converted into a **mesh** or surface models before it is useable in **CAD software**. This is achieved by converting the point cloud to **triangular or quad meshes** that are conducive for CAD modelling. Most IOS produce the generic **.stl (STereoLithography) 3D file format** that is readily imported into CAD software, and can be stitched with different datasets including DICOM or 2D digital photographic files. However, other formats such as **.obj (object)** and **.ply (polygon)** offer additional **colour and texture** information with **improved accuracy**.

Accuracy, trueness, precision and resolution

The choice of IOS is increasing at a staggering rate to keep up with the paradigm shift from analogue to digital dentistry. There are several properties of a scanner to consider before making a decision as to which is suited for a specific practice or discipline. A foremost feature to consider is accuracy, i.e. recreating reality with fidelity. The terms accuracy, precision and trueness are often used synonymously and indiscriminately. The **accuracy** of intra-oral scans, as described by ISO 5725-1, is determined by **trueness and precision. Trueness** is the difference between the original reference model and the 3D image representation of that model. The difference between the two is the unwanted visual noise that deteriorates the signal of the true value, i.e. the higher the signal-to-noise ratio, the higher the accuracy. **Precision** is the second determinant of accuracy and defined as the repeatability or consistency of a measurement performed multiples times. Precision has several variables including the technology of the scanner, calibration, time between scans, operator experience and the humidity, air pressure and temperature of the surrounding environment. **Trueness ranges from 20 µm to 48 µm**, and **precision from 4 µm to 16 µm**. Ideally, a scanner should posses both high trueness and precision to be classed as accurate. **Resolution** is the ability to distinguish detail or the smallest distance between two points in space. This property in unchangeable since it is an inherent **feature of the hardware** (lens and sensor). The smaller the distances that a device can discern, the higher its **spacial resolution.** While accuracy is a comparison between two values, resolution is an absolute value. However, accuracy and resolution are linked; the greater the resolution of an IOS the more accurately it can record an image. The reported resolution of an IOS is similar to a **microCT device**, which has a sensor composed of **pixels of 9.21 µm**. The accuracy of IOS is usually quoted as the difference in µm or percentages, but to date, there is no accepted consensus on how these values should be assessed. In reality, most scanned images have missing data or 'gaps', which are 'closed' by software mathematical algorithms to 'fake' resolution and produce sharp, crisp images. This process is termed **interpolation**, which compensates for shortcomings of the native hardware resolution.

Accuracy can arbitrarily be classified as **local** or **general**. The former is applicable to scanning a single tooth or abutment, while the latter refers to multiple units, quadrants or full arch digitisation. It should be remembered that the morphology of the tooth also influences the degree of accuracy, and teeth displaying pronounced curvature are difficult to reproduce accurately. Furthermore, the type of material being scanned (e.g. teeth, soft tissues, amalgam, cast metal, composite or ceramics) influences the degree of accuracy. In addition, the type of restoration, i.e. inlay, crowns or FPD, also determine the degree of trueness. Since scanning errors are 'stitched' together in the software, each stitched part introduces a small error. Therefore, a 3D image of a single tooth has fewer stitched parts, and therefore, less errors, compared to an entire arch that has multiple stitched parts, and hence, more errors. Generally, hard tissues scans are more accurate that those of soft tissues, which is particularly relevant when providing complete full–full dentures, or designing removable partial denture (RPD) frameworks.

Key points

- Digital impressions are rapidly replacing analogue impressions.
- Hand-held IOS are capable of digitising the oral cavity with clinically acceptable accuracy.
- In general, smaller scans of a few teeth are more accurate than larger scans of full arches or quadrants.

Digital acquisition: EOS (extra-oral scanners) and facial scanners

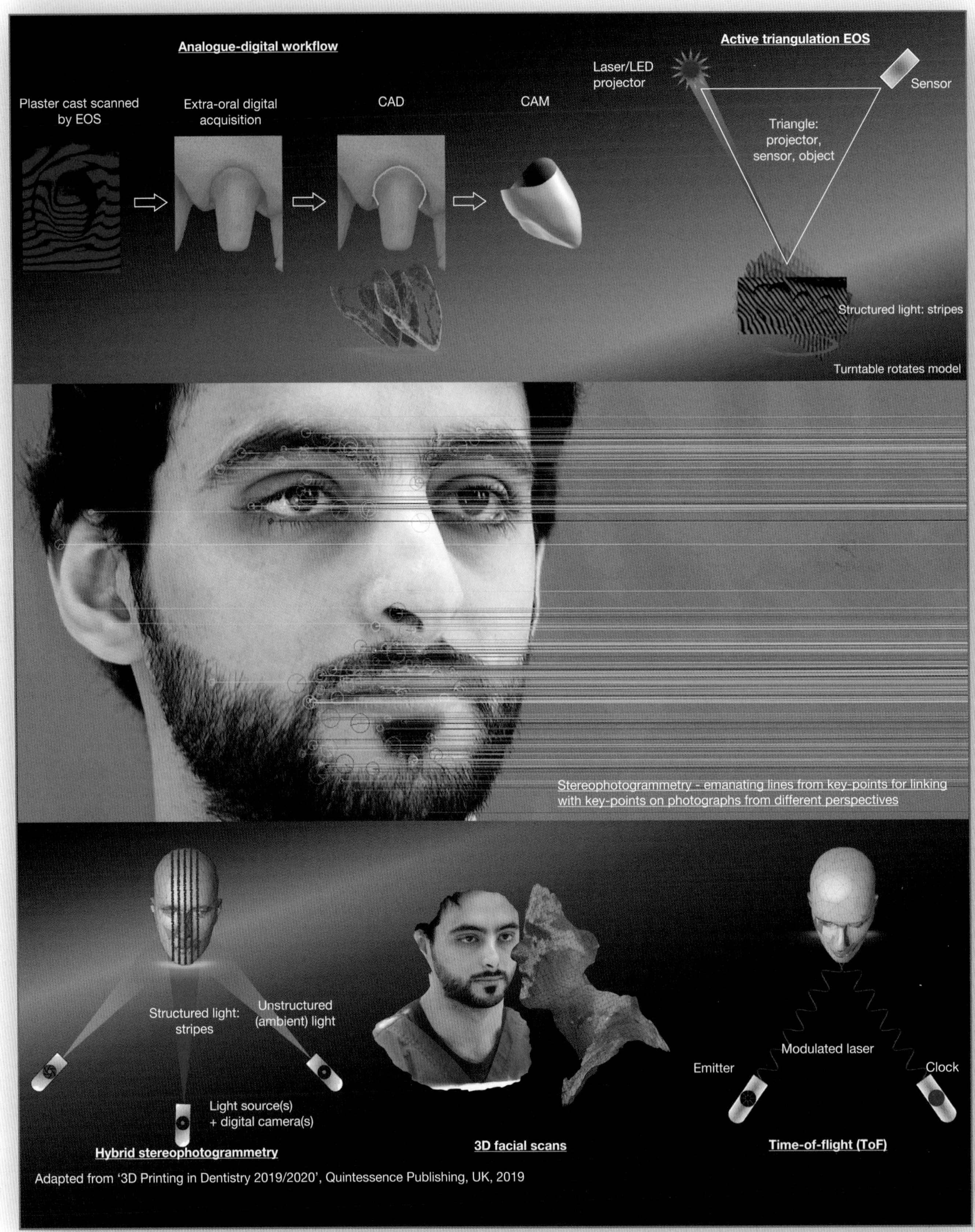

Analogue-digital workflow

Plaster cast scanned by EOS

Extra-oral digital acquisition

CAD

CAM

Active triangulation EOS

Laser/LED projector

Sensor

Triangle: projector, sensor, object

Structured light: stripes

Turntable rotates model

Stereophotogrammetry - emanating lines from key-points for linking with key-points on photographs from different perspectives

Structured light: stripes

Unstructured (ambient) light

Light source(s) + digital camera(s)

Hybrid stereophotogrammetry

3D facial scans

Modulated laser

Emitter

Clock

Time-of-flight (ToF)

Adapted from '3D Printing in Dentistry 2019/2020', Quintessence Publishing, UK, 2019

Prosthodontics at a Glance, Second Edition. Irfan Ahmad.

EOS (extra-oral scanners) or dental laboratory scanners create a digital impression using an indirect method by scanning a plaster cast poured from convention tray/material impressions, or scanning the impression itself to create a 'positive' model. This adds another step and resulting in an analogue–digital workflow. Facial scanners are used for digitising the surface topography of facial landmarks, as well as snapshots of facial movements.

EOS (extra-oral scanners)

Current **EOS non-contact optical scanners** nearly all use **active triangulation** for producing a 3D representation of an object. An EOS consists of a light emitter and a camera(s) or sensor. The light source is either a laser or LED that projects structure light patterns, such as stationery or oscillating lines. Unlike hand-held IOS, which are moved across the teeth and dental arches, EOS have a **turntable that rotates the cast model** in different directions for capturing its surface from various angles. The principle involves either **appending various views** to form a 3D image, or **stitching overlapping 2D images** using reference points. Examples of some EOS [laboratory] scanners are R700 (3 Shape®, Copenhagen, Denmark), Kavo ARCTICA Auto Scan (KaVo® Dental Excellence, Biberach, Germany), CEREC inLab MCXL (Sirona® Dental Systems GmbH, Bensheim, Germany) and Identica T500 (Medit Corp., Seoul, Korea), which claims to scan an entire arch model in 12 seconds with an accuracy of 7 μm.

EOS vs. IOS

The **dilemma between choosing an IOS or EOS** is perplexing. Currently, EOS have the greater market share simply because they were the first type of scanners, and often linked with proprietary CAD software and CAM milling machines. However, this dominance is rapidly being eroded as newer, more reliable, more accurate, faster and user-friendly IOS are being introduced. Furthermore, **IOS allow a complete digital workflow**, without resorting to analogue impressions, which are a potential source of errors due to distortions of the impression and plaster materials. The **accuracy of EOS** is a contentious issue, with ambivalent research results and few guidelines for performance or comparison between different manufacturers. As a general rule, EOS potentially have greater accuracy compared to IOS as the **scan is performed in a controlled environment** without contamination by oral fluids or involuntary movements of the patient and operator. Furthermore, a controlled environment also favours **faster scan speeds** compared to IOS. However, the important point is knowing the **discrepancy between the original and digital scan**. This allows the CAD designer to **compensate for any discrepancy**, e.g. incorporating an appropriate cement space between the prostheses and abutment to ensure a more accurate fit of the restoration.

Facial scanning

3D facial analysis is beneficial for several disciples including **cranio-maxillofacial surgery, plastic surgery, orthodontics,** assessing **dysmorphia**, **monitoring facial growth**, **correcting deformities** (e.g. facial asymmetries or congenial defects) and **evaluating synkinesis** following surgery. There are several methods for producing a three dimensional representation of the face, including **non-contact optical** or **laser scanning**, **stereophotogrammetry** and **time-of-flight (ToF)**.

- A **laser-based facial scanner** consists of a light source and a sensor. The emitted light reflects off the surface and is detected by a sensor. Using the triangulation method, a point cloud is generated, which is subsequently converted by appropriate algorithms to a mesh for **surface reconstruction** of the **facial topography.** Laser scanners cost a few hundred dollar to more than ten thousand dollars. The simpler **hand-held** devices are suited for hobbyists, but the results are often unpredictable. The professional or industrial scanners, are more reliable and available for a wide range of applications such as prototype designs, medicine, architecture, engineering and cartography. The companies supplying **professional imaging** and **facial recognition** equipments include Creaform, Open Technologie, Shining 3D, Artec, AIO Robotics, RangeVision, GOM, Surphaser, ZEISS Optotechnik, etc.
- **Photogrammetry** dates back to the 19th century, and is derived from 'photo' (light), 'gram' (drawing) and 'metry' (measurements), collectively describing the process of taking measurements from a photography. Photogrammetry is based on the triangulation principle of ascertaining the surface topography by calculating the distance formed by a triangle consisting of a light source, object and sensor. **Stereophotogrammetry** is a specific type of photogrammetry in which two or more images of an object, photographed from different angles, are combined to form a 3D image. **Digital stereophotogrammetry can be passive, active and hybrid.** For all three methods, the sensor (usually a high-resolution digital camera) captures the object or scene from different angles and the software subsequently combines the images to form a 3D model. Stereophotogrammetry offers wide, **360° coverage**, which is advantageous for scanning an abject in its entirety. The accuracy of the image depends on both the hardware specifications and software algorithms. However, current devices are capable of delivering **geometric accuracies ranging from 0.1 mm to 0.2 mm**; a 0.2 mm error is regarded as clinically acceptable for contactless anthropometric measurements for cranio-maxillofacial surgery, mammography and facial recognition. In addition, some software is capable of **combining CBCT, intra-oral and facial scans** for producing a comprehensive visualisation of the both the soft tissue and skeletal anatomy. Another emerging development is the **4D surface motion technique** that is capable of capturing **facial expressions** for analysing palsies, involuntary twitches and mood temperaments. Manufacturers supplying professional stereophotogrammetry equipment include 3dMD, Cognitec, Siemens, Canfield, Technest Holdings, Emotient, Motion View and Pritidenta, to name a few.
- The principle of **ToF** is measuring the **time delay between an emitted and reflected light** for calculating the depth or topography of a surface. The emitted source can either be pulsed, or modulated (phased) using acoustic (ultra-sound) or electromagnetic sources such as laser or infra-red. The salient **difference between triangulation** and **ToF principles is that the former measures distance, while the latter measures time.** The emergence of sophisticated ToF technology is developing new applications such as **gesture recognition**, which could prove valuable for assessing dental and facial aesthetics and phonetics, as well as erratic changes in facial expressions for potential intervention by corrective plastic surgery.

Key points

- EOS or dental laboratory-based scanners have a combined analogue–digital workflow.
- Methods for facial scanning include optical, stereophotogrammetry and time of flight.
- Facial scans stitched with CBCT and intra-oral captures allow visualising of both skeletal and soft tissue anatomy.

Dental photography: equipment and principles

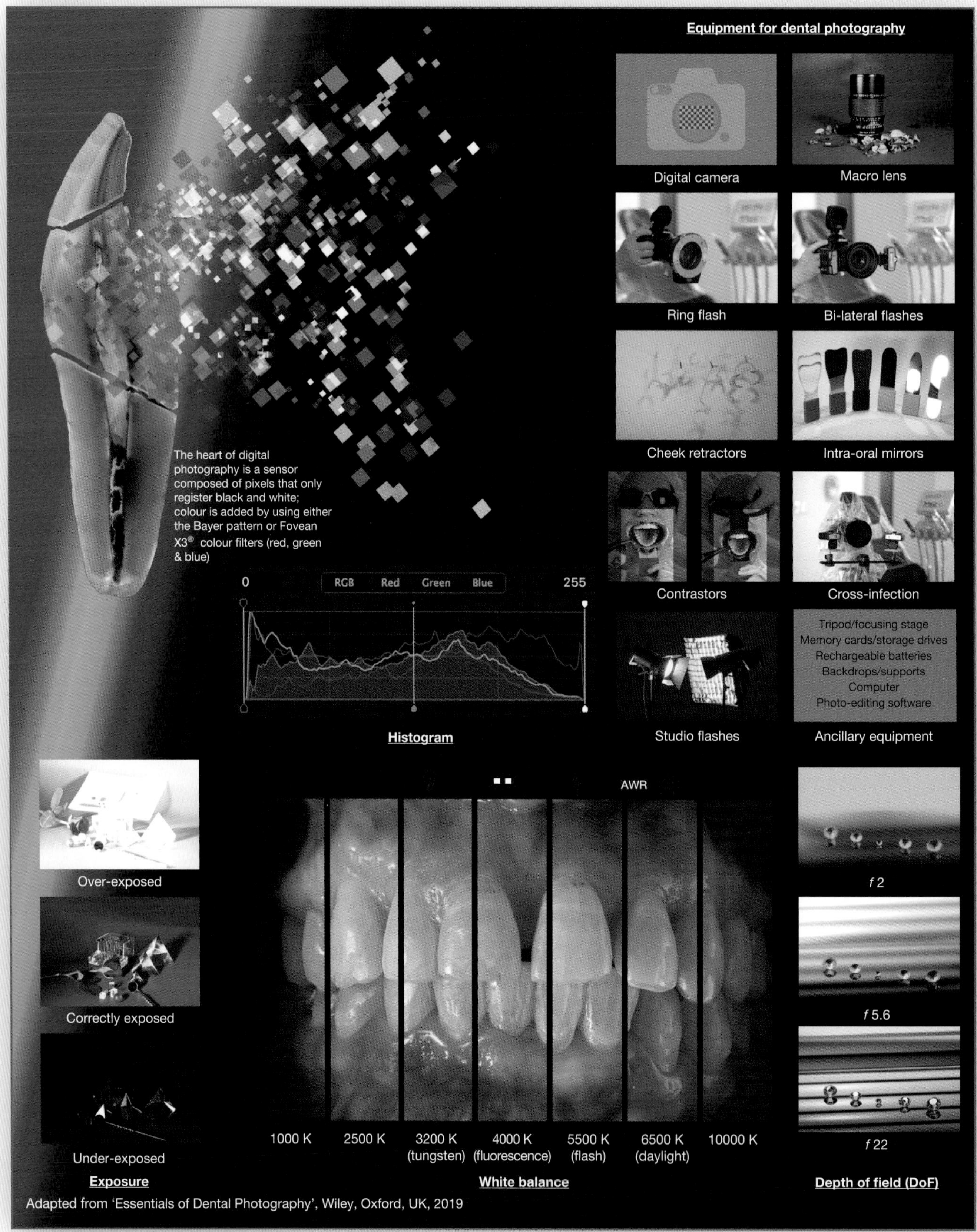

The heart of digital photography is a sensor composed of pixels that only register black and white; colour is added by using either the Bayer pattern or Fovean X3® colour filters (red, green & blue)

Equipment for dental photography

Digital camera

Macro lens

Ring flash

Bi-lateral flashes

Cheek retractors

Intra-oral mirrors

Contrastors

Cross-infection

Studio flashes

Tripod/focusing stage
Memory cards/storage drives
Rechargeable batteries
Backdrops/supports
Computer
Photo-editing software

Ancillary equipment

0 RGB Red Green Blue 255

Histogram

Over-exposed

Correctly exposed

Under-exposed

Exposure

AWR

1000 K | 2500 K | 3200 K (tungsten) | 4000 K (fluorescence) | 5500 K (flash) | 6500 K (daylight) | 10000 K

White balance

f 2

f 5.6

f 22

Depth of field (DoF)

Adapted from 'Essentials of Dental Photography', Wiley, Oxford, UK, 2019

Prosthodontics at a Glance, Second Edition. Irfan Ahmad.

Dental photography is increasingly becoming an integral part of modern dental practice for improving patient care. Its uses extend far beyond **photodocumentation**, e.g. during the **treatment** process (planning, progress and outcome), education (patient and staff), **communication** (with patients, staff, ceramists and specialists), **marketing** (practice literature and brochures) and **dento-legal** records (particularly for elective therapies such as bleaching or aesthetic/cosmetic dentistry).

Equipment

The requirements of photographic equipment for dentistry are two-fold: first for taking **close-up or macro images**, and second, for **portraiture**. The permutations for dental photography are enormous including **different cameras** (smartphones, compact, rangefinders, digital single-lens-reflex [dSLR], mirrorless and medium format), lenses (prime, zooms), lighting (ring, bilateral), framing (rule of thirds, Fibonacci spiral), supports (tripods, stages), etc. The items discussed below are tried and tested, producing **high-quality, repeatable, reliable and consistent results.**

- **Digital camera** – most mid-range dSLR or mirrorless cameras have almost identical specifications, and therefore, choosing a specific brand is almost irrelevant. However, the salient features should include interchangeable lenses, >18 MP (megapixels) sensor, TLL (through-the-lens) flash and a remote shutter release
- **Sensors** – a digital sensor consisting of pixels ((abbreviation of 'picture elements') comes in various sizes. Although a full frame is the ideal, a minimum APS-C size will suffice
- **Macro-telephoto lens** – dual purpose for close-up images and portraiture. It is worth purchasing the highest resolution lens that a budget allows, ideally a prime (fixed focal length) rather than a zoom lens
- **Electronic flashes** – compact flashes (either ring or bi-lateral units – with or without reflectors) for close-up intra- and extra-oral images, and studio flashes, with appropriate trigger mechanism, for portraiture
- **Tripod** (optional) – for mounting camera and flashes
- **Cheek retractors** – either plastic variety for comfort, or steel for steam autoclaving
- **Front-coated intra-oral mirrors** – glass (rhodium coated) or metal
- **Contrasters** – to hide extraneous anatomy, e.g. nostrils or for creating a uniform black background for enhancing translucency within teeth
- **Storage cards/devices** – e.g. SD, SDHC, SDXC, CF cards, external hard drives or cloud storage (with the caveat of using **HIPPA [Health Insurance Portability and Accountability Act]** guidelines for protecting patient confidentiality)
- **Rechargeable batteries** for camera and flashes
- **Backdrops** for portraits, neutral colours for clinical images (18% neutral grey or sky blue), but any colour for promotional images
- **Computer**
- **Photo-editing software**, e.g. Apple® or Microsoft® Photos, Adobe® Photoshop Elements, Adobe® Creative Cloud, Capture One, etc.
- **Moisture control** – saliva ejectors, cottonwool rolls, rubber dam, warm air from six-in-one dental syringe
- **Cross-infection measures** – routine procedures in a dental practice, e.g. disinfection, disposable paper and plastic drapes for covering photographic equipment

Photographic principles

The **requirements** of a dental image is that it should be **correctly exposed**, **in focus,** and convey **colours with fidelity**. There are several factors that interplay to achieve these goals, but the most important are **exposure**, **white balance** and **depth of field (DoF)**:

- **Exposure** determines whether an image is too dark, too bright or just right. It is influenced by the intensity of the light source (flashes) and three cameras settings; **aperture (f number)**, **shutter speed (fraction of a second)** and **ISO number** (sensitivity of the sensor to incoming light). However, with **TTL flash metering,** setting the aperture and shutter speed is all that is necessary, as the camera controls the duration of the flash burst to ensure that the image is properly exposed. For intra-oral images, the aperture is set to ***f* 22** to obtain maximum DoF, and the shutter speed is the **flash synchronisation**, usually 1/125s or 1/250s. Since the **ISO** number influences visual noisy, a low number is advisable to avoid grainy images, e.g. **50–200**. Another method for gauging exposure is using the **histogram**, which is displayed on the LCD (liquid crystal displays) on camera backs, and also in photo-editing software.
- **Depth of field (DoF)** is the range, or linear distance, in front and behind the point of focus that appears sharp. The significance of DoF for dental photography is that a **macro lens** is extremely close to the subject for intra-oral images, which diminishes the area of sharpness, limited to only a few millimetres (shallow depth of field), approximately **one-third in front and two-third behind the point of focus**. Therefore, to achieve a deep DoF, a large *f* number (or small aperture) is necessary, e.g., *f* 22
- **White balance (WB)** is simply 'telling the camera' about the quality, or **colour temperature of light**. The term 'white balance' is used because any 'white' part in a scene should be faithfully reproduced as 'white' in the image, without unwanted colour casts. There are three methods for setting the WB, automatic (AWB), manually inputing **5500 K representing photographic daylight** or using an **18% neutral density reference grey card** for a particular setup, and subsequently correcting the white balance in photo-editing software.

Processing images

If proper guidelines are followed, little processing should be necessary in the photo-editing software. It is crucial to minimise the amount of eating for the following reasons. First, since dental images are a photodocumentation record, **tampering is unethical**. Second, any alteration, no matter how insignificant, **degrades image quality**. Nevertheless, some editing is alway necessary and even desirable to enhance, **not manipulate**, the final image. The permissible factors that are beneficial include sequential adjustments starting with colour spaces, white balance, exposure, orientation and cropping, removing artefacts (dust particles), local adjustments (layers) and lastly, sharpening. Ideally, all capture should be performed with the propriety **RAW format** of a specific camera brand, and after editing exported to high-quality **TIFF** (Tagged Image File Format) for archiving, presentations or publishing. The **JPEG** (Joint Photographic Experts Group) image file format is ideal for e-mail attachments, web publishing and social media.

Key points

- Photodocumentation is an integral part of practicing dentistry.
- Dental photographic equipment serves a dual purpose, macro and portraiture.
- The key factors are high quality, sharpness, exposure, white balance and depth of field.
- Processing images should be kept to a minimum.

Dental photography: EDP and EPP

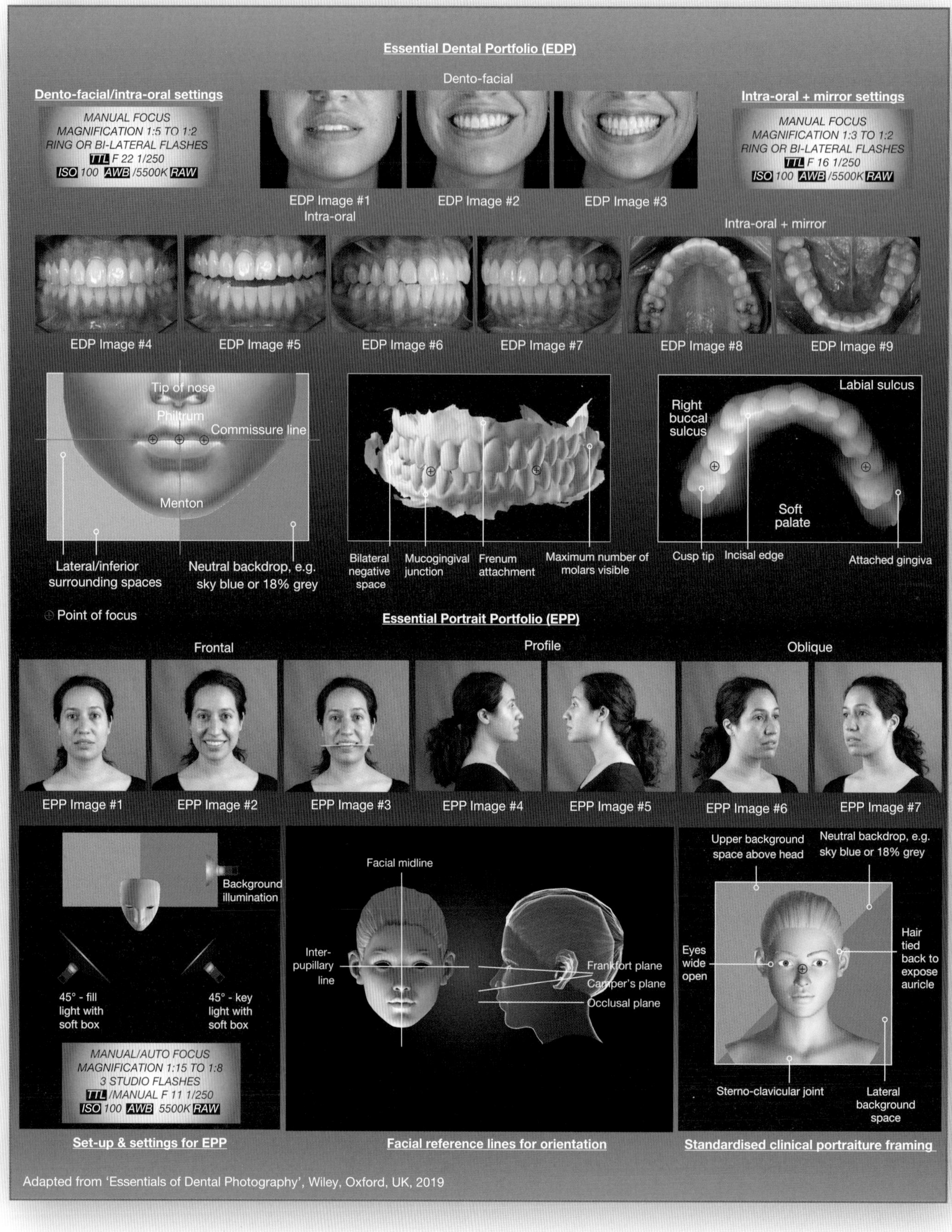

Essential Dental Portfolio (EDP)

Dento-facial/intra-oral settings

MANUAL FOCUS
MAGNIFICATION 1:5 TO 1:2
RING OR BI-LATERAL FLASHES
TTL F 22 1/250
ISO 100 AWB /5500K RAW

Dento-facial

EDP Image #1
EDP Image #2
EDP Image #3

Intra-oral + mirror settings

MANUAL FOCUS
MAGNIFICATION 1:3 TO 1:2
RING OR BI-LATERAL FLASHES
TTL F 16 1/250
ISO 100 AWB /5500K RAW

Intra-oral

EDP Image #4
EDP Image #5
EDP Image #6
EDP Image #7

Intra-oral + mirror

EDP Image #8
EDP Image #9

Tip of nose
Philtrum
Commissure line
Menton
Lateral/inferior surrounding spaces
Neutral backdrop, e.g. sky blue or 18% grey

Bilateral negative space
Mucogingival junction
Frenum attachment
Maximum number of molars visible

Labial sulcus
Right buccal sulcus
Soft palate
Cusp tip
Incisal edge
Attached gingiva

⊕ Point of focus

Essential Portrait Portfolio (EPP)

Frontal

EPP Image #1
EPP Image #2
EPP Image #3

Profile

EPP Image #4
EPP Image #5

Oblique

EPP Image #6
EPP Image #7

Background illumination
45° - fill light with soft box
45° - key light with soft box

MANUAL/AUTO FOCUS
MAGNIFICATION 1:15 TO 1:8
3 STUDIO FLASHES
TTL /MANUAL F 11 1/250
ISO 100 AWB 5500K RAW

Set-up & settings for EPP

Facial midline
Inter-pupillary line
Frankfort plane
Camper's plane
Occlusal plane

Facial reference lines for orientation

Upper background space above head
Neutral backdrop, e.g. sky blue or 18% grey
Eyes wide open
Hair tied back to expose auricle
Sterno-clavicular joint
Lateral background space

Standardised clinical portraiture framing

Adapted from 'Essentials of Dental Photography', Wiley, Oxford, UK, 2019

Prosthodontics at a Glance, Second Edition. Irfan Ahmad.

The realm of dental photography is diverse, ranging from **clinical reality** to **seductive promotional imagery**. Therefore, before embarking on a photographic session, it is important to decide on the intended use of the images. The array of uses includes **photo-documentation** (dento-legal and treatment planning/monitoring), **communication** (e-mail attachments, sharing pictures on mobile devices), **marketing** (web-publishing, e-marketing, social media, office stationery and treatment portfolios) and **education** (lecturing, training). The discussion below is limited to the **EDP (essential dental portfolio**) and the **EPP (essential portrait portfolio)**, which cater for most clinical needs. However, **additional images** for specific disciplines may be required consisting of bench images or **close-up macrophotography**, which is ideally suited for analysis, graphically showing techniques or simply having artistic flare with high visual impact. The possibilities offered by dental photography are truly endless for the imaginative and creative mind.

Standardisation

Dental photography is basically visual dental documentation; its value lies in **comparison for self- and peer-critique** of the same or different patients, and historical cohort studies for monitoring as well as **research**. To realise these objectives, some form of **standardisation** is prerequisite by establishing guidelines for consistency, comparison and communication. Furthermore, standardisation starts at the **capture stage** when an image is composed and ends at the **processing/display stage** when the image is edited using computer software and reproduced with the chosen media (monitor, projector, print). There are certain aspects of dental photography that can be standardised including predefined positions of the patient, photographic equipment and operator, and configuring photographic and ancillary equipment to specific settings. However, some factors, predominantly hardware-related, **cannot be standardised**. These include photographic equipment that is unique to a particular manufacturer, which is rarely interchangeable or intercompatible with other brands. Therefore, the factors that are standardisable will produce comparable and consistent images for **interpatient and intrapatient documentation**, but are limited to an individual dental practice or institution with specific brands of photographic equipment.

EDP (essential dental portfolio)

As well as gaining appropriate **consent**, it is essential that **confidentially is safeguarded** and dissemination is according to stringent security such as using encrypted e-mails and adhering to **HIPAA (Health Insurance Portability and Accountability Act of 1996)** guidelines. Since the intended use of an EDP is clinical photodocumentation, **standardisation is mandatory**. The EDP consists of **nine basic dental** views, **three extra-oral (dento-facial) and six intra-oral compositions**, as follows:

EDP Image # 1: Extra-oral, frontal habitual or 'rest' lip position
EDP Image # 2: Extra-oral, frontal relaxed smile
EDP Image # 3: Extra-oral, frontal laughter
EDP Image # 4: Intra-oral, frontal view in maximum intercuspation (MI)
EDP Image # 5: Intra-oral, frontal view with separated teeth
EDP Image # 6: Intra-oral, right lateral view in MI
EDP Image # 7: Intra-oral, left lateral view in MI
EDP Image # 8: Intra-oral, occlusal full-arch maxillary view
EDP Image # 9: Intra-oral, occlusal full-arch mandibular view

The setup for these images is almost identical, with similar equipment settings, but the intra-oral views require **check retractors** and **intra-oral mirrors**. The occlusal views of each arch are accomplished by capturing the reflected images in the intra-oral mirrors, with or without **contrastors. DoF** for dental photography is that a macro lens is extremely close to the subject for intra-oral images, which diminishes the area of sharpness, limited to only a few millimetres (shallow depth of field), approximately one-third in front and two-third behind the point of focus. Therefore, to achieve a deep DoF, a large f number (or small aperture) is necessary, e.g.***f* 22**

EPP (essential portrait portfolio)

While the essential dental portfolio (EDP) concentrates primarily on the teeth, the essential portrait portfolio (EPP) consists of basic full face images and the relationship of the teeth to the face. The **EPP is quintessential for a variety of dental disciplines** including orthodontics, prosthodontics, periodontics, restorative dentistry, implantology, peadodontics, smile analysis, smile design, and facial enhancement and cranio-maxillio-facial procedures. The **clinical portraits** are excluded from the EDP since some patients are reticent to give **consent** to photograph their face due to personal, social, cultural or religious reasons. However, if this is not a concern, and appropriate consent is obtained, the EPP can be added to the EDP making a complete set of 16 images. The **EPP consists of seven views** as follows:

EPP Image # 1: Fontal view with interlabial separation
EPP Image # 2: Fontal view – relaxed smile
EPP Image # 3: Fontal view – biting wooden spatula for assessing the incisal/occlusal plane alignment to the inter-pupillary line
EPP Image # 4: Profile right side – interlabial separation
EPP Image # 5: Profile left side – interlabial separation
EPP Image # 6: Oblique right side – interlabial separation
EPP Image # 7: Oblique left side – interlabial separation

Three are several **reference lines** that are utilised for orientating the head in the vertical and horizontal planes. However, it is important **not to rely on the incisal or occlusal plane as a reference**, as this may be eschewed and result in pseudo alignment. The ideal location for portrait photography is a dedicated, or make shift studio using studio flashes with the patient seated on a revolving chair.

Key points

- Dental photography offers a wide scope for both clinical and non-clinal uses.
- Standardised is essential for clinical photodocumentation.
- The EDP and EPP cater for most dental disciplines.
- Addition photographs may be necessary for specific treatment modalities.

15 Occlusal analysis

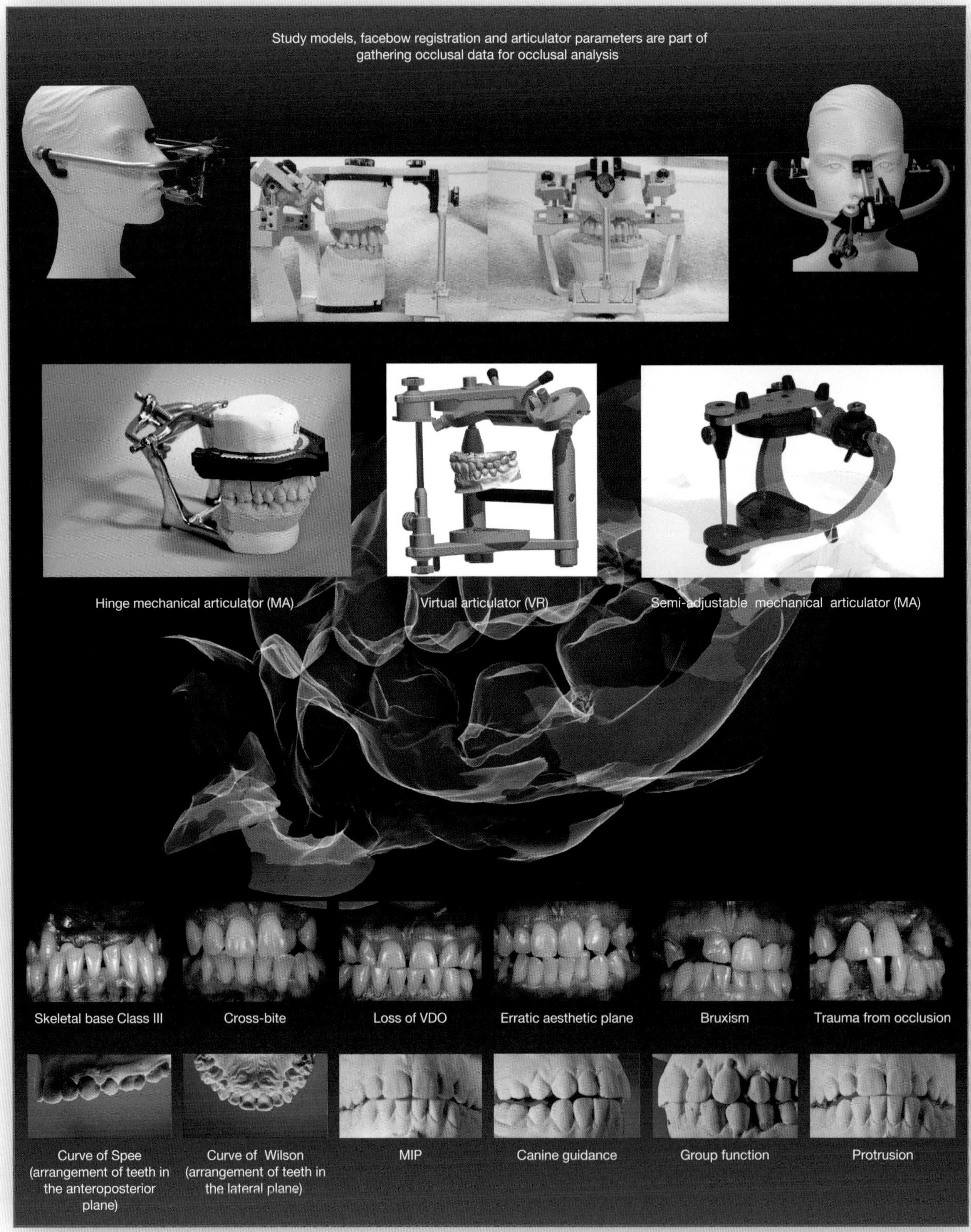

Study models, facebow registration and articulator parameters are part of gathering occlusal data for occlusal analysis

Hinge mechanical articulator (MA)

Virtual articulator (VR)

Semi-adjustable mechanical articulator (MA)

Skeletal base Class III

Cross-bite

Loss of VDO

Erratic aesthetic plane

Bruxism

Trauma from occlusion

Curve of Spee (arrangement of teeth in the anteroposterior plane)

Curve of Wilson (arrangement of teeth in the lateral plane)

MIP

Canine guidance

Group function

Protrusion

Prosthodontics at a Glance, Second Edition. Irfan Ahmad.

Occlusal analysis assesses **dysmorphology** and **dysocclusion,** and is a prerequisite before starting prosthodontic treatment, ensuring correct function and satisfactory occlusal schemes that are essential for aesthetics and long-term harmony of the **stomatognathic system**. This chapter is an introduction to occlusion as part of the Diagnostic Section of this book, and is further elaborated in Chapters 21 to 24. It should be remembered that there are numerous **occlusal philosophies**, with varying subjectivity and bias.

Occlusal data registration

To diagnose a patient's **occlusal status,** and formulate a treatment plan, information needs to be **transferred from the patient to an extra-oral simulating device**, which can either be a mechanical or virtual articulator. **Dental articulators** are devices to visualise both **static and dynamic occlusion**. The data required depend on the chosen type of articulator and includes:

- **Study models** – either plaster casts poured from accurate impressions of the maxillary and mandibular arches or 3D printed models from IOS digitisation of the maxillary and mandibular arches
- **Facebow transfer** – locating the maxillary arch to the condylar hinge axis
- **Occlusal records** – locating the mandibular cast to the maxillary cast. Check bite records, using wax or rigid addition silicone impression materials; may be required for **maximum intercuspation (MIP), centric relation (CR)** and **anterior and lateral excursions**, and **vertical dimension of occlusion (VDO)** or occlusal vertical dimension (OVD)
- **Articulator parameters** – Bennett angle (average 15°) and condylar angles, intercondylar distance and spacial relationships of craniomandibular geometry
- **Mandibular movements** – instrumental measurements using pantographs, Gothic arch tracing or computer-assisted jaw-tracking systems
- **Articulator-related registration** – rather than transferring data from the patient to an articulator, articulator registration works the opposite way. The articulator geometry is virtually transferred to the patient, using an electronic recording system, and the articulator adjusted accordingly
- **Digital scans** – digitising the dentition using a 3D scanners (IOS or EOS), and subsequently outputting the data into appropriate computer software for virtual articulation

Mechanical articulators (MA)

Numerous types of **mechanical articulators (MA)** are available with varying complexity:

- **Hand-held or hinge** – suitable for single tooth restorations that integrate with the existing occlusal status
- **Fixed condylar path** (average value with a condylar angle of 30°) – similar to hinge types, for single-tooth restorations and maintaining the existing occlusal status quo
- **Semi-adjustable with fixed or average parameters** (condylar and arcon types) – suitable for most full-arch rehabilitation requiring a change of occlusal status
- **Fully adjustable** – for complex analysis of jaw movements, occlusal equilibrium and a diagnostic aid for temporomandibular disorders (TMD), assuming there is no muscular spasm or TMJ pathology

Virtual articulators (VA)

Presently, MAs are the most prevalent device for occlusal analysis. However, these devices are limited in their applications and do not represent dynamic occlusion. Furthermore, mobile teeth, deformation of the mandible during function and the influence of the soft tissues and muscles cannot be simulated. Other shortcomings are technique-sensitive methods for collating data, and errors in laboratory protocols that contribute to decreased accuracy for representing the clinical situation. The concept of **virtual articulator (VA)** is **digital acquisition** of the maxillary and mandibular arches with an IOS, and **recording jaw movements** with devices such as the JMAnalyser+ (Zebris Medical GmbH, Isny, Germany). The jaw recording devices use different technologies such as ultrasound or a combination of LED with CCD digital cameras to record **protrusion**, **retrusion**, **laterotrusion**, **Bennett angle**, **collision detection**, etc. The collated data are input to a VA software such as DentCAM® (Kavo, Germany), and using algorithmic dental occlusion (ADO), simulates occlusal contacts with corresponding jaw excursions. The information is combined by software to create a 3D VA offering the following advantages:

- **Sectional slices of individual teeth** for assessing flowing and sliding contacts and interferences
- **Protrusive and lateral movement** analysis
- **Dynamic occlusion** assessment by animations of jaws in 'real time', e.g. simulated mastication
- VR is more precise than MA for reproducing jaw movements and **collision detection**
- **Designing restorations** with correct cuspal and ridge inclines that 'fit' into a patient's occlusion
- **Fabricating CAD/CAM restorations** by transferring data to a milling machine or 3D printer
- **Deciphering TMJ pathologies** during functional movements
- **Avoiding facebow transfer,** plaster casts and measuring articulator paravmeters
- **Communicating information** with patients, dental laboratories and specialists
- **Plug-in modules** for orthodontics, tooth wear and **holoperspective** display environment for **virtual teaching** via the Internet

Occlusal analysis

A systematic occlusal analysis should consider the following items:

- **Skeletal and dental bases** – classes I, II or III
- **Cross-bites**
- **VDO** – e.g. loss of vertical dimension due to tooth wear
- **Functional and aesthetic occlusal planes**
- **Vertical or horizontal chewing patterns** (evidence of bruxism)
- **Curves of Spee, Wilson and Monson** (3D combination of curves of Spee and Wilson)
- **MIP,** also known as centric occlusion (CO) – habitual maxillary and mandibular teeth interdigitation
- **CR** – the condyle are in the most posterior retruded position in the glenoid fossa (independent of tooth contact)
- **Lateral excursions** – group function, canine protected (guidance), working and non-working (balancing) contacts
- **Protrusive excursions** – steep or shallow anterior guidance
- **Trauma from occlusion** – e.g. fractured fillings and/or teeth, or increased tooth mobility

Key points

- Occlusal analysis is essential for successful prosthodontic treatment.
- Articulation can be mechanical or virtual.
- Virtual articulators offer promise for detailed occlusal analysis and may eventually replace mechanical devices.

Colour and shade assessment

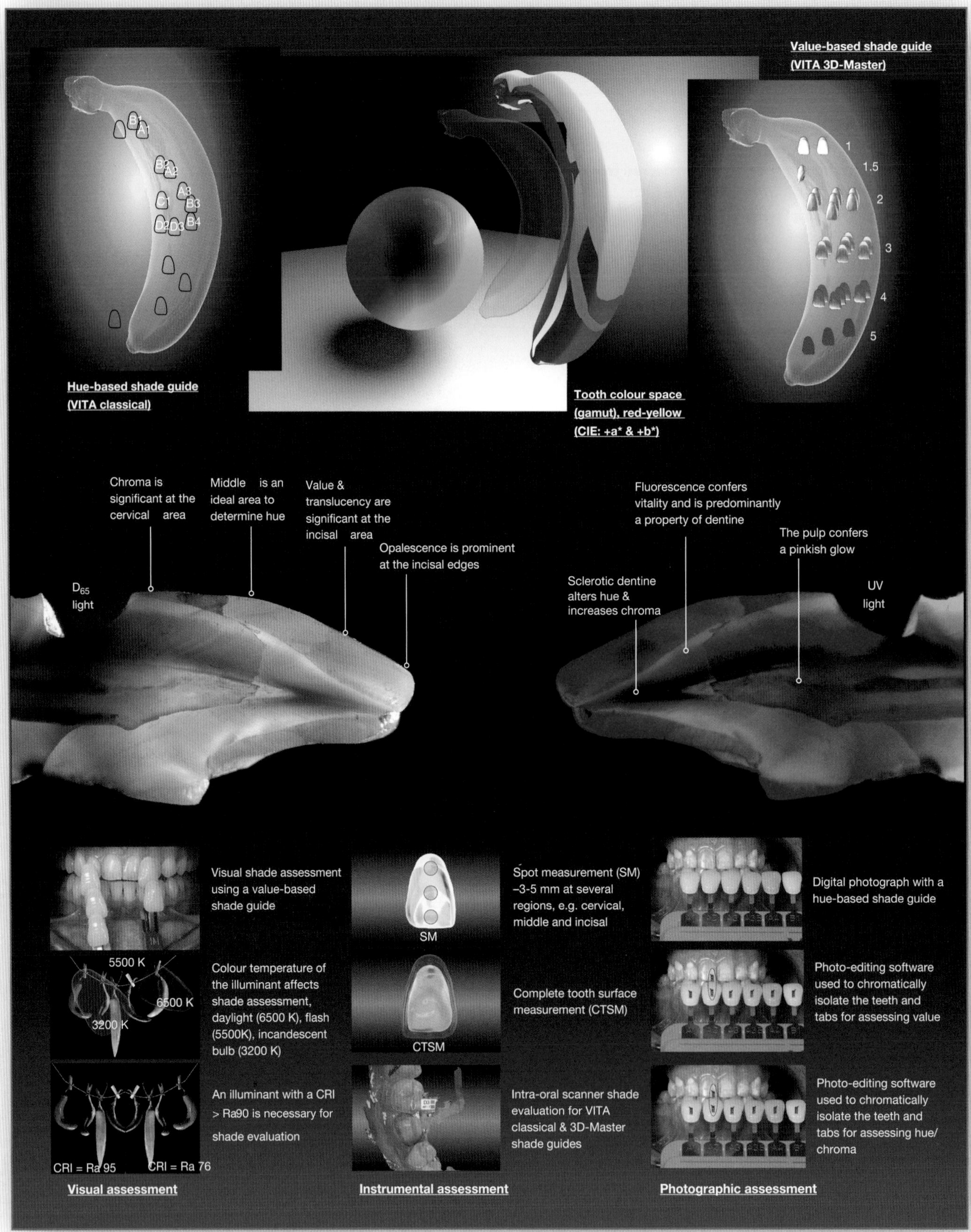

Value-based shade guide (VITA 3D-Master)

1
1.5
2
3
4
5

Hue-based shade guide (VITA classical)

B1 A1
B2 A2
A3
C1 B3
D2 D3 B4

Tooth colour space (gamut), red-yellow (CIE: +a* & +b*)

Chroma is significant at the cervical area

Middle is an ideal area to determine hue

Value & translucency are significant at the incisal area

Opalescence is prominent at the incisal edges

D_{65} light

Fluorescence confers vitality and is predominantly a property of dentine

The pulp confers a pinkish glow

Sclerotic dentine alters hue & increases chroma

UV light

Visual assessment

Visual shade assessment using a value-based shade guide

5500 K
6500 K
3200 K

Colour temperature of the illuminant affects shade assessment, daylight (6500 K), flash (5500K), incandescent bulb (3200 K)

CRI = Ra 95
CRI = Ra 76

An illuminant with a CRI > Ra90 is necessary for shade evaluation

Instrumental assessment

SM

Spot measurement (SM) –3-5 mm at several regions, e.g. cervical, middle and incisal

CTSM

Complete tooth surface measurement (CTSM)

Intra-oral scanner shade evaluation for VITA classical & 3D-Master shade guides

Photographic assessment

Digital photograph with a hue-based shade guide

Photo-editing software used to chromatically isolate the teeth and tabs for assessing value

Photo-editing software used to chromatically isolate the teeth and tabs for assessing hue/chroma

Prosthodontics at a Glance, Second Edition. Irfan Ahmad.

The purpose of **shade analysis** is to **chromatically integrate** an artificial restoration with the surrounding dentition. **Colour theory** and shade assessment are complex subjects involving both **scientific disciplines** and **artistic flair**.

Chromatic properties of natural teeth

The **constituents of colour** are **hue** (wavelength of light), **value** (brightness or darkness) and **chroma** (intensity or depth). Natural tooth colour is represented by a **banana-shaped envelope** on the **psychometric colour space**. The starting point for shade assessment is understanding the **chromatic and optical properties of natural teeth**. Light interacts with the **enamel surface** by reflection, transmission and refraction depending on the superficial **macromorphology**, **micromorphology** (or texture) and **lustre**, and influences **value**. A highly polished surface encourages **specular reflection** (aged teeth), while a matt surface promotes **diffusion** (youthful teeth), while **translucency** is evident at the interproximal and incisal edges/cusp tips areas. Other optical phenomena are **opalescence**, (which confers an orange aura with transmitted light, and a bluish glow with reflected light) and **goniochromism**, or iridescence (akin to 'mother of pearl', peacock feathers or rainbow appearance on soap bubbles). Goniochromism is the ability of an object to appear differently depending on the angle of view or the angle of incidence of the illumination. Practically, this means that viewing a tooth from various angles (or varying the position of the light source) can **conceal or make a restoration more conspicuous,** and obscure or display tooth characterisations. The **dentine and pulp** mainly absorb light and influence the **degree of chroma**, which is more apparent at the cervical regions, while value is lowest due to a thinner enamel overlay. Conversely, at the incisal edges, chroma is less significant compared to value due to the thicker enamel layer. Furthermore, **each tooth in the dental arches has a different hue**, with unique distribution of value and chroma, and is in a state of continual **chromatic flux,** i.e. the shade of a tooth is constantly changing throughout life, and can be transient, such as dietary pigments, or insidious enamel staining due to indelible chromogen discolouration.

Shade evaluation

Any system or device that assess shade should ideally represent the entire colour space of natural teeth. Shade matching is essentially making a **comparison between the specimen or target (tooth) and a reference (shade tab)**, and the difference is represented by the CIE (Commission Internationale de l'Eclairage) **L*a*b* chromaticity (or colour) coordinates** using the following formula:

$$\Delta E^*_{ab} = \left[(\Delta L^*)^2 + (\Delta a^*)^2 + (\Delta b^*)^2 \right]^{1/2}$$

where ΔE * ab is total colour change, ΔL is difference in lightness (0 for white, 100 for black), and Δa* and Δb* are differences in the chromaticity (or colour) coordinates a* and b*.

The **a* coordinate** represents red–green: a **positive value is red**, while a negative value is green. Similarly, the **b* coordinate** represents yellow–blue: **a positive value is yellow**, while a negative value is blue. A **perfect match** between the specimen and a reference equates to **ΔE = 0**, where 'Δ' is the difference and 'E' represents 'Empfindung', the German for sensation or perception. At present, there is no concord in the dental literature about colour difference that is clinically acceptable for a restoration to be classed as a good match. The **perceptible threshold (PT)** and **acceptable threshold (AT)** is sui generis, but the general agreement is that a ΔE = 1 for PT for 50% of observers, and the AT of ΔE = 3.7 for 50% of observers is satisfactory. Unlike monolithic solid objects, for which shade selection is fairly straightforward, shade analysis of teeth presents a formidable challenge due to their unique structure and optical properties, i.e. **multilayered, semi-translucent, anisotropic, curvaceous, fluorescent, opalescent and iridescent.** There are two methods for **shade evaluation: visual and instrumental** (digital); the former is subjective, while the latter objective.

Visual assessment

The visual method relies on the principle of **chromatic differentiation** by comparison using shade guides. The main issue with shade guides is that they do not cover the entire **tooth colour gamut,** which varies according to patient ethnicity, disparate materials of tabs and teeth, and translucency. Two types of **guides** are available; **hue-based** (e.g. VITA classical) or **value-based** (e.g. VITA 3D-Master) that follow the Munsell three-dimensional colour system, and assess shade by sequentially determining value, followed by chroma and, lastly, hue. It is worth noting that the **majority of human dentition (greater than 80%) is located within the VITA classical A shade tabs**, and 50% within the value group 3 of the VITA 3D-Master guide. If shade evaluation remains elusive with commercial guides, bespoke shade guides can be fabricated with either composite or porcelain using My Shade Guide Mini or Master Kits, which is theoretically more precise since the tabs can be of the same material as the definitive restoration. For most circumstances, visual shade assessment produces acceptable matches, but depends on a wide range of variables including **operator factors** (temperament, training, colour blindness, afterimages and chromatic adaptation), **illuminant** (colour temperature for avoiding metamerism, colour rendering index [CRI] for preventing colour distortions, correlated colour temperature [CCT], intensity), **dehydrated teeth, position of shade tabs** (ideally in same optical axis as target tooth), **vectoring** for assessing goniochromism, **distance of viewing** (1 m for value, and 30 cm for hue/chroma) and background colour (ideal 18% neutral grey card), to name a few.

Instrumental (digital) assessment

The instrumental approach measures **absolute colour** without making a comparison to a reference. This is accomplished by using colour **measuring devices, digital photographs** and **intra-oral scans**. The devices record CIE L*a*b* colour coordinates or **L*C*h* parameters (SM or CTSM),** which are subsequently converted to shade tab equivalent of a specific shade guide. The technologies include filter **colorimeter** (e.g. ShadeEye-NCC), **reflectance spectrophotometers** (e.g. Easyshade V) or spectrocolorimeters. Although digital methods are precise and have high agreement rates, the drawbacks are lack of vectoring, poor translucency assessment and require periodic calibration to ensure accuracy. Assuming standardisation, digital photographs are useful for individually assessing value and creating **chromatic maps** showing colour distribution and characterisations for both direct and indirect restorations. Lastly, intra-oral scanners (IOS) can simultaneously assess colour with the in-built software tool/function for shade evaluation while taking a digital impression.

Key points

- Knowledge of the chromatic and optical properties of natural teeth is essential for shade matching.
- Colour consists of hue, value and chrome, but translucency, fluorescence, opalescence and goniochromism also require evaluation.
- Shade assessment is visual or instrumental (digital).
- It is prudent to combine visual and instrumental shade assessments.

17 Dental simulations

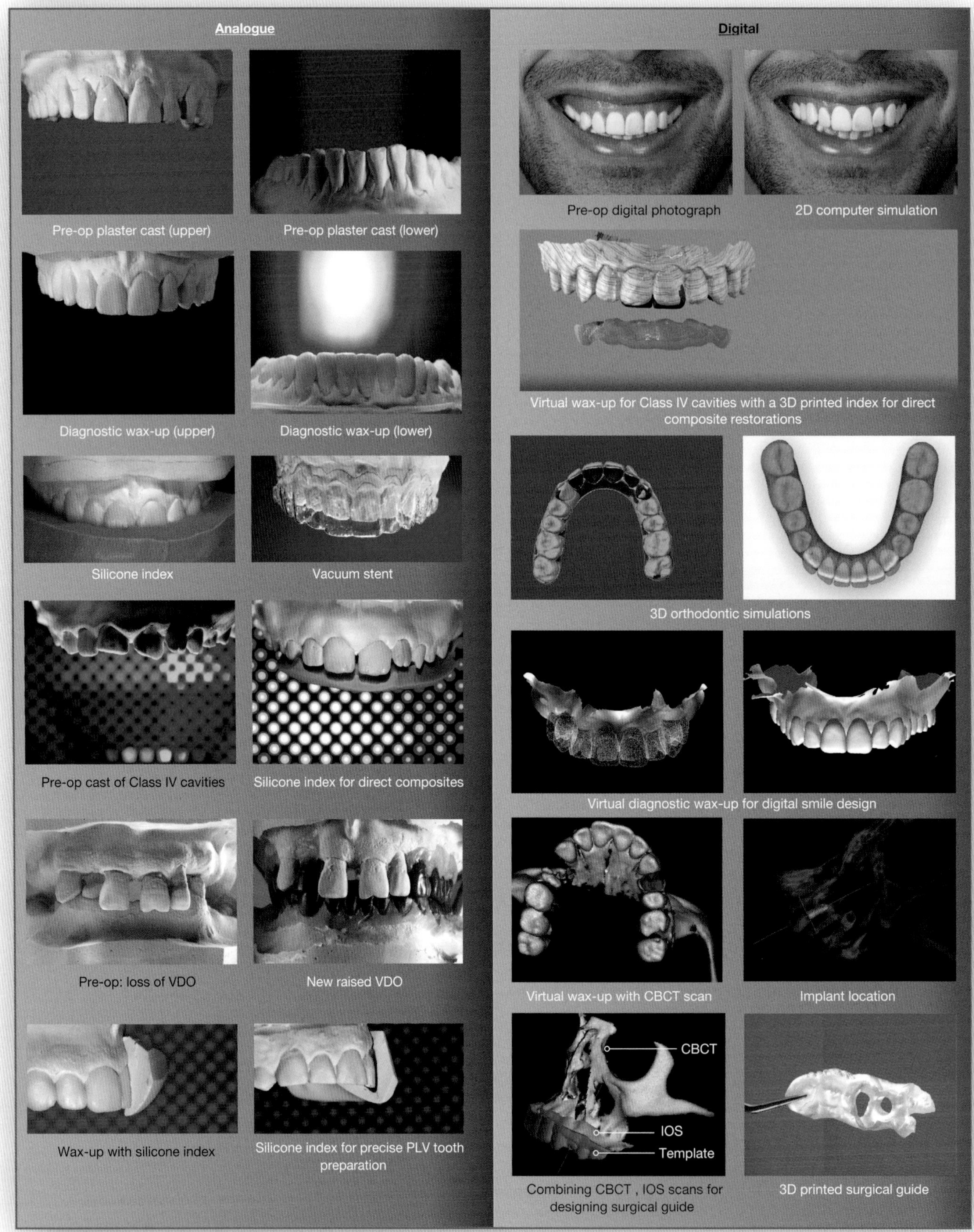

Analogue
Pre-op plaster cast (upper)
Pre-op plaster cast (lower)
Diagnostic wax-up (upper)
Diagnostic wax-up (lower)
Silicone index
Vacuum stent
Pre-op cast of Class IV cavities
Silicone index for direct composites
Pre-op: loss of VDO
New raised VDO
Wax-up with silicone index
Silicone index for precise PLV tooth preparation
Digital
Pre-op digital photograph
2D computer simulation
Virtual wax-up for Class IV cavities with a 3D printed index for direct composite restorations
3D orthodontic simulations
Virtual diagnostic wax-up for digital smile design
Virtual wax-up with CBCT scan
Implant location
CBCT
IOS
Template
Combining CBCT , IOS scans for designing surgical guide
3D printed surgical guide

Prosthodontics at a Glance, Second Edition. Irfan Ahmad.

Dental simulations are pivotal for diagnosis, **treatment planning, treatment acceptable** as well as **monitoring and reviewing** outcomes. In addition, simulations provide essential information regarding tooth number, alignment and morphology as well as arch form and relation of the dentition to adjacent soft tissues and the jaws. There are two methods for simulation: **analogue** and **digital**.

Dental simulation uses

Dental simulations, either analogue or digital, have many uses including:

- **Documentation** of the proposed therapy
- Ability to **discuss different treatment options** before irreversible treatment is initiated
- **Comprehensive evaluation** by combining intra-oral scans (Chapters 10 and 11), CBCT data (Chapter 9) and facial scans (Chapter 12) to visualise the dentition, intra-oral soft tissues, skeletal anatomy and facial soft tissue landmarks
- **Digital smile design** (Chapter 33)
- **Communication** between patient, ceramist and specialists for multidisciplinary collaboration
- **Vacuum stents** made of transparent acrylic for intra-oral composite mock-ups for aesthetic approval, chair-side temporary restorations for assessing occlusal scheme changes, e.g. increasing the vertical dimension of occlusion (VDO)
- **Indices** (silicone or 3D printed) for direct composite fillings – using the simulation as a guide for restoring a fractured tooth, e.g. class IV cavity
- **Indices for guided tooth preparation** to ensure sufficient and precise tooth preparation and prevent inadvertent removal of tooth substrate, and retaining enamel that is crucial for adhering porcelain laminate veneers (PLV)
- **Surgical guides** in conjunction with cone beam computed scans (CBCT) and IOS for guided implant placement
- **Laboratory-fabricated provisional restorations** for resilient long-term temporary restorations
- **Template for definitive restorations** copying morphology and alignment of a simulation for the permanent restorations

Analogue simulation

The **analogue simulation** approach involves pouring plaster casts from tray/material impressions to recreate the dental arches and surrounding anatomy. **Unmounted casts** (without an articulator) serve as essential pretreatment documentation. In addition, teeth can be visualised from all angles, which is usually difficult during an intra-oral examination. Hand-held pairing of the maxillary and mandibular casts permits a limited assessment of occlusion, and a thorough analysis is only possible when the casts are mounted on a dental articulator. **Mounted casts** are an ideal method for carrying out a detailed analysis of **static occlusion,** and **dynamic occlusion,** by simulating mandibular movements in various excursions. The type of **mechanical articulator (MA)** on which to mount the casts depends on the extent of analysis and complexity of the treatment. For most purposes, a **semi-adjustable MA** is the recommended choice. A useful method for visualising proposed restorative prostheses is by additive simulation in wax or composite, referred to as **additive diagnostics wax-up** or **composite-up**, depending on the material used. Waxes are available in various colours, and tooth-coloured varieties are ideal for anterior teeth simulations. Diagnostic wax-ups can be utilised to restore the **curves of Spee and Wilson** to their correct inclinations, and to ensure a smooth and unimpeded mandibular disclusion. A worn **incisal plane** can be restituted with correct tooth proportions (**width/length ratio**) and morphology. Also, eccentric and harmful **tooth contacts** during excursions can be eliminated with **correct cusp/ridge inclinations.** Finally, teeth can be added to or removed from the wax-up (e.g. prior to a **full arch rehabilitation**), to help discussion about various treatment options before any irreversible procedure is carried out in the mouth.

Digital simulation

The **digital approach** can be either be **2D simulation**, or **3D simulation**. For the 2D method, a digital photograph is taken (Chapters 13 and 14), and imported into photo-editing software, e.g. Adobe® Photoshop, or dedicated dental software, e.g. a smile design programme. The pre-operative image is then manipulated to the desired objectives. Although 2D simulations are tantalising and ideal for promotion or treatment acceptable, caution is necessary. It is of course expedient to use computer software to show patients the immediate aesthetic improvements of their anterior teeth. However, **the proposed 'virtual' treatment may not be clinically feasible** because little information regarding arch form or occlusion is incorporated into a 2D computer photo manipulation. Hence, committing to this pseudo-outcome can be catastrophic, especially if the proposed treatment involves considerable expenditure.

The second method is 3D simulation that involves obtaining files from **IOS, CBCT and facial scans**, which can be used alone or **stitching together,** and with **virtual articulation (VA)**, is a far more realistic representative of the clinical environment compared to a 2D simulation. A **virtual diagnostic wax-up** is relatively easily to perform using **CAD software** (Chapter 55), and can be altered as necessary according to the occlusion, alveolar anatomy and surrounding soft tissues. This is particularly useful for positioning teeth correctly for **orthodontics** and **dental aesthetics**, so that they harmoniously integrate with surrounding soft tissues and facial features. Afurther benefit of a virtual diagnostic wax-ups is obviating the need for impressions, pouring plaster models and building up with wax or composite. Finally, **CAD/CAM technologies** allow fabrication of **temporary** or **permanent restorations**, a**crylic indice**s for direct composite build-ups or mock-ups, **sequential aligners for orthodontic clear aligner therapy** (CAT) and **surgical guides** for guided implant placement.

Key points

- Dental simulations are essential for diagnosis, treatment planning and reviewing outcomes.
- Simulations can either be analogue or digital, e.g. diagnostic 'wax-ups'.
- Digital files from IOS, CBCT and facial scans can be 'stitched' together to allow visualisation of tooth roots, facial skeleton and soft tissues.
- Simulations serve many purposes such as fabricating indices, surgical guides, as well as templates for temporary and permanent restorations.

Treatment planning

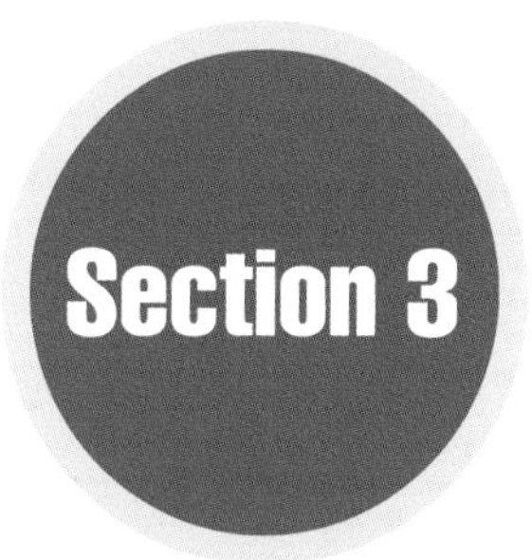

Chapters

18 Treatment planning: evidence-based treatment

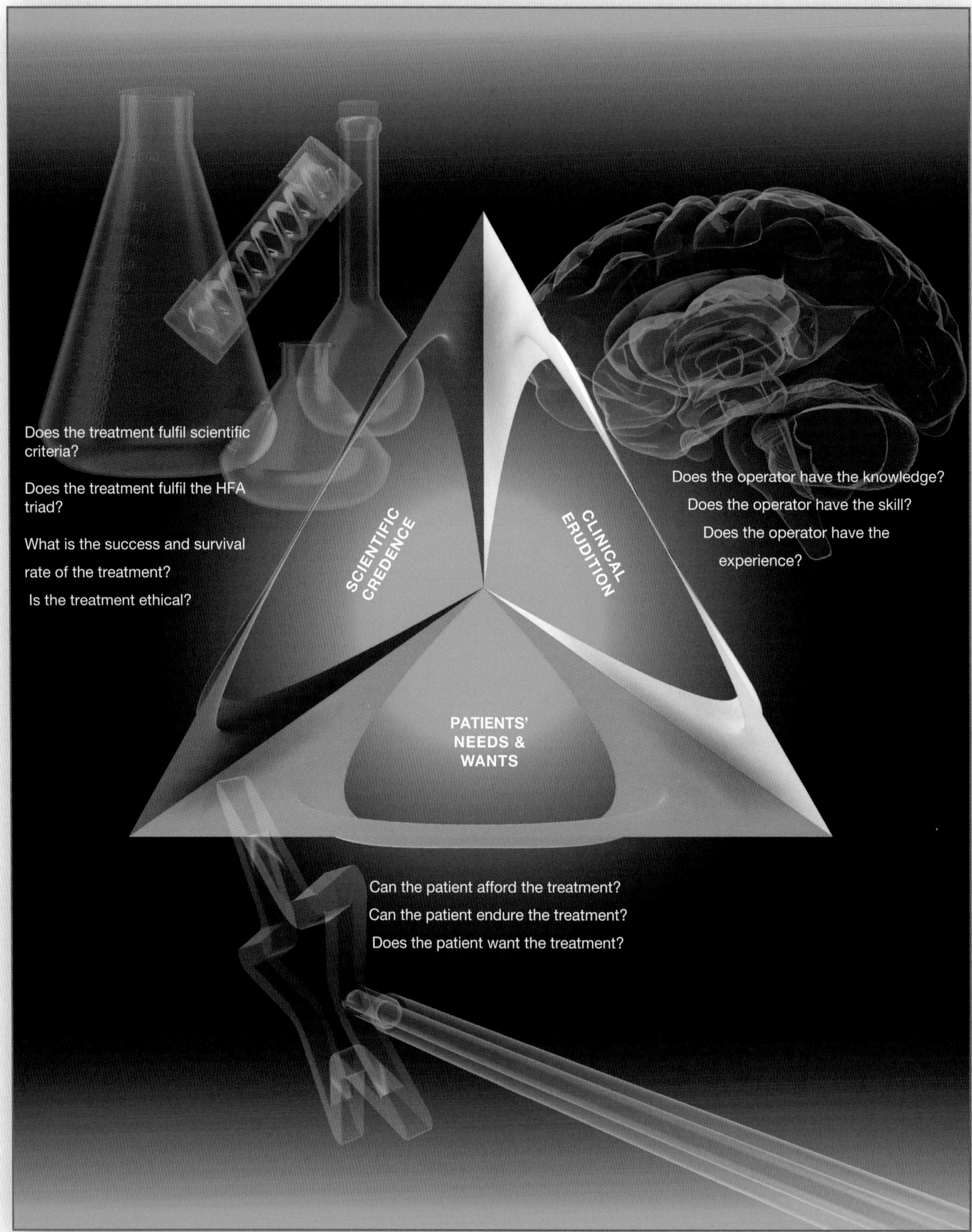

Prosthodontics at a Glance, Second Edition. Irfan Ahmad.

After arriving at a **working**, **provisional** or **definitive diagnosis** from the information gathered by an examination and requisite tests, the next stage is preparing **treatment option(s)** for therapy. Ideally, the proposed treatment should sequentially restore **health, function and aesthetic (the HFA triad).** The HFA triad is a sequence, where health is the primary goal, followed by function and aesthetics. Therefore, if conditions are not optimal, achieving health is the priority, at the sacrifice of function and aesthetics. However, in reality, achieving this Utopian goal is challenging and often a compromise may be the best possible outcome. It is essential to recognise and **communicate compromises to the patient at the outset** of treatment, rather than waiting for complications to arise. **Evidence-based treatment (EBT)** planning is not only a sound **scientific model**, but also a **systematic approach to decision-making**. EBT consists of three elements:

- **Scientific credence**
- **Clinical erudition**
- **Patients' needs and wants**

Scientific credence

Before considering a specific treatment option, it is important to arrive at a **definitive diagnosis.** If the diagnosis is incorrect, the therapeutic options will also be incorrect. Hence, **differential diagnosis** is essential to eliminate doubts and confirm aetiology before commencing therapy. In some circumstances, there may be more than one **treatment option**, and each choice should be assessed to ensure there is sufficient research and clinical trials evidence to support its long-term efficacy. Besides scientific validity, the patient should be informed of the likely **survival or success rate** of each treatment option. Survival and success rates are not synonymous. **Survival** implies that a restoration of prostheses has endured, but may be functionally and aesthetically inadequate. For example, a crown with defective margins causing chronic periodontal inflammation together with tooth mobility is neither aesthetic nor functional. Conversely, **success** implies that a treatment option has not only endured, but is also fulfilling all the intended requirements. The next item to consider is **ethics** (Chapter 3), which comprises:

- **Nonmalfeasance** – 'doing no harm' (the Hippocratic principle)
- **Beneficence** – well-being of patients
- **Autonomy** – veracity in clinician–patient relationships
- **Justice** – fairness

At times, the clinician is faced with the dichotomy of clinical necessity and the patient's desires for a particular treatment. This scenario frequently arises when a patient requests elective aesthetic (or cosmetic) treatment. Ultimately, the decision to provide or refuse treatment resides with the clinician. However, when marketing and actively promoting cosmetic dentistry, it is worth remembering that there is a **fine line between persuasion and coercion**.

Clinical erudition

The second part of EBT planning is **operator factors** (both clinician and ceramist, if using a dental laboratory). The first aspect to consider under this heading is knowledge. **Knowledge is acquired**, not innate or possessed. To learn any technique or procedure requires a certain degree of knowledge to perform a given task. As well as undergraduate education, postgraduate training is essential for gaining insight of a particular discipline. Attending conferences, reading journals and participating in hands-on courses are mandatory to keep abreast of recent scientific research and updates on new techniques. Besides attaining knowledge, it is essential to possess the **skill and manual dexterity** to perform a procedure. Knowledge alone is insufficient for clinical practice. Furthermore, **clinical self-deprecation** is paramount for delivering successful treatment. If the proposed treatment plan is beyond one's capabilities or beyond one's **comfort zone**, it best to refer to a specialist at the beginning before embarking on procedures that may end in failure. **Referral** as a last resort is not only embarrassing, but can result in justifiable **litigation**. Having gained knowledge and skills does not automatically equate to success. In addition, experience is necessary for ensuring predictability. **Experience is the result of making and learning from mistakes.** It is an entity that develops over time and as a result of repetition. Experience is also important for making judgements regarding specific treatment options. A protocol or material that works for one clinician may be a disaster for another.

Patients' needs and wants

Often, an elaborate treatment is rejected by the patient, not because it is scientifically unsound or from lack of trust or confidence in the practitioner, but because of **financial constraints**. However, offering **alternative treatment options** that achieve only health may be at a fraction of the cost compared to a treatment plan that ideally incorporates function and aesthetics. **Sometimes, a compromise is the only option that a patient can afford.** Another reason why patients may reject therapy is a protracted treatment plan spanning several months or years. This is especially true for medically compromised or infirm elderly patients. **Dental phobias** or simply **indifference to oral health** are other reasons for reluctance to accept dental treatment, and counselling and educating is the best way forward. Finally, aesthetic dentistry is a unique clinical situation. As opposed to other forms of modalities, the **success of aesthetic or cosmetic dentistry involves patient participation.** Even if all clinical procedures are executed meticulously, adhering to sound scientific principles, the patient may judge the treatment outcome a failure. Dental aesthetics is fraught with **subjectivity**, and it is imperative to understand the patient's desires and wishes before starting therapy. It is also important to **clarify and discuss foreseeable compromises,** since failure to do so will inevitably be costly and disappointing.

Key points

- EBT planning avoids a haphazard approach at the treatment planning stage.
- EBT has three constituents: scientific credence, clinical erudition and patient needs and wants.
- It is prudent to inform patients of compromises before starting treatment, especially that involving aesthetic or cosmetic dentistry.

19 Treatment planning: decision-making

Review: caries

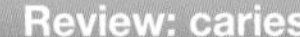

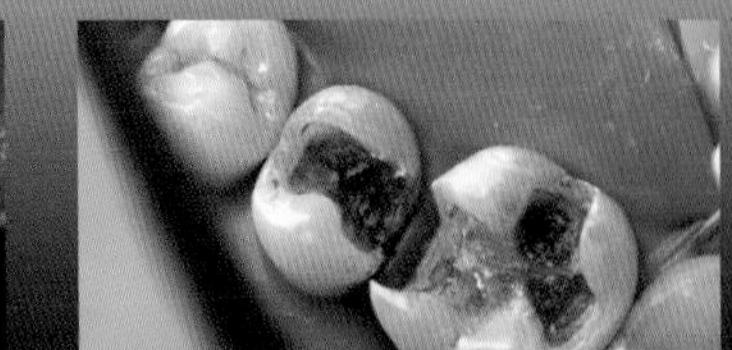

Caries presenting as hard tissue lesions can be left in situ and monitored

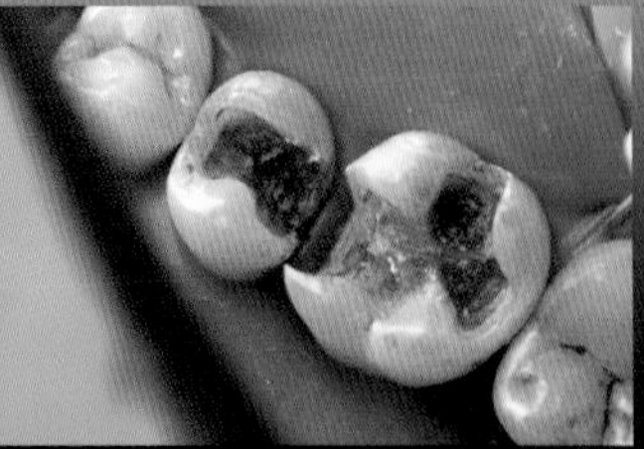

It may be possible to leave caries-infected soft dentine if a peripheral enamel/ filling seal is achievable

Shortened dental arch (SDA) concept

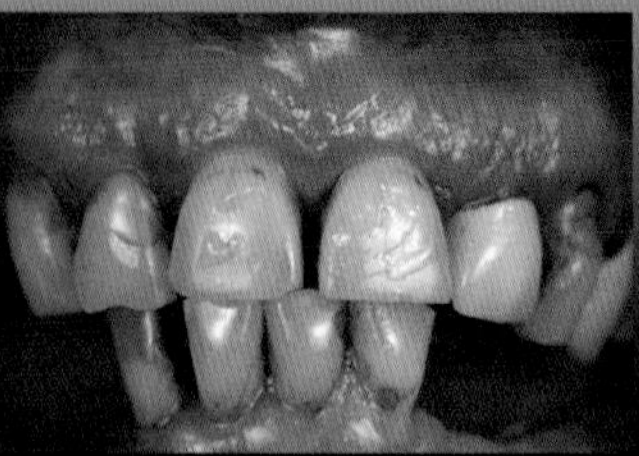

Assuming health can be restored to 10 anterior occluding teeth (SDA concept), missing molars do not need replacing for oral health and comfort

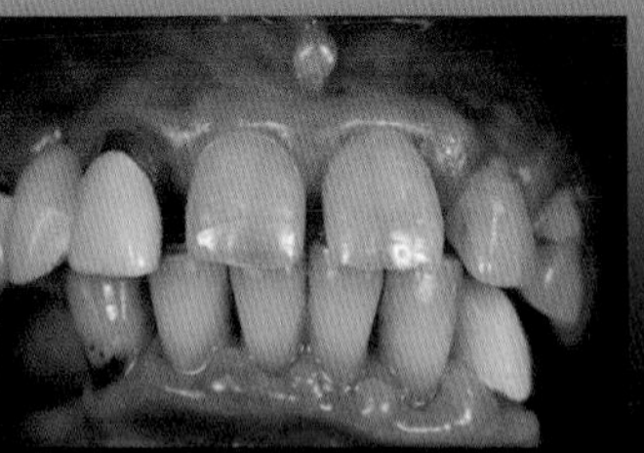

According to the SDA concept, if the missing lower premolars can be replaced (e.g. with implants), the missing mandibular molars do not need to be replaced

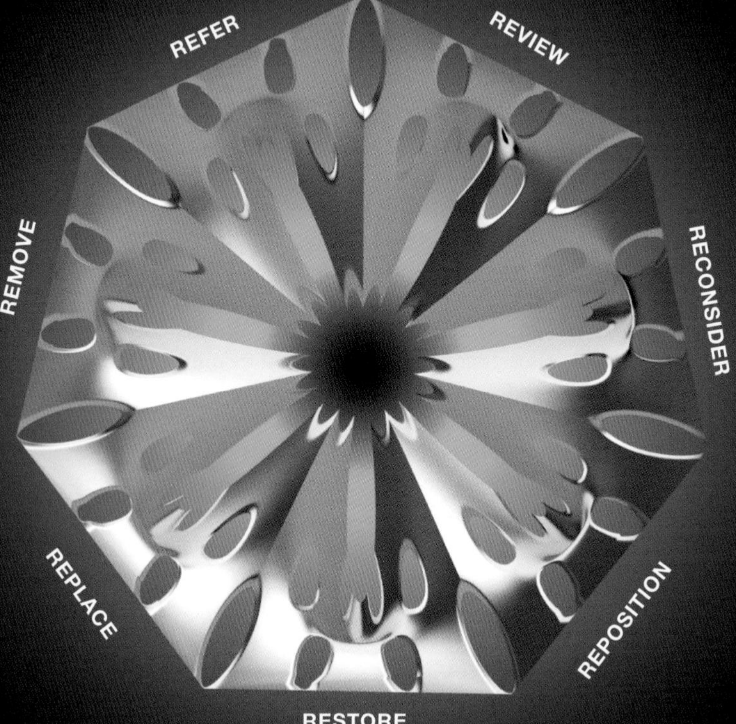

Reposition teeth by orthodontic therapy to...

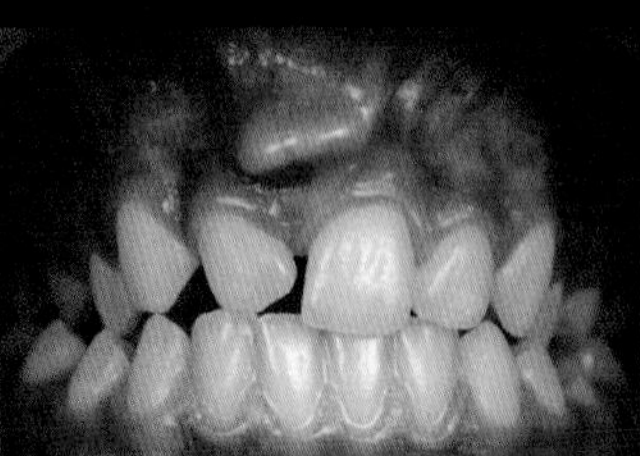

...create space for prosthetic unit(s)

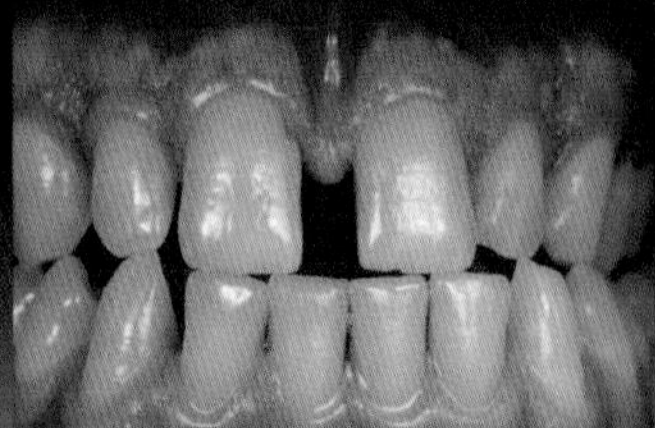

...close diastema

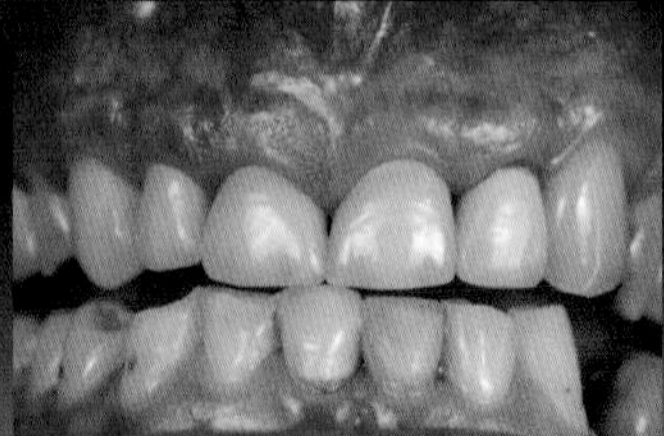

...create space for restorations by intrusion of the mandibular anterior teeth

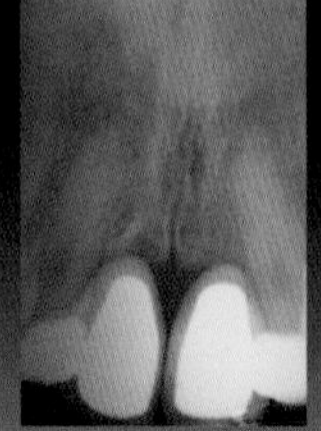

...upright roots to create space for implants

Prosthodontics at a Glance, Second Edition. Irfan Ahmad.

Decision-making is crucial at the treatment planning stage. When presented with oral disease (of the hard or soft tissues), the options available are:

- **Review** – e.g. caries or periodontal disease
- **Reconsider** – e.g. retain edentulous spaces (shortened dental arch [SDA] concept)
- **Reposition** – orthodontic appliances for realignment, closing or gaining space
- **Restore** – with direct or indirect restorations, root canal therapy, etc.
- **Replace** – replace existing restorations, or close edentulous space(s) with removable, fixed or implant-supported prostheses
- **Remove** – extraction, with or without bone and soft tissue grafting
- **Refer** – to specialist for advice or treatment if the therapy is complex, the patient is medically compromised, the patient wishes to be treated by a specialist and the clinician does not feel he/she has the knowledge, training, skill or experience to manage the condition

Very often, a combination of the above is indicated to arrive at a treatment plan with a **multidisciplinary approach**. Many of the options listed above are discussed in subsequent chapters. This chapter concentrates on a few issues that should be addressed during the planning process.

Review (monitor) caries

Traditional teaching is dogmatic about removing all carious lesions, whether they present as hard or soft enamel/dentine lesions. However, research has shown that **hard lesions can be left in-situ** and monitored for progression before considering a filling. For example, non-cavitated occlusal caries can either be fissure sealed, or periodically coated with chlorhexidine/fluoride varnish to arrest the lesion or allow remineralisation.

Similarly, a shift in attitude is beginning to emerge regarding caries that presents as soft dentine lesions. The conventional approach is that caries-infested soft dentine be 'completely' removed until sound or hard dentine is reached, and restored with a suitable filling. The new approach is that **infected soft dentine can be left in situ,** and the cavity restored with a filling. The rationale for this is that it is impossible to remove all bacteria from a lesion, and attempting to do so may result in pulpal exposure. So long as the cavity margins have intact enamel (decay-free and not hypocalcified), a marginal seal with a dental adhesive and a resin-based composite filling will deprive any remaining bacteria of nutrients and retard their proliferation. This allows time for formation of a **secondary dentine** barrier to protect the dental pulp. Although considered heretical by some at present, further research may confirm the validity of this protocol.

Shortened dental arch (SDA) concept

Contrary to popular belief, it is not always necessary to restore a partially edentulous dentition to a full complement of teeth, the so-called **'28-tooth syndrome'**. The **SDA concept,** although not without its critics, states that **10 occluding pairs of teeth** (six anterior teeth and usually the four premolars) are sufficient to ensure oral aesthetics and function. Both cross-sectional and longitudinal studies have concluded that the SDA concept is within the **adaptive capacity of the stomatognathic system**, with little variability (compared to a full dentition) in masticatory ability, signs of TMD, tooth migration, periodontal disease and general oral comfort. The ethos of the SDA concept is that efforts should be directed at saving and maintaining the incisors, canines and premolars at the expense of the molars. Also, providing removable dentures for bilateral free-end saddle to restore occlusal function may introduce **iatrogenic insult**, e.g. root caries. Furthermore, restoring missing molars with implants may be clinically superfluous and scientifically unsound. However, to adopt the SDA concept, certain criteria are essential:

- **Aesthetic and functional demands** are satisfied
- The **remaining teeth are periodontally sound**
- **Absence of pathological tooth surface loss (TSL)** (wear)
- **No pre-existing TMD symptoms**
- **No anterior open bite, class III** or **deep class II malocclusions**
- The clinical situation should be **monitored and regularly reviewed** so that the above criteria are maintained

Reposition

In some instances, repositioning teeth to a favourable position may be all that is required for achieving aesthetic and functional objectives, without intervention by irreversible restorative procedures. **Orthodontics movement(s)** can be used to realign teeth and roots, close diastemata, create space for prosthetic units, reduce open and deep overbites (levelling the curve of Spee), rectify dental cross-bites, expand arches and relieve crowding. The **basic movements** include **tipping**, **rotation**, **translation**, **root torquing**, **extrusion**, **intrusion** and **arch expansion**.

The **drawbacks of orthodontics** are protracted treatment times, poor patient compliance, root absorption and indefinite retention (fixed or removable) after the therapy. The choice of orthodontic appliances depends on the complexity of treatment and the type of desired movement. Orthodontic appliances are categorised as follows:

- **Removable** – full-arch acrylic appliances with wires, brackets, screws and springs. Ideal for tipping movements, intrusion/extrusion (Dahl appliance), arch expansion, but limited for complex positioning or root torqueing.
- **Fixed** – wires, springs, elastic bands, etc. held with steel or plastic brackets bonded onto labial or lingual surfaces of teeth. These varieties of appliance are state-of-the-art for the majority of tooth movements.
- **Clear aligner therapy (CAT)** – full-arch acrylic appliances generated from a computer virtual diagnostic setup. Using software simulation, the teeth are positioned to an ideal position, and a series of clear aligners constructed on CAD/CAM 3D printed models of the arches. As tooth movement progresses, the successive appliance in the series is worn until treatment is complete. A wide range of movements are possible, especially in combination with fixed appliances. The use of clear aligners is relatively new, introduced in 1999; and future developments are perpetually emerging to allow more complex movements using auxiliaries such as anchorage attachments, buttons with cutouts and elastic hooks.

Key points

- Decision-making is summarised as review, reconsider, reposition, restore, replace, remove or refer.
- Current paradigm shifts should be considered and incorporated into treatment planning options, e.g. leaving caries in situ, SDA concept and orthodontic repositioning.

20 AI (artificial intelligence)

Terminology	
Big data	Vast amount of data in the form of images, sound, text, numerics, time series
Data science	Utilises big data and machine learning to interpret data for decision-making purposes
Algorithm	Set of instructions to execute or solve a computational task
Data mining	Analysing data sets to reveal causal relationships and helps explain/understand trends or correlations
ANN (artificial neural networks)	Often synonymously referred to as neural network (NN) – core of deep learning, representing a set of algorithms that recognise patterns, similar to the human brain neural networks. Recent variations include CNN (convolutional neural networks), which are extensively used in dental & medical AI applications for analysing visual imagery, and DCNN (dilated convolutional neural networks) for predicting dose of medication
ML (machine learning)	Ability of a machine to make informed decisions from what it has learnt from data input and is classified as supervised and unsupervised learnings
RL (representation learning)	(or feature learning), subset of ML that automatically learns features required for classification of raw data
DL (deep learning)	Subset of ML, and the latest generation of AI, consisting of multiple layers of ANN, i.e. it structures algorithms in interconnecting layers to create a deep neural network that can learn and make intelligent decisions on its own without human intervention
Fuzzy logic	Assumes that tackling real-time problems, similar to conventional logic, are pragmatic rather than dogmatic

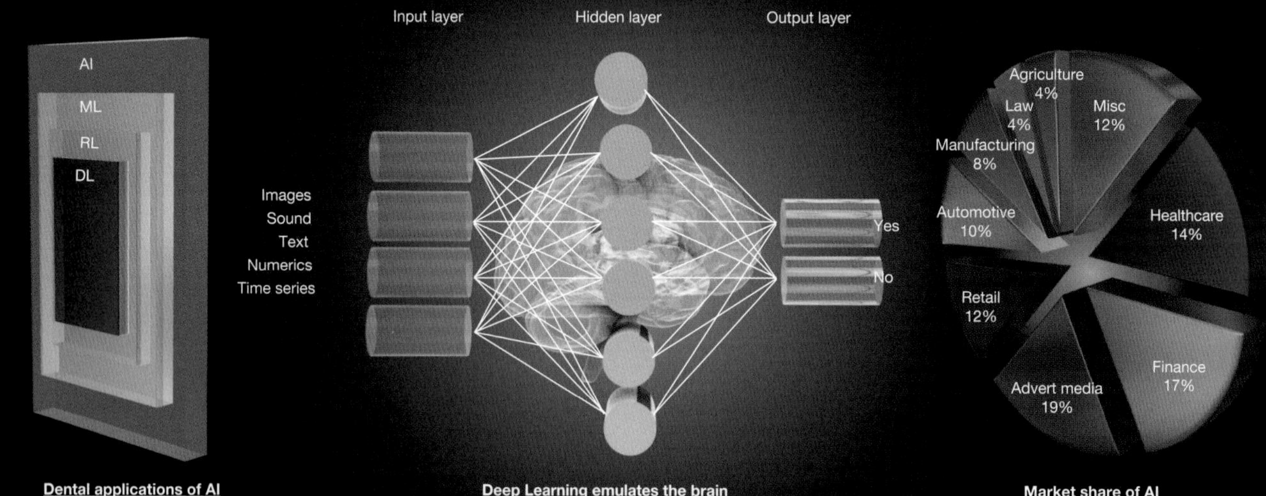

Dental applications of AI | Deep Learning emulates the brain | Market share of AI

Application	Procedure	AI technology
Administration	Appointments scheduling according to work, family and social commitments, automatically replenishing stock, education (staff, patients, undergraduate, postgraduate) , assess staff or student performance, prevent insurance claim fraud	ML, DL, virtual and augmented reality , machine vision
Equipment	Voice activated dental chair functions and ancillary equipment. Memorised chair positions for individual patients	NLP, ML, DL
Diagnosis	Caries detection, vertical root fractures, chronic/aggressive periodontitis, forensic odontology, cephalometric analysis of skeletal abnormalities (facial asymmetries), pre-cancerous lesions	Machine vision, data mining, DL, machine vision, CNN, DCNN, GA, SVM
Treatment planning & treatment	Treatment pre-visualisation, motivation, acceptance, triage, benefits and limitation. Robot-assisted implant surgery, fabrication & precision fit of indirect restorations, 3D bioprinted scaffolds for replacing hard tissue, locating tooth preparation margins, design indirect restoration for CAM milling or 3D printing, digital smile design and virtual/intra-oral mock-ups, implant surgical guides	DL, virtual and augmented reality
Perioperative	Apex location during endodontic therapy, demarcating lesion margins for excision, nerves & vital structures recognition	ANN, machine vision
Prescience/ prognosis	Predicting oral cancer, BRONJ/MRONJ, bone density, hard/soft tissue loss after surgery, dental decay, apthous ulceration, toothache, cariogenic bacteria, size & location of impacted canines/3rd molars, number of extractions required for orthodontics, outcome of aesthetic/orthodontic/surgical treatments, longevity of restorations, TMD, peri-implantitis, tooth surface loss (TSL), tooth shade following bleaching, and analysing patient '-omics' data (e.g. genomics, microbiomics, metabolomics)	ML, ANN, CNN, DCNN, Bayesain network, SVM, logistic regression, decision tree, NLP

Prosthodontics at a Glance, Second Edition. Irfan Ahmad.

Artificial intelligence (AI) is not science fiction, but science fact which is pervading our world at a breathtaking pace. Since the beginning of the 21st century, AI has been **abstrusely integrated into many aspects of our daily lives**, e.g. the Apple® A13 Bionic chip in mobile phones, online customer targeting by Amazon®, Netflix® recommendations, weather forecasting, interactions with Siri and Alexa (NLP – natural language processing), traffic control (machine vision) and even calculating delivery times of UberEats. AI is also the driving force behind self-driving cars that are literally around the corner and powers robotic automation for innumerable industries.

What is AI?

AI is a rapidly evolving technology, broadly describing a variety of **intelligent tasks performed by machines**. AI is capable of learning to **mimic intelligent tasks**, similar to **natural intelligence**, with a synergy of hardware and software using a variety of algorithms. This involves **cognitive processing,** such as **reasoning**, **decision-making** and **conclusion drawing** that are essentially human traits.

Although the term 'artificial intelligence' was coined by John McCarthy in 1956, but it was the **British polymath, Alan Turing**, in the 1940s, who is regarded as the **pioneer of AI**. The basic precept of the Turning machine, termed **strong AI**, assumes that human cognition is exclusively mathematical. In reality, human cognition is based on previous experiences and learning, and decisions are often haphazard, irrational and not purely mathematical. This approach is termed **weak AI** and forms the basis of modern AI developments such as Google® DeepMind's AlphaGo, IBM Watson®, Teslar® Auto Pilot, Softbank Robotics' Pepper and David Hanson's Sophia that not only 'thinks', but possess human abilities of **learning from experience**.

AI technology

AI is computational understanding for analysing large data sets (**big data**) using algorithms. The simplest form of AI is **machine learning (ML)** that requires **structured or labelled data** to perform its task, and therefore only suitable for relatively **basic tasks** and handling small amounts of data. The processing power and storage requirements are minimal and the computations quick. ML uses various training models or algorithms such as **genetic algorithm (GA), artificial neural network (ANN)** and the **support vector machine** (SVM). This type of learning is referred to as **'shallow learning'** as it uses few layers of ANN, whereas **'deep learning'** uses many interconnected ANN layers for complex tasks.

Deep learning (DL) is the most sophisticated AI capable of handling vast amounts of **unlabelled data** and is better suited for **complex query solving**, but computations take more time. **DL emulates the functioning of the human brain** and, compared to ML, requires greater processing power with large storage capacities necessitating **parallel and/or cloud computing**. The core of DL is ANN, consisting of a set of nodes forming the hierarchical input, hidden and output layers. The nodes interconnect or link each layer to form a **deep neural network** to **'self-learn'** from repeated varying weighted input. DL uses intuitive algorithms such as self-learning **backpropagation algorithms** for refining data. The two main programming language used in AI are Prolog and Lisp, resulting in an impressive number of algorithm, e.g. adaptive neuro-fuzzy inference system (ANFIS) or **fuzzy logic**, Bayesian inference models, interactive backward chaining inference, decision tree, infrastructure expert system (for medical use), generative adversarial networks (GANs), Genetics Nanotechnology and Robotics (GNR), knowledge-enabled mass destruction (KMD), CRISPR-Cas9 (for modifying human DNA), etc. Finally, many AI are based on **hybrid intelligent systems** that complement each other rather than relying solely on one system.

Healthcare applications

Besides administrative tasks, AI offers clinical **decision support systems (CDSS)** for diagnosis, disease prescience (ectopic pregnancy, onset of arthritis, macular degeneration, metastasises, and cardiovascular, stroke), treatment options, perioperative, drug prescribing, robot-assisted surgery, prognosis (post-surgical morbidity), epidemiology and research (translational medicine).

Benefits and concerns

The main benefit is **standardisation**, **efficiency** and **accuracy**, which should be **98–99%** for clinical applications. **Although they lack emotions and feelings, machines have the advantages of not suffering from fatigue, boredom, bias and idiosyncrasies.** The concerns are litigation for misdiagnosis due to AI, quality of data input (photographs, radiographs, intra-oral scans, MRI, ultrasound and CBCT images). Also, **algorithms are inaccessible** and unchangeable, making it difficult to understand or tweak the criteria for diagnosis. Finally, adherence to **HIPPA guidelines** is imperative for confidentiality.

Emerging and future developments

The ultimate gain of AI, at both the administrative and clinical levels, is delivering **personalised dentistry** according to the genome of the individual. For example, research into oral multifactorial diseases to help isolate **susceptible individuals**, and using the **collective knowledge for risk assessment** and **early intervention**, plus personalising treatment depending on medical history, economic status, previous dental history and compliance. Also, **nanomachines** for creating medical micro-robots and self-healing materials that repair themselves without human intervention.

AI will assist technicians to design and fabricate restorations with ideal emergence profiles and form that integrate harmoniously into the dentition with respect to **health, function and aesthetics**. In **implantology**, automatic merging intra-oral and CBCT scans will allow **robot-assisted implant placement** according to bone architecture and tissue biotypes.

Teaching institutions will download and incorporate the latest developments into their expanding big data libraries to **increase knowledge base** for training AI machines. In addition, intra-oral scans of **students' work will be accessed objectively** without bias of a faculty member. AI will also **provide transparency** for **insurance claims** with standardised assessment criteria. Finally, **patient preferences** for chair position, room temperature, ambient lighting, genre of music, beverage penchant and duration of dental treatment can be set-up beforehand to **enhance the dental experience**.

Key points

- AI is an all-encompassing term defining the ability to substitute human intelligence by artificial means, irrespective of the methods used to achieve this objective
- The main subsets of AI are machine learning and deep learning
- AI is well established in many sectors of industry
- In dentistry, AI augments administrative and clinical tasks
- Ethical guidelines are required to prevent subversive abuse of this revolutionary technology

Occlusion

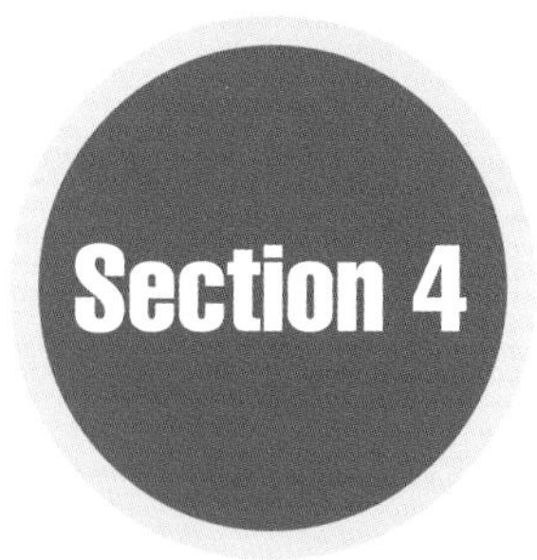

Chapters

Occlusion: terminology and definitions

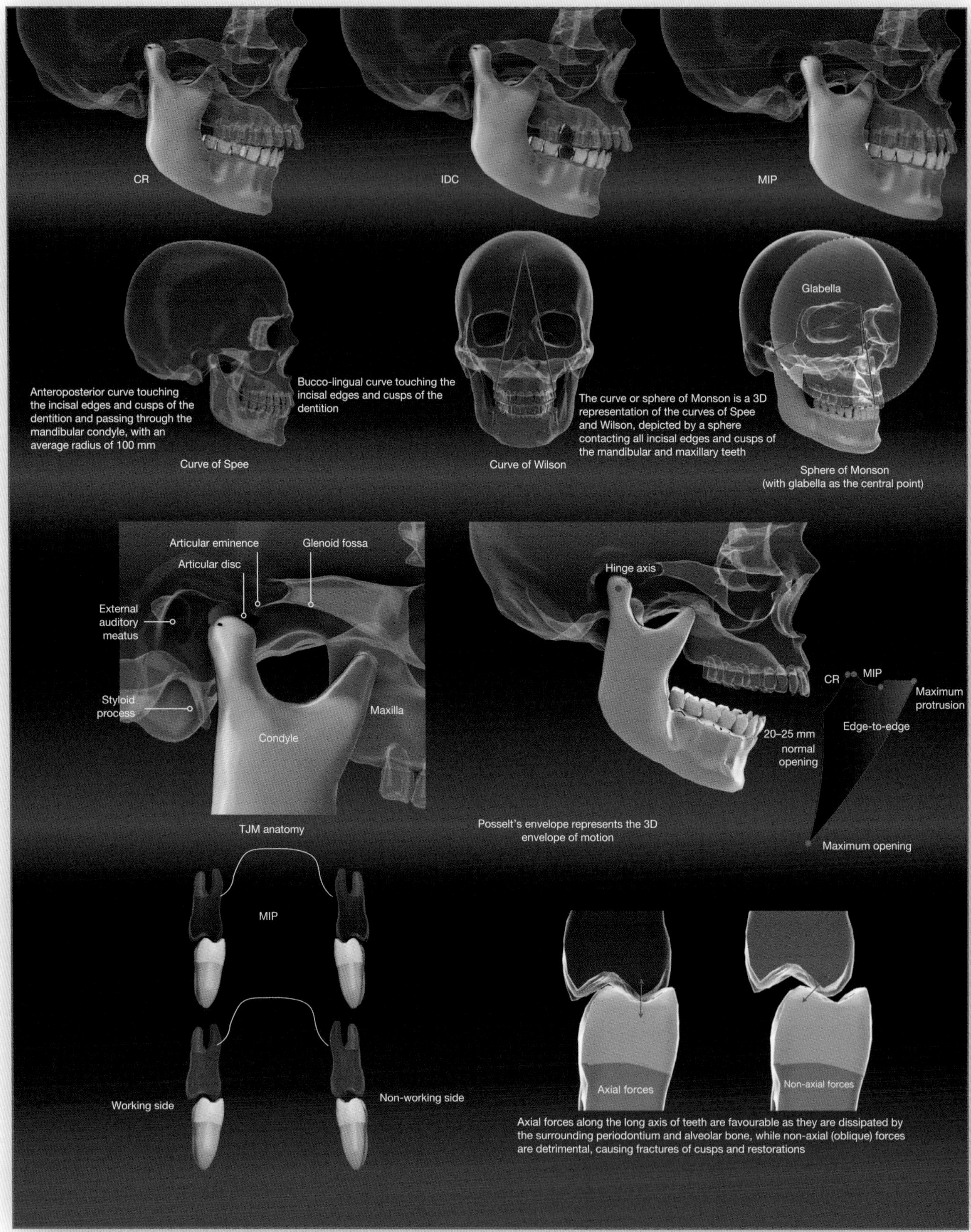

Occlusion simply means surface contact of the maxillary and mandibular teeth. Although the definition is straightforward, there are few topics in dentistry that are more shrouded in mystery than the subject of occlusion. Furthermore, definitions and synonyms for describing occlusal terms add to the confusion. There has been much speculation, and various theories have been put forward, but **opinion remains fragmented**. However, there are basic principles that are undisputed, and the ensuing chapters cover these points, offering a practical approach for prosthodontic treatment.

Curves of Spee, Wilson and Monson

The significance of these curves is that, in an unworn dentition, the **anteroposterior** and **bucco-lingual curvature** allows **unimpeded mandibular lateral and protrusive excursions**. However, disruption of these curves due to tooth wear, migration or tooth loss causes occlusal disharmonies that require addressing to re-establish these curves.

CR, RCP and MIP

Centric relation (CR) is a dynamic state when the mandibular condyles are maximally seated in their fossae, i.e. the **terminal hinge axis (THA)** position and the muscles are relaxed. This is an **anatomical bone-to-bone position** not influenced by the dentition. The **initial deflective contact (IDC)** is a **static position** when one or two teeth contact at the **retruded contact position (RCP)**. From this location, the mandible slides laterally or anteriorly (0.25 mm to 2.25 mm) to **MIP (maximum intercuspation)**, also known as the intercuspal position (ICP) or centric occlusion (CO). **MIP** is a **static habitual position** influenced by genetics, tooth shape, neuromuscular 'memory', pathological or iatrogenic factors. **MIP is tooth-to-tooth contact**, irrespective of the position of the condyles. MIP and CR may or may not coincide depending on the position of the condyles. In the minority of the population (10%), CR and MIP are coincident, without any slide (or deflective contacts). When the teeth are **at MIP, the occlusal forces are in an ideal vertical direction**, directed through the long axis of the teeth, and subsequently dissipated by the periodontal ligament and alveolar bone. In most cases, artificial restorations are tailored to 'fit' this occlusal status quo, referred to the **confirmative approach**, or alternately, restored to the CR position, known as the **reorganised approach**. Without clinical symptoms, a slide from CR to MIP is not detrimental to health, and occlusal adjustments to eliminate defective contacts are unjustified since it may create unwanted forces on teeth which were previously not subjected to occlusal forces, causing fracture of teeth and fillings that become subjected to occlusal stress, and are perceived as 'high'. This also applies to providing new restorations that **alter MIP**, which can result in similar consequences, such as causing **anterior tooth wear**, **loss of face height**, **fractured teeth and fillings** or **TMJ problems**. The clinical relevance of CR, RCP and MIP is as follows:

- When the **tooth to be restored is the IDC at CR or RCP**
- If **anterior teeth require restoration** and there is a **substantial shift in CR** against the teeth that require artificial restorations
- A **new vertical dimension of occlusal (VDO) is planned**, e.g. following tooth wear. Anterior tooth wear is accompanied by **dentoalveolar compensation** to maintain VDO but result in insufficient interocclusal space to accommodate restorative materials to restore the incisors. Two methods are available to create interocclusal clearance. The first is to **reposition the mandible in CR** using an anterior deprogrammer (assuming there is a horizontal shift from CR to MIP). The rationale for this is that **tooth wear causes the mandible to reposition itself in an anterior and superior direction.** An anterior deprogrammer, e.g. Lucia jig, helps relocate the mandible to its original CR position, i.e. posterior and inferior directions, and thereby creating interocclusal clearance for the restorative materials. The second method is using a **Dahl orthodontic appliance to allow periodontal growth (overeruption)** of the posterior teeth and intrusion of the anterior teeth.

Guidance

The above discussion has focused on static occlusion consisting of IDC, RCP and MIP. During **dynamic occlusion**, **posterior guidance is provided by the TMJ (posterior determinant)** and **anterior guidance by the teeth (anterior determinant)**. **Posterior guidance** is limited by the shape of the temporomandibular joints (**TMJ**), while anterior guidance can be by any teeth (anterior or posterior). The forces generated during excursions are **oblique, and** these **lateral forces (non-axial loading)** are more detrimental than the vertical forces observed in MIP, a point worth remembering when restoring guiding teeth with artificial restorations. **Mutual protection** is when the posterior teeth contact in MIP to **protect the anterior teeth**, and the anterior teeth and canines disclose the mandible in protrusion and lateral excursions, respectively, to **protect the posterior teeth**. In **protrusion**, the **incisors usually** act as the guiding teeth. The so-called **anterior guidance** may be **steep** or **shallow** depending on the degree of overbite. This is significant when choosing restorative materials, i.e. a steep anterior guidance places greater stress on artificial restorations, requiring more resilient materials, e.g. metal rather than all-ceramic. In **lateral excursions,** the guiding teeth are the canines in isolation (**canine protected or canine guidance**), or the canines in combination with other teeth, usually the premolars (**group function**). Group function allows **lateral forces** to be distributed among several teeth, placing less demand on the restorative material.

Interferences

Any contact that impedes mandibular excursions or reaching MIP is termed an interference. A **working side interference** is on the side to which the mandible is moving, while a **non-working side interference** is on the opposite side. In effect, these posterior teeth interferences provide undesirable anterior guidance. Interferences can potentially cause inflammatory changes of the TMJ, and periodontium, as well as fractures of the teeth and/or restorations. However, most interferences are insignificant, since the stomatognathic system adapts or avoids them during function. Nevertheless, interferences are relevant when considering prosthodontic treatment, e.g. a non-working side contact may cause cross-arch pivot, lifting the teeth on the working side, and should be eliminated before starting restorative treatment, and new interferences not introduced by new prostheses (especially those with steep cusps). Furthermore, **dynamic occlusal changes** should be rehearsed on articulated models before considering intra-oral adjustments or grinding teeth. Alternately, occlusal splint or stabilising appliances can be provided to safeguard interfering teeth and the TMJ.

Key points

- Both static occlusion (IDC, MIP) and dynamic occlusion (guidance and interferences) should to considered before prosthodontic therapy.
- There is no justification for indiscriminate pursuit of occlusal equilibrium to achieve an 'ideal occlusal scheme'.

22 Occlusion: clinical procedures

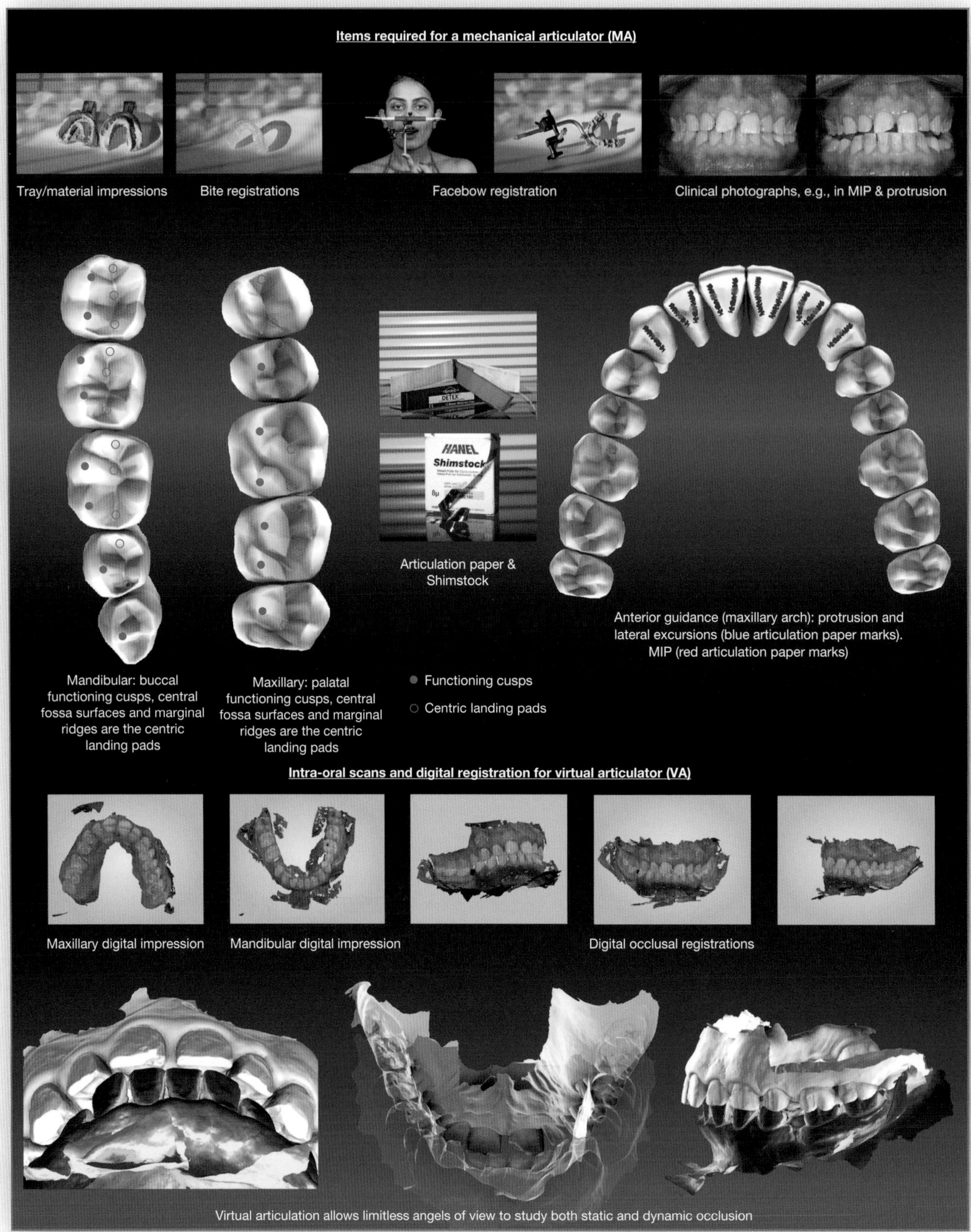

Items required for a mechanical articulator (MA)
Tray/material impressions
Bite registrations
Facebow registration
Clinical photographs, e.g., in MIP & protrusion
HANEL
Shimstock
Articulation paper & Shimstock
Anterior guidance (maxillary arch): protrusion and lateral excursions (blue articulation paper marks). MIP (red articulation paper marks)
Mandibular: buccal functioning cusps, central fossa surfaces and marginal ridges are the centric landing pads
Maxillary: palatal functioning cusps, central fossa surfaces and marginal ridges are the centric landing pads
● Functioning cusps
○ Centric landing pads
Intra-oral scans and digital registration for virtual articulator (VA)
Maxillary digital impression
Mandibular digital impression
Digital occlusal registrations
Virtual articulation allows limitless angels of view to study both static and dynamic occlusion

Prosthodontics at a Glance, Second Edition. Irfan Ahmad.

Even if an occlusal status quo is envisaged, a **preoperative static and dynamic occlusal assessment** is worthwhile. Furthermore, it is instructive to know the patient's occlusal status so that the treatment provided does not disrupt the existing occlusal equilibrium. This chapter describes the salient clinical procedures of an **occlusal examination and assessment.**

MIP and CR

To observe **maximum intercuspation position (MIP)**, the patient is asked to bite on their posterior teeth, so that there is **maximum interdigitation** of the teeth. In this position, there should be maximum contact between opposing teeth, which is dependent on tooth shape and neuromuscular 'memory'. **Centric relation (CR)** is an **anatomical dynamic state**. To place the mandible in CR, a **transient neuromuscular amnesia** is necessary so that the mandible can be freely guided into its most posterior and superior location, rather than its habitual MIP. Methods to place the mandible in CR include:

- **Bimanual mandibular manipulation**
- **Anterior deprogramming with a jig (e.g. Lucia jig)**
- **Gothic arch tracing**

Visual and tactile inspection

A **visual examination** requires the following armamentarium: **photographic documentation**, **Shimstock foil**, **articulation paper** and **study models** to view the teeth from the lingual perspective. Placing the mandible in CR allows the initial deflective contact (**IDC**) to be observed, and subsequent slide (if any) into **MIP**. Articulation paper of one colour is used to mark tooth contact in MIP (**static occlusion**). Another paper of a different colour is used to superimpose contacts during various mandibular excursions (**dynamic occlusion**). This allows clear distinction between MIP and guiding contacts, as well as discriminating eccentric contacts or **interferences**. The **supporting or functional cusps** in both arches are verified, i.e. palatal cusps of maxillary teeth and buccal cusps of mandibular teeth. The visual inspection should also detect degree of mandibular movement, trismus, wear facets and shifts, and clicking of the TMJs (temporomandibular joints). Finally, the curvature of the occlusal planes is noted, and whether these conform to the **curves of Spee, Wilson and Monson**. In addition, digital photographs serve as a reminder of the occlusal status for reference.

Tactile examination includes palpation of the **major muscles of mastication, i.e. masseter, temporalis, and medial and lateral pterygoids.** The TMJs are also palpated for tenderness or eliciting a painful response, especially if the patient reports a history of temporomandibular disorders (**TMD**). Differential diagnosis of TMD includes symptoms arising from bruxism, of myogenous or articular origin. Palpation is also useful for ascertaining the degree of **tooth mobility** and **fremitus** during mandibular movements.

Facebow transfer

A facebow transfers the orientation of the maxillary arch relative to the condylar hinge axis or **terminal hinge axis (THA)**. It simply informs the technician about the **intercondylar width** and where to mount the maxillary model on a mechanical articulator (MA), but **does not convey any information about the occlusion**. The facebow can either be an **earbow**, or a **kinematic type**, depending on the chosen articulator. The **basic elements of a facebow** are:

- **Bite fork** to register the cusp tips and incisal edges of the maxillary teeth
- **Two posterior reference points**, e.g. external auditory meati for orientation of the transverse condylar axis. If the right and left external auditory meati vary in height, it is better to align the facebow (earbow type) so that its horizontal plane coincides with the interpupillary line to avoid canting of the maxillary model when mounted onto the articulator
- **One anterior reference point**, e.g. the ala-tragus line or an arbitrary point 43 mm superior to the maxillary lateral incisor

Impressions and occlusal records

Accurate and precise full arch impressions and subsequent mounted plaster casts are essential for extra-oral visual inspection. Alternately, **digital acquisitions of the arches with an IOS can be used to 3D print models** of the arches. It is important to decide at **which vertical dimension of occlusion (VDO), the models are to be mounted,** irrespective of whether they are mounted in MIP or CR. Usually, the models are mounted to the VDO at which the patient is to be restored. **If MIP is obvious, and the treatment relatively simple, occlusal records are superfluous**, since they may prevent accurate location of the opposing model. **If MIP is not obvious, the models must be mounted in CR at the chosen VDO. Lateral excursion records are only necessary to set the condylar angles** instead of using average values on the articulator, and **protrusive registration to verify that the articulator is set-up correctly**. Many materials are available for recording occlusal positions, e.g. wax, acrylic, zinc-oxide eugenol or addition silicone bite registration formulations. It is advisable to use similar materials for impressions and occlusal records, since differences in material accuracies may prevent accurate location of the bite records onto the plaster casts.

Articulators

The choice articulator is determined by the complexity of treatment (see Chapter 15).The most widely used is a **semi-adjustable MA**, with **average articulator parameters, i.e. Bennett and condylar angles, intercondylar distance and spacial relationships of craniomandibular geometry** are pre-set to average values. Although not a true representation of the clinical situation, **a semi-adjustable articulator is satisfactory for the majority of prosthodontic treatment**. If a **fully adjustable articulator** or articulator-related registration devices are chosen, further parameters are required, and greater adjustment possible, e.g. intercondylar distance, condylar and Bennett angles, upper and lower rear wall inclinations and fossae morphology. As discussed in Chapter 15, occlusal analysis can also be performed in a virtual environment by **virtual articulators (VA)** using intra-oral scans, jaw movements and **algorithmic dental occlusion (ADO)** for simulating occlusal contacts with corresponding jaw excursions.

Key points

- An occlusal inspection includes visual, tactile, study models and articulation.
- Articulation can be mechanical or virtual.
- For most prosthodontic treatment, a semi-adjustable MA with average values is adequate.

23 Occlusion: laboratory procedures

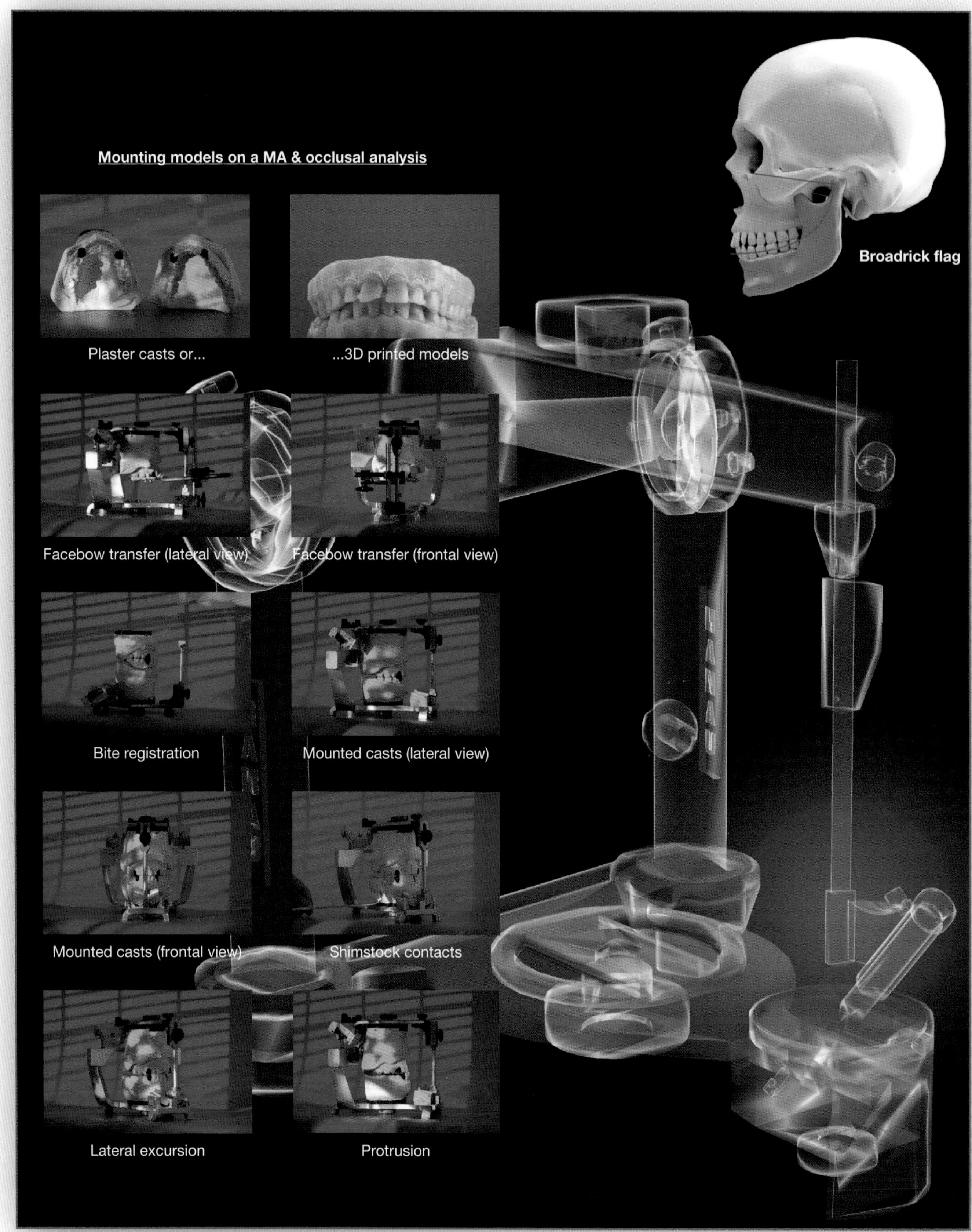

Mounting models on a MA & occlusal analysis
Plaster casts or...
...3D printed models
Facebow transfer (lateral view)
Facebow transfer (frontal view)
Bite registration
Mounted casts (lateral view)
Mounted casts (frontal view)
Shimstock contacts
Lateral excursion
Protrusion
Broadrick flag
HANAU

Prosthodontics at a Glance, Second Edition. Irfan Ahmad.

The **analogue laboratory process** of **mechanical articulation** involves mounting plaster casts or 3D printed models onto a simulating device for reproducing, in three spatial planes, the occlusal situation of the patient's mouth. The degree of sophistication to which this is achieved depends on the chosen type of **mechanical articulator (MA)**, and the meticulous steps taken to avoid introducing errors at each stage of the mounting process. As discussed in Chapters 15 and 22, hinge and fixed value articulators assume no semblance to the relationship of the jaws, while fully adjustable types allow a wider range of adjustable values that are more representative of jaw movements. For most prosthodontic treatment, the most popular type of **MA is the semi-adjustable** (e.g. Denar or Hanau) with accompanying **earbow type of facebow** transfer.

Pouring/printing models

The first stage is pouring casts from the impressions using high-quality, minimum distortion **hard plaster** or **printing models** with a 3D printer. Any aberration of tooth anatomy will detrimentally distort the clinical scenario, leading to misleading interpretations and incorrect treatment planning.

Maxillary model location

The **facebow transfer**, with the bite fork, **locates the maxillary model within the articulator to the hinge axis** and ensures its **orientation to the horizontal plane** (external auditory meati or interpupillary line of the patient). The **anterior reference pointer,** 43 mm above the maxillary lateral incisor, ensures that the reference plane is adjusted accordingly.

Mandibular model location

The **mandibular model** is located to the maxillary cast in either **CO or CR**, at the chosen **vertical dimension of occlusion (VDO)** using the occlusal records.

Mandibular excursions

Once both models of the arches are correctly and accurately mounted, **protrusive and lateral excursions** can be assessed. **Photographic documentation** showing articulation paper marks are useful for the technician to verify initial contact in **CR**, **slide from CR to MIP, non- working side interferences** and guiding teeth in protrusion and lateral excursions, i.e. **canine guidance or group function.**

Adjusting contacts and VDO

Depending on the treatment plan and clinical prescription, any trial **selective occlusal adjustments** can be performed on the casts, and analysed, before carrying out irreversible adjustments in the mouth. Similarly, the **VDO can be increased**, and either an occlusal splint or a temporary prosthesis fabricated to the new VDO for assessing intra-oral occlusal tolerance.

Custom incisal guidance table

A custom **incisal table** is used to **copy either the preoperative** or the **proposed anterior guidance** of the **temporary or definitive restorations.** An incisal table is indicated if the **VDO is to be altered**, several **anterior teeth are to be restored**, the **canine or supporting teeth require restorations,** and to **prevent wear of the diagnostic plaster casts**. Cold-cured acrylic resin is placed on the guide table, and the articulator pin is moved in all excursions until the material has set to create a record of mandibular movements. When the working cast of the definitive restorations is mounted on the articulator, the table acts as a guide to **shape the palatal surfaces of the restorations** to conform to the mandibular movements.

Anterior diagnostic wax-up

If anterior aesthetics are to be restituted, additive diagnostic procedures such as **diagnostic wax-ups** are invaluable for assessing appearance and gaining the patient's acceptance. From the diagnostic wax-up, a **vacuum stent** can be made, which serves as an excellent template for **intra-oral mock-ups** with composite resins for assessing aesthetic parameters such as:

- **Degree of tooth display at rest**
- **Amount of the tooth display** during smiling
- **Parallelism of maxillary incisal plane** with **curvature of mandibular lip during a relaxed smile**
- **Shade assessment**
- **Tooth morphology**

In addition, diagnostic wax-ups are ideal for **prosthetically driven implant treatment planning**. The wax-up can be scanned and the 3D files 'stitched' with DICOM files from a CBCT scan to fabricate **surgical guides** for precise placement of implant fixtures, and/or assess the need for **augmenting the site** prior to implant placement.

Broadrick flag

If the **posterior dentition requires rehabilitation**, a diagnostic wax-up can be carried out using the **Broadrick flag** to **restore the curves of Spee, Wilson and sphere of Monson**, thereby allowing posterior tooth disclusion during mandibular excursions.

Using the Broadrick flag technique assumes correct functional and **aesthetic position of the mandibular incisors**. An anterior survey point is chosen, usually the mandibular incisors, and using a compass (opened 100 mm), an arc is drawn on the 'flag'. The **posterior reference point** is either a molar, or if none is present, the condylar part of the articulator is selected, and another arc drawn to intersect the first. Using the two arcs as reference curves, wax is curved to **restore the occlusal plane in three dimensions (sphere of Monson)**. The completed wax-up can be used in a similar manner to the anterior wax-up as a template for temporary prostheses and surgical guides.

Key points

- A semi-adjustable MA is commonly used for occlusal analysis and prosthodontic treatment.
- Mounting models on a MA is carried out with a facebow transfer and interocclusal registration records at the correct VDO.
- A custom incisal table is used for copying anterior guidance for the definitive restorations.
- Anterior diagnostic wax-ups are ideal for scrutinising aesthetics.
- The Broadrick flag technique is used for restoring the 3D sphere of Monson.

24 Occlusion: adjustment and splints

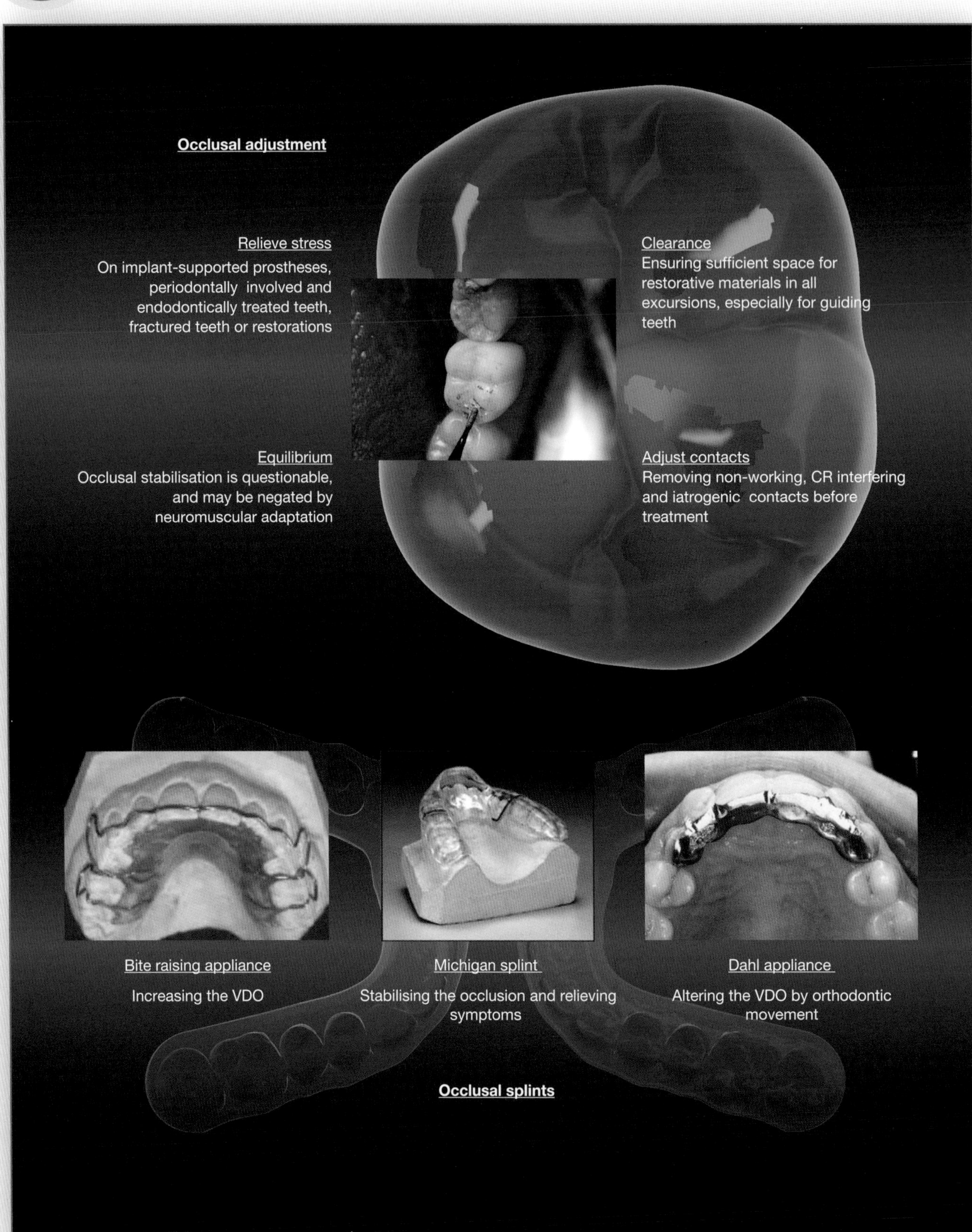

Prosthodontics at a Glance, Second Edition. Irfan Ahmad.

After analysing the occlusion by performing a clinical examination and laboratory assessment, the next step is deciding whether any occlusal adjustments or occlusal splints are necessary before starting prosthodontic therapy.

Occlusal adjustment

Occlusal stabilisation by **occlusal adjustment (OA)** is a controversial topic. Before discussing opposing theories, if **TMD** (temporomandibular disorder) is suspected, differential diagnosis is essential to elucidate whether TMD symptoms originate due to **myogenous** or **bruxism** origins, or **pathology** of the mandibular articular region. If the latter is suspected, occlusal adjustment is futile.

However, if TMD problems originate from myogenous or bruxism causes, OA may or may not alleviate symptoms. There are **two schools of thought regarding OA**. The first states that **neuromuscular feedback will adapt** to any adjustments, and therefore, negate its effect. The second opinion is that **OA can stabilise the occlusion**, removing interferences that impede physiological mandibular excursions, and hence provide symptomatic relief. Whichever opinion one holds, to prevent irreversible occlusal destruction, it is probably prudent to avoid OA until further conclusive research is forthcoming.

Besides TMD reasons, **selective OA is justified before starting restorative treatment.** Preoperative adjustments can be invaluable in saving time and avoiding disappointment as treatment progresses, especially at the cementation stage to 'grind in' the restoration(s), for example:

- **Removing non-working side interferences** causing lifting of the mandible on the working side
- Ensuring sufficient **occlusal clearance for restorative materials** in all excursions (particularly for guiding teeth)
- If the tooth to be restored is the **initial contact in CR**
- **Eccentric contact(s)** preventing closure in MIP
- **Extruded teeth**
- **Preventing** undue **stress on implant-supported prostheses**
- **Relieving occlusal stress on fractured teeth or restorations**
- **Eccentric contacts exacerbating bruxism**
- **Iatrogenic interferences** introduced by existing artificial prostheses
- **Relieving** periodontal **trauma due to occlusion**
- **Reducing stress on endodontically treated teeth** that are more susceptible to occlusal bite forces

Alternately, if the defective filling was in **intra occlusion** or had an inclined contact causing oblique forces, this can be corrected by shaping the new filling that has occlusal contact or the cuspal contact is **directed axially**, respectively.

Occlusal stabilising splints

Various designs of splint are advocated depending on the clinical manifestations. The most popular is the full arch splint, e.g. **Michigan**, normally worn at night. The construction is of heat-cured acrylic, 2 mm in thickness, with either anterior or canine disclusion. The important factor is that the interocclusal device be **periodically adjusted** until symptoms subside, or the treatment objective is achieved. Other varieties include partial coverage types that are contraindicated because they permit **unwanted orthodontic tooth movement**, while the soft varieties (or vacuum-formed splints) are less efficacious than the Michigan type. The disadvantage of splints is lack of patient compliance, which diminishes the potential beneficial effects of these appliances. Innumerable studies have confirmed the efficacy of occlusal stabilising appliances for **reducing parafunctional and electromyographic activity** in conjunction with mandibular repositioning. Occlusal splints are prescribed for a variety of reasons including:

- **Tooth wear** (or tooth surface loss – TSL) and bite-raising appliances (see below)
- **Protecting fragile or susceptible restorations** (especially all-ceramic prostheses)
- **Retainers** following orthodontic or periodontal therapy
- **Differential diagnosis of TMDs** (myogenous, bruxism or articular origin)
- **Reducing clenching, bruxism,** cheek biting, fractured teeth/restorations
- **Controlling stresses on implant-supported prostheses,** trauma from occlusion
- **Tempering bruxism** coexisting with comorbid syndromes (e.g. Parkinson's disease)
- **Supportive treatment for secondary otalgia** associated with clenching
- **TMJ disk derangement**, clicking, locking, arthralgia, arthritis and myalgia
- Symptomatic **relief** in certain types **of migraine**
- **Relief of** smarting symptoms associated with **burning mouth syndrome (BMS)** using lingual splints

Bite-raising appliance

TSL is accompanied by compensatory growth of the alveolus, termed **dentoalveolar compensation**, that maintains the VDO but leaves little or no interocclusal space for replacing the lost enamel and dentine. One method for gaining interocclusal clearance is using a **bite-raising appliance** for assessing whether the patient can tolerate an increase in the VDO, before providing reparative restorations.

The Dahl appliance

The principle of the **Dahl orthodontic appliance** is to allow periodontal growth of the posterior dentition and intrusion of the anterior teeth, thereby creating room in the anterior region for restorative materials to replace the lost tooth substrate **at a new VDO**. This was originally achieved by a removable palatal bite-raising platform on the anterior teeth, causing posterior disocclusion and allowing overeruption of the posterior teeth (periodontal growth) for re-establishing the bite. However, **to overcome poor patient compliance, direct or indirect fixed restorations** (either temporary or permanent), can instead be cemented onto the palatal surfaces of the anterior teeth to achieve a similar objective, with better outcomes.

Key points

- Occlusal stabilisation by occlusal adjustment (OA) is contentious.
- Selective OA before starting treatment is prudent and avoids future complications.
- Occlusal splints are inexpensive and non-invasive treatment modalities.
- Occlusal splints can alleviate parafunctional habits and reduce muscular spasms.
- Bite-raising or Dahl appliances are useful for establishing a new VDO by creating interocclusal clearance for restorative materials following tooth wear.

Periodontal aspects

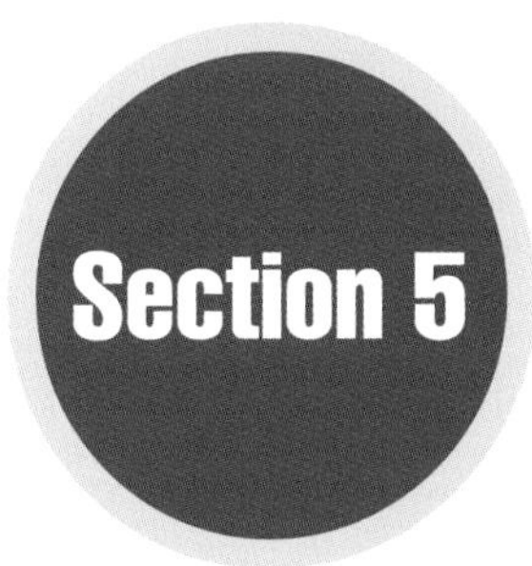

Chapters

Periodontal: dentogingival apparatus

Superficial anatomy of the dentogingival apparatus

Attached gingiva
Free gingival groove
FGM
Alveolar mucosa
Muco-gingival junction
Interdental papilla
Gingival stippling

Free gingival margin
Sulcular epithelium (SE)
Rete pegs
Free gingival groove
Junctional epithelium (JE)
CEJ
Connective tissue attachment (CTA)
Cementum
Alveolar bone crest (ABC)
Muco-gingival junction
Periodontal ligament (PDL)
Alveolar mucosa

JE
CTA
JE

Cross-section anatomy of periodontium

Biologic width (BW) = JE + CTA

Long JE

Biologic width (BW) variations...

Bone sounding with local anaesthesia to ascertain alveolar crest dimension for calculating BW

...smaller around anterior teeth

...established at apical location due to trauma from defective crown margin on the left lateral incisor

...wider around teeth with altered passive eruption (short clinical crowns)

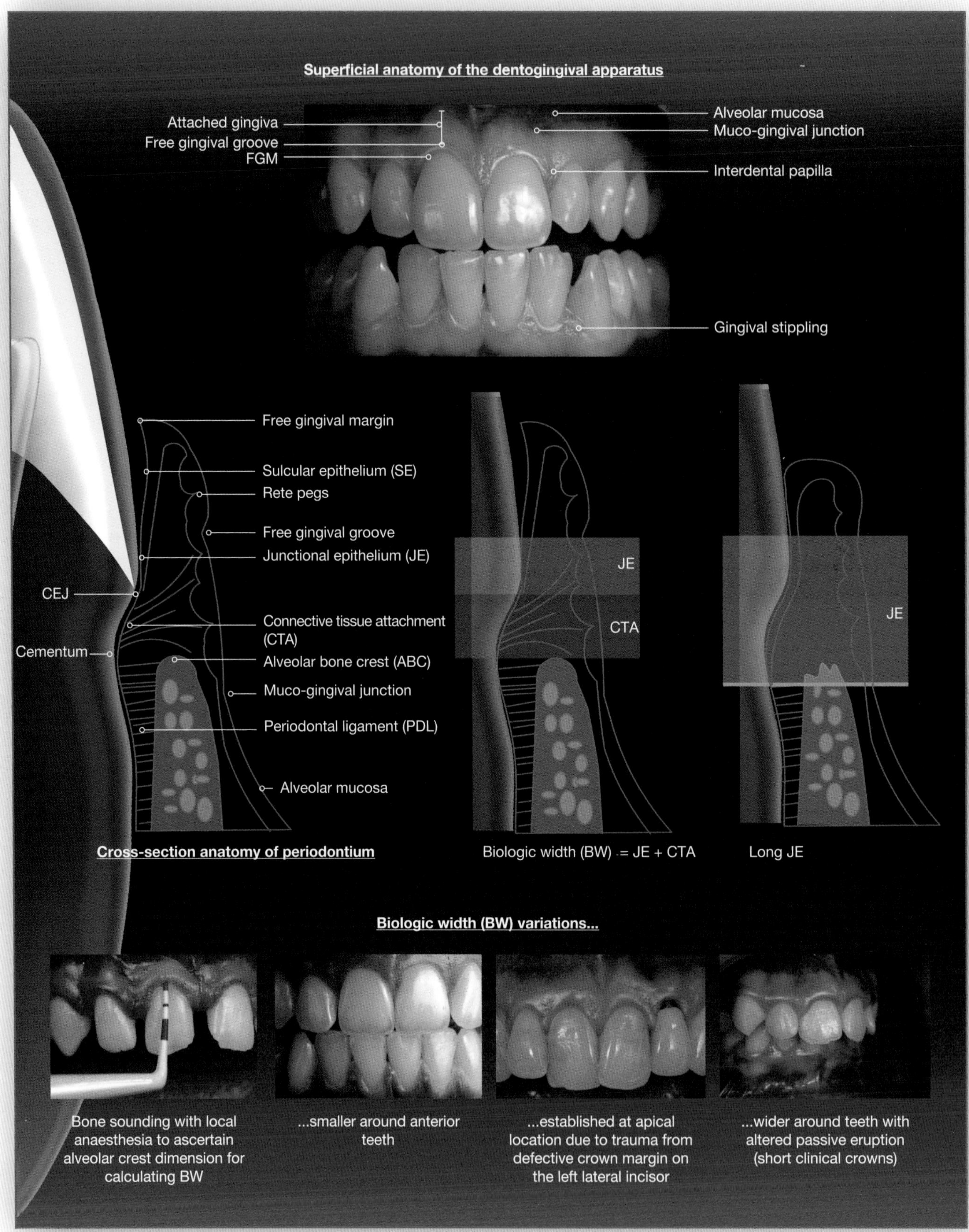

Prosthodontics at a Glance, Second Edition. Irfan Ahmad.

Periodontal health is essential for successful prosthodontic treatment outcomes. This chapter describes basic periodontal aspects that require consideration before embarking on restorative treatment.

Superficial anatomy of the periodontium

The **periodontium consists of five tissues**: **gingiva**, **alveolar mucosa**, **periodontal ligament (PDL)**, **cementum** and **alveolar bone**. Viewed from the facial or buccal aspect, the soft tissue envelope around the teeth is distinguished into the gingiva and alveolar mucosa. Starting from the tooth junction, the gingiva is further divided into the **free gingival margin (FGM)**, **interdental papilla** and **attached gingiva,** terminating apically at the **mucogingival junction** with the **alveolar mucosa**. The **location of the FGM** is determined by active eruption, passive eruption, altered passive eruption (APE) and gingival recession. The interdental gingiva site concavity, known as the **col (non-keratinised),** is the starting area for gingivitis with possible progression to periodontitis.

The **attached gingiva is keratinised**, tenacious and resilient to withstand masticatory function, while the alveolar mucosa is unattached and non-keratinised. The **dimensions and texture of the attached gingiva (AG)** vary enormously, not only between individuals, but also around specific teeth. The width **(apico-coronal dimension)** varies from **0.5 mm to 8 mm**, and the average thickness **(bucco-lingual dimension) is 1.4 mm.** It is narrowest near frenal attachments, around canines and premolars, and widest around the buccal aspect of the incisors. On the lingual aspect, AG is widest around the molars and narrowest around the incisors. However, the minimum width of the AG required for health is unknown, but its absence, especially around implants, has been shown to increase the propensity to inflammation. Finally, the texture of the AG can be **stippled** (orange peel appearance) **or smooth.** It should be noted that the absence of stippling is not necessarily indicative of disease.

Dentogingival apparatus

In cross-section, the **dentogingival apparatus** can be divided into three major components: **epithelium, connective tissue and bone**. In a healthy periodontium, the sulcus starts at the FGM and ends at the **junctional epithelium (JE)**. The depth of the **sulcus** (or gingival crevice) varies from 0.3 mm to 6 mm depending on numerous factors such as location on the tooth (deeper sulcus interproximally). The JE extends apically to the **cemento-enamel junction (CEJ)**, ranging from 0.3 mm to 3.3 mm. The **connective tissue attachment (CTA)** is apical to the JE and terminates at the **alveolar bone crest (ABC)** housing the teeth. The CTA shows the least variance of the dentogingival apparatus, i.e. 0.3 mm to 1.8 mm. The **combined linear measurements of the JE and the CTA are termed the biologic width** (**BW**), averaging **2.04 mm**.

Biologic width

The frequently quoted measurement of the biologic width (BW) as 2.04 mm is based on **average measurement** of the dentogingival apparatus from cadavers:

- Sulcus depth = 0.69 mm
- EA = 0.97 mm
- CTA = 1.07 mm
- JE + CTA (biologic width) = 2.04 mm

The **significance of the BW** is that it is nature's approach to protecting the most important part of the dentogingival apparatus, i.e. the periodontal ligament and the ABC, which ensures survival of a tooth. This **soft tissue shield** guards against mechanical and bacterial insult. However, as for any shield, its efficacy is diminished if violated or damaged, placing the tooth (together with any restorations) in a precarious situation. The salient points about the BW can be summarised as follows:

- **Present around every tooth**
- Nature's **soft tissue shield** for ensuring tooth survival
- **2.04 mm is an average dimension**, not applicable to every patient or every tooth
- It is **essential to preserve the BW a**nd prevent its violation during clinical procedures
- **Differential diagnosis is necessary for BW variations**

BW variations

The biologic width is a physiological **3D concept**, sometimes referred to as the **biologic space**. At present, **the minimum dimension of the BW for health is unknown** and can be as small as 0.6 mm. The **dimension of the BW varies** depending on the type of tooth and the location around a tooth; some differences are listed below:

- Type of tooth
- Incisors and canines = 1.75 mm; Premolars = 1.97 mm; Molars = 2.08 mm.
- Population variations
- 85% normal relationship of ABC and EA to CEJ;
- 13% ABC and JE in an apical position to norm – larger BW; 2% ABC and JE in a coronal position to norm – smaller BW
- Apical position of JE (long JE) – pseudo-healing following episodes of periodontitis and/or mechanical or surgical trauma
- Passive (apical location of BW), and altered passive eruption or APE (coronal location of JE with short clinical crowns)
- Restored teeth have a larger BW
- Implants – BW is located more apically compared to natural teeth

Methods for determining BW dimension

Since it is impossible to determine the BW by visual inspection, the methods available include:

- **Tactile** – most popular method by **sounding bone** (along long axis of tooth) and transgingival probing (perpendicular to tooth). Requires local anaesthetic, invasive, erratic reading in presence of inflammation or presence of a long JE
- **Parallel profile radiography** – questionable unnecessary radiation exposure
- **Ultrasound** – non-invasive, variable readings, which are averaged for a given tooth
- **Soft tissue cone beam computed tomography** (ST-CBCT) CBCT scan taken with photographic cheek retractors to displace lips and cheeks, and requesting patient to place tongue to floor or back of the mouth to allow visualisation of the gingival soft tissues (buccal and palatal/lingual). Non-invasive, precise measurements of both soft tissues and bone in both axial and perpendicular axis to tooth. The drawbacks of this method are unnecessary radiation exposure, and unable to distinguish between JE and CTA or inflamed and healthy tissues.

Key points

- The dentogingival apparatus consists of epithelium, connective tissue and bone, and its health is paramount for successful prosthodontic treatment
- It is essential to determine dimension and location of BW before starting restorative treatment
- The most popular methods for determining BW are tactile and ST-CBCT

26 Periodontal: prosthodontic considerations

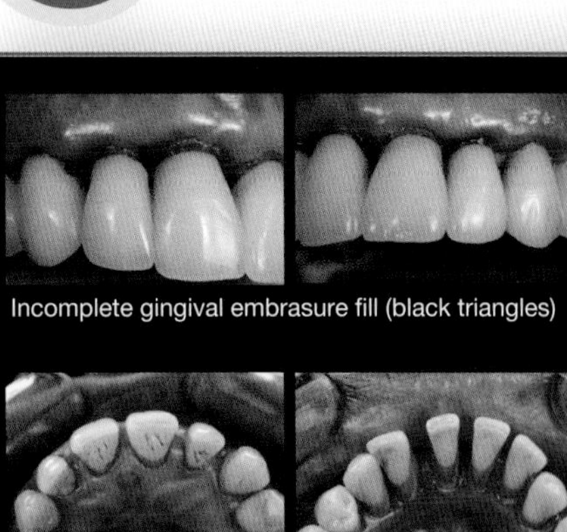

Incomplete gingival embrasure fill (black triangles)

Migration & flaring due to periodontal disease

Tooth shape	Gingival scallop	Distance from interproximal bone crest to mid-facial bone crest (mm)
Square	Flat	2.1
Oval	Scalloped	2.8
Triangle	Pronounced scallop	4.1

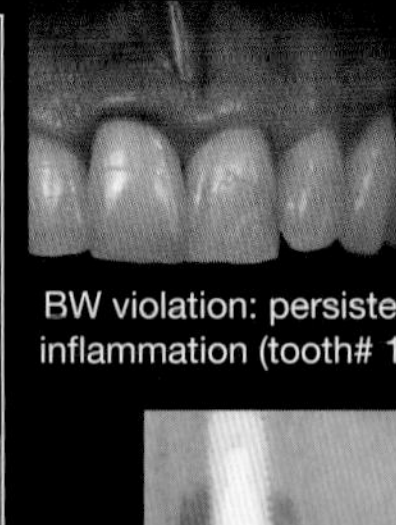

BW violation: persistent inflammation (tooth# 11)

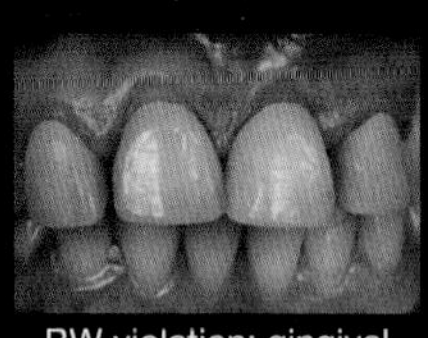

BW violation: gingival recession

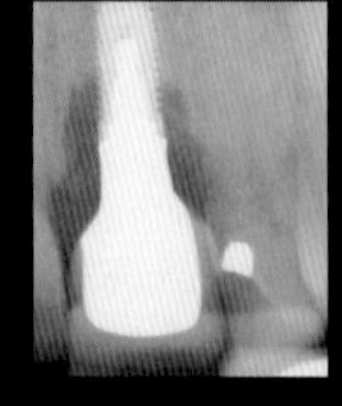

Peri-implantitis (pre-op)

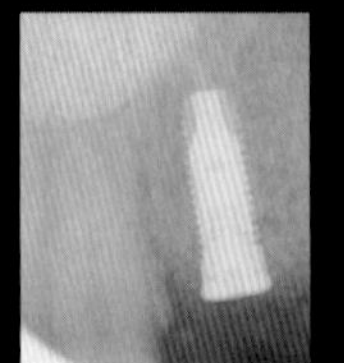

Peri-implantitis (resoultion)

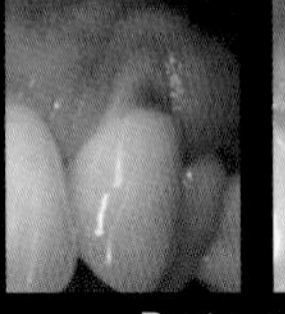

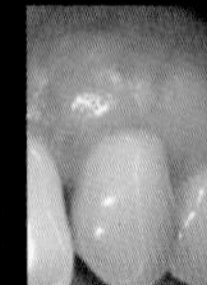

Root coverage

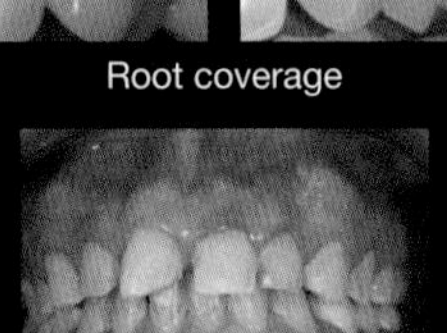

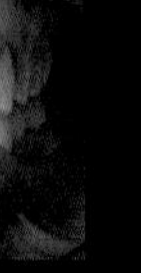

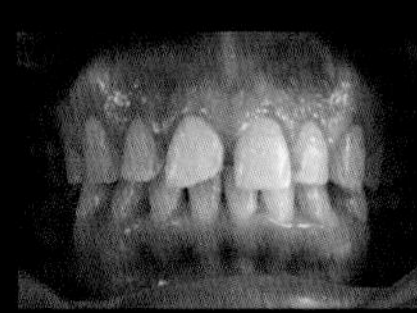

Aesthetic crown lengthening

PPS

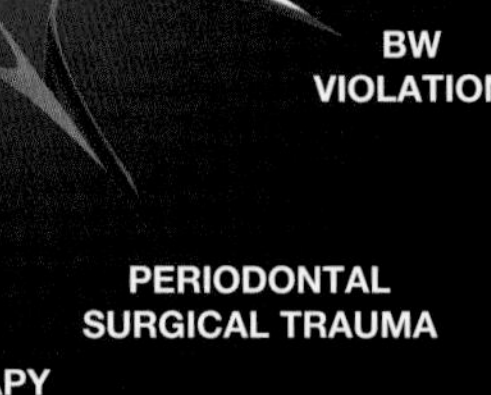

Determinants of periodontal health

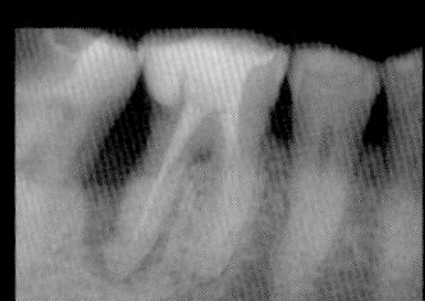

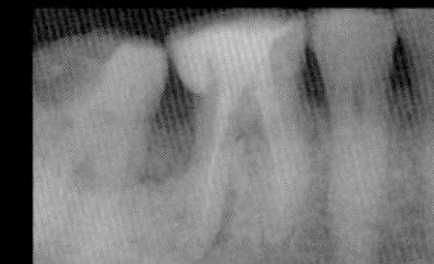

GBR to fill-in bony defects

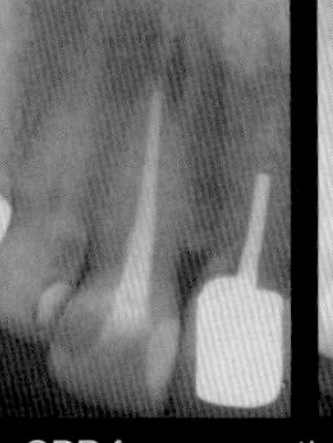

GBR for augmenting extraction sites

Guided bone regeneration (GBR)

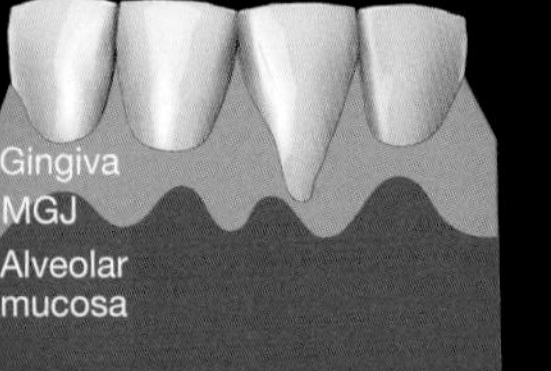

Class I

Gingival recession is on facial aspect and does not extend to muco-gingival junction (MGJ), without interproximal bone or soft tissue loss. Complete root coverage possible

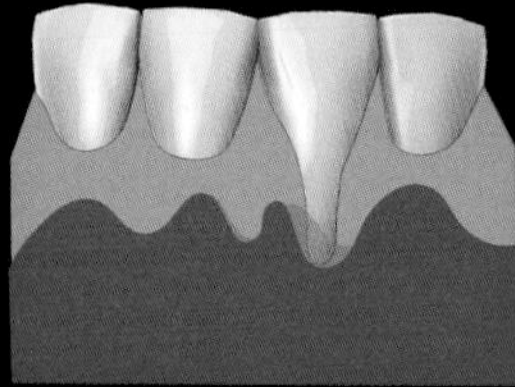

Class II

Gingival recession extends to, or beyond MGJ, without interproximal bone or soft tissue loss. Complete root coverage possible

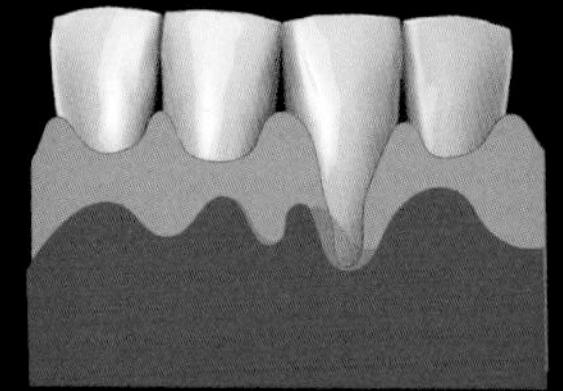

Class III

Gingival recession extends to, or beyond MGJ, with interproximal bone & soft tissue loss. Partial root coverage possible

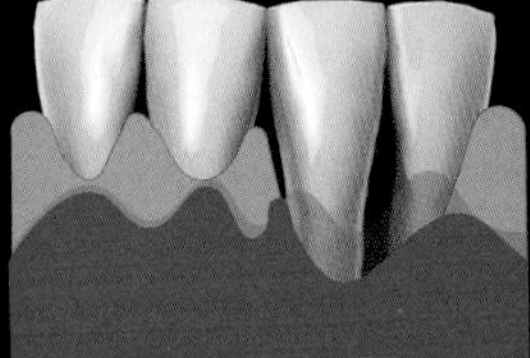

Class IV

Gingival recession beyond MGJ, with exposure of more than one proximal root surface, gross bone & soft tissue loss. No root coverage possible

Miller's classification of gingival recession

Prosthodontics at a Glance, Second Edition. Irfan Ahmad.

Achieving and **maintaining periodontal health** is **influenced by numerous factors**, including disruption of the biofilm by scaling/root surface debridement (formerly root planing), periodontal surgical trauma, chemotherapy (local and systemic), patient factors (local factors, oral hygiene, constitutional [immune response], stress, family history, systemic illness, habits [smoking]) and degree of trauma during operative procedures. Also, it is important to realise that managing periodontal disease is a team approach, consisting of professionals and the patient, and the **treatment plan is bespoke depending on an individual's risk factors**. A paradigm shift is also emerging regarding the treatment of periodontal disease. Conventional scaling, root surface debridement and surgery are being replaced by a more minimal, non-invasive approach of full-mouth **ultrasonic** and **laser debridement** (Chapters 43 and 44) for **disrupting the biofilm**, and thereby achieving disinfection of the root. Periodontal health is an essential constituent of the health, function and aesthetic (**HFA**) triad.

Periodontal biotypes and bioforms

Periodontal biotypes represent gingival texture and architecture around teeth, play a significant role when planning prosthodontic and implant therapies, and are classified as:

- **Thin-scalloped** (< 1.5 mm bucco-ligual thickness) – delicate, prone to gingival recession, dehiscences and fenestrations, prevalent in 15% of population (high risk to gingival trauma or inflammation)
- **Thick-flat** (> 2 mm bucco-ligual thickness) – fibrotic, resilient, prone to periodontal pocket formation
- **Medium** – intermediate between the above two extremes

The **periodontal bioform** describes the degree of gingival scallop around teeth, which is dictated by tooth shape, tooth alignment, size and location of the contact areas and can broadly be categorised as square, oval or triangular, corresponding to the flat, scalloped or pronounced scalloped bioforms, respectively.

Contact areas

The relationship of the **contact areas** (either of natural teeth or artificial prostheses) **to the interproximal alveolar bone crest determines the amount of interproximal gingival papilla fill**. If the distance is **5 mm or less, total papilla fill** is evident in the gingival embrasures. If the distance is greater than 5 mm, incomplete papilla fill is observed, especially with thin biotypes, colloquially referred to as 'black triangles'. However, to achieve complete **papilla fill between two adjacent dental implants**, the distance required is less than for natural teeth, i.e. < **3 mm**.

Trauma from occlusion

Trauma from occlusion is a major contributing factor in periodontal disease and can present as **bone loss without periodontal pocket formation**. Trauma from occlusion can be:

- **Primary trauma** – with an adequate (healthy) periodontium
- **Secondary trauma** – inadequate (diseased) periodontium, resulting in teeth that are incapable of withstanding occlusal forces in an axial direction, leading to **migration**, fremitus and **flaring**.

The treatment depends on the severity of trauma and includes orthodontic alignment (to correct osseous defects and improve crown-to-root ratios), occlusal adjustment, occlusal stabilising splints, periodontal splints, bone regenerative therapies and implants (replacing strategic teeth for occlusal stabilisation).

Biologic width violation

Many clinical procedures can potentially violate the biologoic width (BW), and therefore compromise a healthy periodontium and influence the success of an artificial prosthesis. The consequences of **BW violation** depend on the host response and include:

- **Adaptation** – formation of a new BW in a more apical position to restore health of the periodontium
- **Persistent inflammation** – requires orthodontic extrusion, or bone resection by a surgical approach to restore the BW
- **Gingival recession** – causing asymmetrical gingival zeniths, 'black triangles', especially with thin-scalloped biotypes
- **Pocket formation** – common with thick-flat biotypes
- **Perio-endodontic lesions** – abscesses or chronic periapical pathology

Peri-implantitis

Periodontal diseases also plague dental implants. Inflammation around implants is classified as:

- **Mucositis** – is reversible inflammation without bone loss
- **Peri-implantitis** – inflammation combined with irreversible bone loss around implants, more prevalent with partially dentate ridges due to cross-infection from adjacent periodontally involved teeth, compared to edentulous arches. Peri-implantitis is time-dependent, affecting a small number of patients following implant therapy. The **risk factors** associated with this condition are not fully clear, but links have been postulated with systemic illness (e.g. diabetes, osteoporosis, obesity), habits (e.g. smoking, drinking extremely hot fluids), local factors (e.g. bone quality and quantity, reduced blood supply), implant design (microgap between implant fixture and abutment) and implant surface coatings

Periodontal plastic surgery (PPS)

Periodontal plastic surgery (PPS) is indicated for correcting periodontal deformities to restore function, aesthetics and longevity of restorative therapy. PPS is divided into two categories:

- **Exposing tooth** – crown lengthening for improving crown-to-root ratio for restorative procedures, enhancing anterior aesthetics by restituting erratic gingival contours, e.g. due to altered passive eruption (APE) to increase clinical crown length, pocket reduction, re-establishing BW
- **Gingival grafting** – increasing the width of attached gingiva (or root coverage) according to Miller's classification. Soft tissue grafts, e.g. **subepithelial connective tissue grafts (SCTGs)** usually harvested from the palate, or collagen membrane grafts (e.g. acellular dermal matrix [ADM] – Alloderm).

Regenerative therapy

Regenerative therapies involve augmenting bone volume lost as a result of periodontal diseases, or establishing an adequate platform for eventual implant placement. The principles of **GBR** are to retard epithelial growth to allow time for bone formation using a combination of membranes and bone grafting materials, such as **autogenous bone** (from host, e.g. nasal spine, mandible or iliac crest), **allografts** (from animals, e.g. bovine-derived prion-free tissue) and **xenografts** (synthetic materials, e.g. particulate ceramics and hydroxyapatite). In addition, emerging regenerative technologies such as **tissue engineering** and **stem cell therapy** are other options for regeneration (Chapters 74 and 75).

Key points

- Periodontal health is influenced by a variety of factors.
- Corrective measures include regenerative therapies, e.g. PPS and GBR.
- Peri-implantitis significant affects implant survival rates.

Coronal foundation

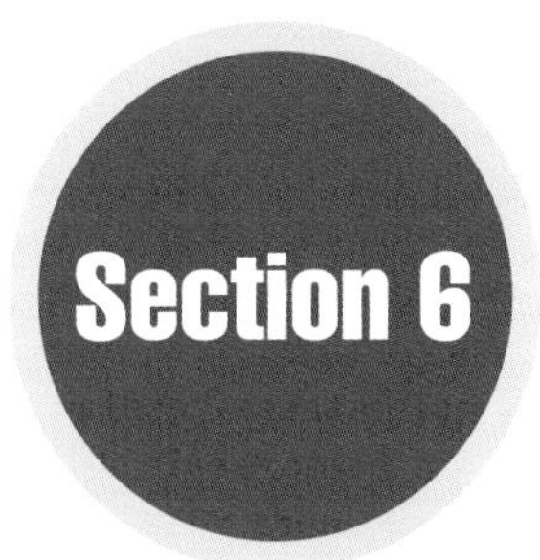

Chapters

27 Coronal foundation: endodontic considerations

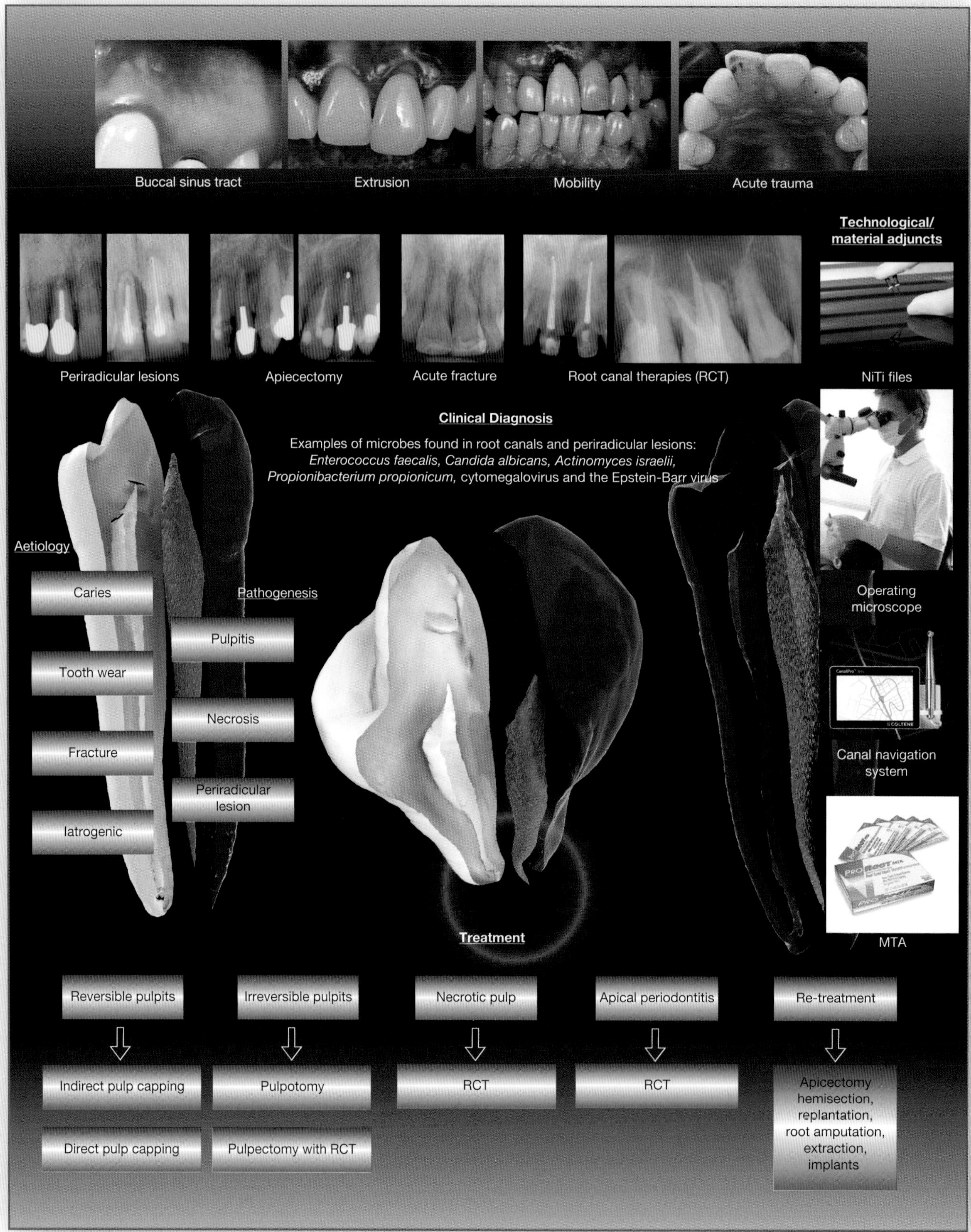

Buccal sinus tract

Extrusion

Mobility

Acute trauma

Periradicular lesions

Apiecectomy

Acute fracture

Root canal therapies (RCT)

Technological/ material adjuncts

NiTi files

Operating microscope

Canal navigation system

MTA

Clinical Diagnosis

Examples of microbes found in root canals and periradicular lesions: *Enterococcus faecalis, Candida albicans, Actinomyces israelii, Propionibacterium propionicum,* cytomegalovirus and the Epstein-Barr virus

Aetiology

- Caries
- Tooth wear
- Fracture
- Iatrogenic

Pathogenesis

- Pulpitis
- Necrosis
- Periradicular lesion

Treatment

Reversible pulpits	Irreversible pulpits	Necrotic pulp	Apical periodontitis	Re-treatment
⇩	⇩	⇩	⇩	⇩
Indirect pulp capping	Pulpotomy	RCT	RCT	Apicectomy hemisection, replantation, root amputation, extraction, implants
Direct pulp capping	Pulpectomy with RCT			

Prosthodontics at a Glance, Second Edition. Irfan Ahmad.

A sound coronal foundation is prerequisite, but may be compromised by endodontic issues discussed below: it require an intra-radicular support or a core build-up, which is discussed in the next two chapters.

Aetiology and pathogenesis

Pulpal diseases are bacterial in origin, either directly or indirectly, from the **resident oral microbiota** due to:

- **Caries** – bacteria or bacterial acid travelling down dentine tubes to the pulp
- **Tooth wear** – eventual pulpal pathosis due to attrition, abrasion, erosion and abfraction
- **Tooth fractures** – pulp exposure due to acute extra-oral accidents or masticatory misadventures
- **Iatrogenic** – pulp exposure caused by restorative procedures

Whatever the aetiology, **micro-organisms and their toxins** initiate an inflammatory response (**pulpitis**). Bacterial toxins precede bacterial invasion, causing a vascular response by releasing **cytokines** and **mediators**. If the bacterial insult is confined to the hard tissues, a reparative and protective **secondary dentine** barrier is formed. If the pulp is exposed, formation of a soft tissue barrier is impossible since the pulp is devoid of epithelial cells. Therefore, the bacterial invasion and proliferation is profuse, leading to colonisation of the root canal system and subsequently the **periradicular** areas. The infected periradicular areas react with a **protective response by bone resorption** to contain and eliminate the infection, which is visible as an **osteolytic bone lesion (periapical radiolucency on a radiograph)**.

Clinical manifestations and diagnosis

Precise and efficient diagnosis is essential for determining the appropriate treatment. **Differential diagnosis** includes **pulpitis** (reversible and irreversible) and **necrosis** (partial or complete) with or without **periradicular involvement**. A major clinical challenge is differentiating between **reversible and irreversible pulpitis**. The symptoms and tests for pulpal diseases include:

- **Pain** – throbbing, lingering, spontaneous, tender to percussion (TTP) or tooth sensitivity
- **Painless** – e.g. total pulpal necrosis
- **Swelling** – intra- and extra-oral
- **Tooth mobility**
- **Extrusion** – combination of periodontal/endodontic lesions (apical periodontitis)
- **Periapical radiolucency** – assessed by radiographic or CBCT evaluation (if necessary and justified)
- **Systemic** – fever, lethargy, malaise and anxiety
- **Pulp vitality tests** – thermal, electrical, chemical and pulse oximetry (Chapter 6)

Treatment modalities

Management of the damaged pulp is predominantly concerned with reducing or eliminating bacteria. Treatment depends on whether the diagnosis is reversible or irreversible pulpitis, and failure of previous endodontic treatment. The **treatment for reversible pulpitis:**

- **Indirect pulp capping** – to avoid pulp exposure, and dressing the thin remaining dentine barrier with a palliate dressing, e.g. calcium hydroxide (**Ca(OH)$_2$**) and cover with glass-ionomer (GI) or resin modified GI (RMGI). Possible stepwise caries excavation after 2–3 months
- **Direct pulp capping** – symptomless pulp exposure, dress with Ca(OH)$_2$ or **MTA** (mineral trioxide aggregate), cover with by GI or RMGI

The **treatment for irreversible pulpitis**:

- **Pulpotomy** (partial or coronal) – indicated for acute traumas of healthy pulps in young individuals with incomplete root formation (with an enhanced regenerative potential), for encouraging pulp regeneration or repair by formation of secondary dentine using Ca(OH)$_2$, MTA, cover with GI or RMGI
- **Pulpectomy** with root canal therapy (RCT) – extirpation of infected pulps followed by RCT, with the objectives of debridement, shaping, disinfecting and obturating the root canal system

Failure of endodontic treatment is attributed to lack of asepsis during treatment, failure to eliminate infection from the root canal and/or periapical areas, or subsequent leakage due to poor obturation or defective coronal restorations. In these circumstances, the treatment options are:

- **Re-RCT** with a new, correctly fitting coronal restoration
- **Surgical endodontics** – apicectomy and retrograde filling, hemisection, replantation, root amputation
- **Extraction** with subsequent **implant(s)**. Implants may also be considered for failed apicectomies or complex re-treatment cases

Technological adjuncts

The last few decades have witnessed a burgeoning of technological advances for improving endodontic therapy outcomes, including the **operating microscope**, **ultrasonic devices**, **electronic apex locators, lasers**, **light-activated disinfection**, **NiTi** (nickel-titanium) files, miniaturised instruments for working with magnifications up to × 32, **automated canal navigation systems** (CanalPro™ Jeni), newer efficacious **dental adhesives** and repair/regenerative **bioactive materials** such as Biodentine and MTA.

Endodontic controversies

As with many medical disciplines, there is a schism between clinicians and researchers. Furthermore, different criteria are used to assess endodontic outcomes or success, e.g. absence of pain, survival of the tooth, survival of a restoration, apical bone regeneration or elimination of infection. Some **current controversies** include:

- **Leave or remove all carries?** – excavating all caries may result in infecting the pulp and lead to irreversible pulpits
- **Direct vs indirect pulp capping?** (step-wise excavation for indirect pulp-caping)
- RCT or conservative approach for ambivalent diagnosis between **reversible and irreversible pulpits?** Immediate RCT is easier, while procrastinating is complicated by tertiary dentine, apical periodontitis
- **Leave or remove the smear layer?**
- **One vs two appointment RCT?**
- Ideal measures for promoting **regeneration (of pulp) or repair by secondary dentine?** (using **bioactive materials** – Chapter 40)
- **Importance of coronal vs apical seal?**
- **Efficacy of disinfecting agents?** (e.g. sodium hypochlorite, chlorhexidine, Ca(OH)$_2$, tetracycline isomer compound
- **Concept of sterile periradicular granulomas?**
- **Apical terminus location** and **healing with cementum-like tissue?**
- **Lateral condensation vs vertical compaction obturation?**

Key points

- Understanding the biological processes ensures correct diagnosis and selection of the most appropriate endodontic treatment.
- Technological and scientific advances have resulted in more predictable therapy, but further research is required to resolve current controversies.

28 Coronal foundation: intraradicular support

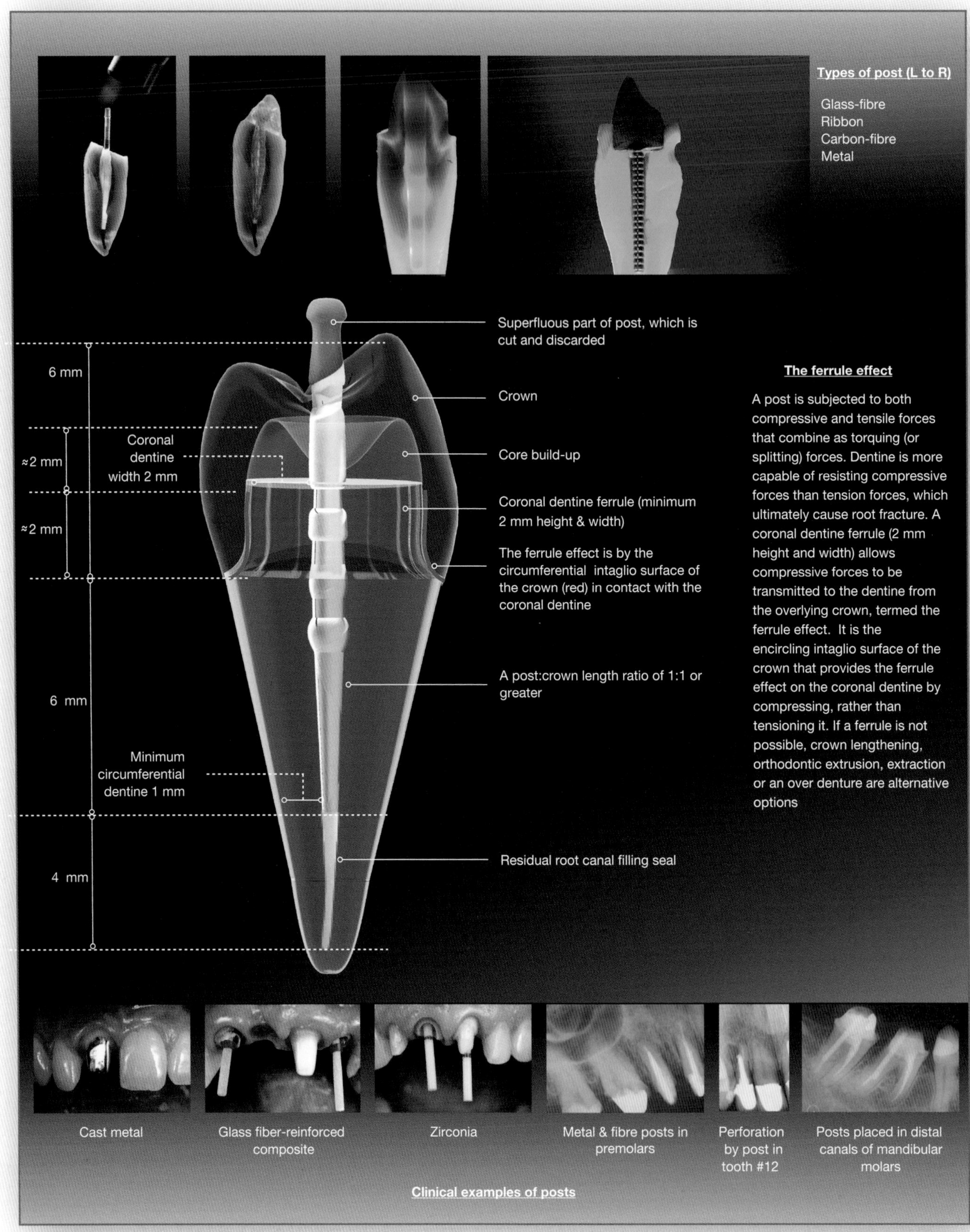

Prosthodontics at a Glance, Second Edition. Irfan Ahmad.

Posts, or **intraradicular supports**, **do not strengthen or reinforce teeth**. In fact, the opposite is true: removal of dentine from a root canal to accommodate a post weakens the structural integrity of the root. Heavily broken teeth due to trauma or caries, with or without a root filling, may present with insufficient coronal foundation to retain an extra-coronal definitive restoration. Therefore, **the purpose of a post and core is to gain intraradicular support for the definitive restoration.**

Indication for posts

If there is sufficient remaining **coronal dentine** to support a restoration, a post is unnecessary. This is especially true for molars with considerable amounts of dentine and large pulp chambers. At the other extreme, the incisors have smaller amounts of coronal dentine, which is reduced following trauma, caries or endodontic access cavities. In these circumstances, a post is essential for retention of a permanent restoration. Furthermore, **root-filled teeth have reduced proprioceptive response**, and are therefore more vulnerable to masticatory and occlusal forces.

Guidelines for post placement

Before placing a post, **certain criteria must be fulfilled** to ensure its survival and that of the overlying extracoronal restoration. Some factors to consider are:

- Tooth **anatomy**:

Molars – choose the largest and straightest canal for post placement, i.e. distal canals of mandibular molars and palatal canals of maxillary molars. Placing posts in curved root canals often results in perforations into the periodontal ligament or alveolar bone

Premolars – smaller pulp chambers, with tapering roots exhibiting thin mesiodistal cross-section with proximal invaginations

Incisors and canines – post is unnecessary if sufficient coronal dentine is present. Mandibular incisors have thin tapering and narrow mesiodistal root morphology

- **Sufficient alveolar bone support** encompassing at least half of post length into the root
- **Minimum 1:1 post length:crown length ratio**
- **Root length** long enough to accommodate a **4–5 mm apical root filing seal** and **½ to ⅔ of the post length**
- **Post width not exceeding ⅓ of root width at narrowest point, and 1 mm of remaining circumferential dentine**
- **Ferrule effect** for bracing a minimum of 2 mm width and height of coronal dentine to mitigate root fracture

Ideal properties of a post

The **ideal properties of a post c**an be summarised as follows. A post should ideally have similar mechanical and physical properties as natural teeth, e.g. **modulus of elasticity**, **compressive strength, coefficient of thermal expansion and optical characteristics.** The post material should be **biocompatible**, **non-corrosive** and **hypo-allergenic**, **minimise microleakage**, **prevent root or restoration fractures** (both cohesive and adhesive fractures) and exhibit favourable clinical handling and **ease of use**. The dental market is inundated with posts of different materials, shapes, configurations, surface finishes and colours. There is no single post that has all the properties for every clinical situation, and often the **choice is empirical**.

Choice of post

Posts can broadly be categorised as **custom-made** or prefabricated. **Custom posts** are usually made of cast metal or ceramics by an indirect technique, including CAD/CAM milling or 3D printing. This is useful for making a unified post and core to replace extensive coronal dentine loss. However, the process involves two visits to the office with the possibility of contamination of the root canal due to provisional cement failure or defective temporary restorations. **Prefabricated posts** are the most popular type, offering expediency, single-visit placement and immediate preparation of core build-ups, and are available in a large selection of materials and designs:

- **Metal**, e.g. stainless steel, brass, titanium. Disadvantages include poor aesthetics, root fracture, corrosion and nickel (Type IV) sensitivity
- **Ceramics**, e.g. alumina, zirconia or porcelain fused to metal. High flexural strength and fracture toughness, favourable aesthetics. However, the drawbacks are difficult retrievability and propensity for root fracture
- **Fibre posts**, e.g. pliable ribbon, glass fibre-reinforced composite, quartz or carbon fibre. Flexible, similar physical properties to dentine, e.g. modulus of elasticity of dentine (15 GPa). Highly aesthetic (light-transmitting), easily retrievable, bonding to dentine with dental adhesives and mitigate root fracture
- **Design** – tapered types require less dentine removal, but offer poorer retention compared to parallel designs. The surface finish can be smooth or serrated and may incorporate cement vents for luting agents. The threaded or screw posts (active posts) offer enhanced retention, but at the expense of root fracture susceptibility due to dentine stresses

Canal preparation and post cementation

Placing a post requires shaping the canal to accommodate the post geometry by removing a part of the root filling (usually gutta-percha). **A thorough knowledge of root anatomy is essential before canal preparation.** The **two methods** for gutta-percha removal are **thermal** and **mechanical**. The thermal approach is tedious but less traumatic. The mechanical approach involves using rotary instruments such as Gates-Glidden burs or P-type reamers, which may inadvertently disrupt the apical seal or result in **lateral perforation.** The majority of posts are passive, requiring a luting agent for cementation into the root canal. Although zinc phosphate cement has the longest clinical history but is prone to leakage, and is now superseded by **glass ionomers** that offer dentine adhesion, but their poor mechanical properties may cause cement failure leading to microleakage. Resin-based composite cements (self-adhesive or in conjunction with a dental adhesive) have high compressive strength and offer dentine adhesion, but are technique sensitive.

Key points

- Posts weaken teeth, and careful consideration is required beforehand placing a post for intraradicular support for the definitive restoration.
- There is no ideal post system, and a pragmatic approach is necessary to choose an appropriate post for a specific tooth and clinical scenario.
- Meticulous root canal preparation and choice of cement are essential for long-term survival of the post and definitive restoration.

29 Coronal foundation: core build-up

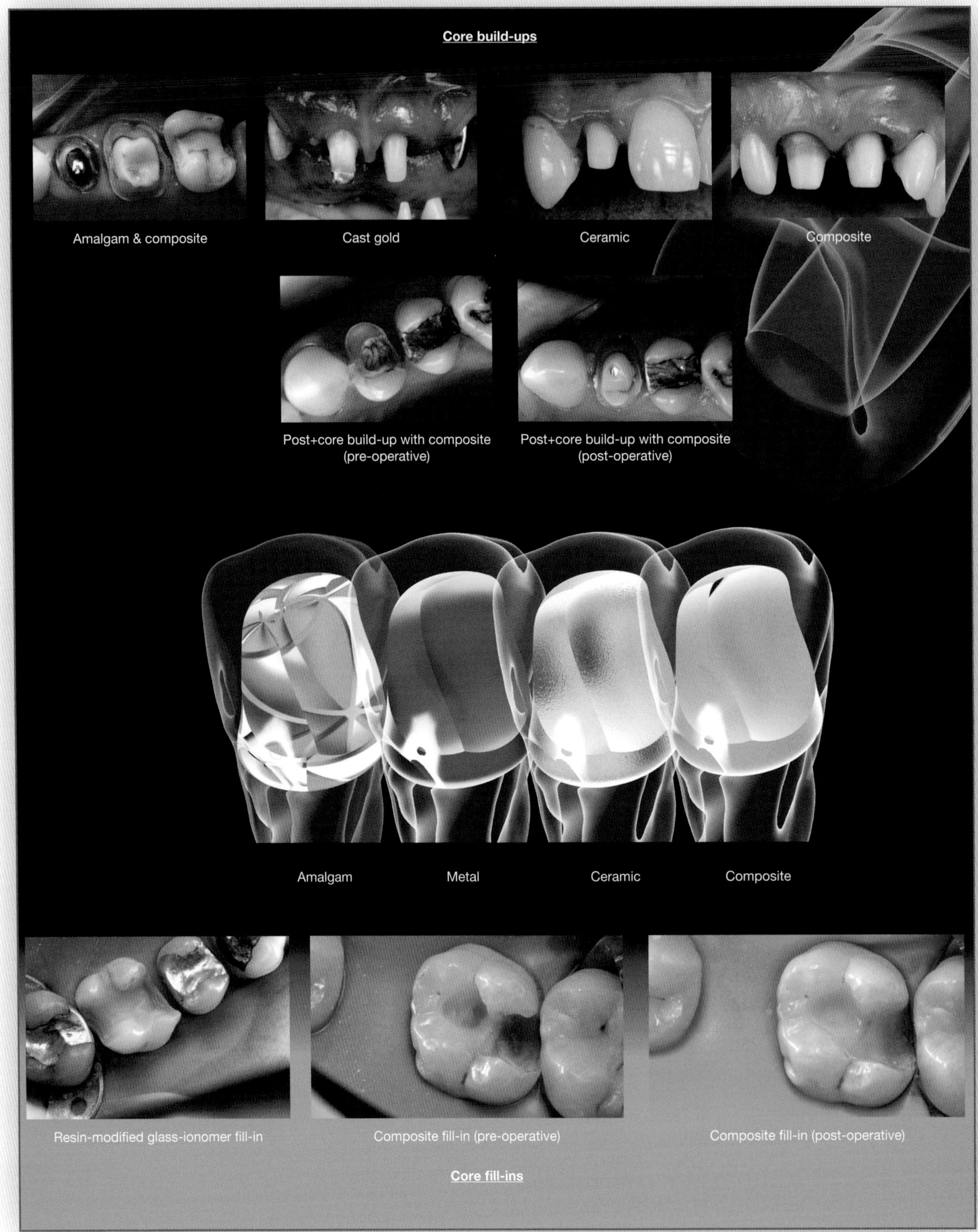

Core build-ups

Amalgam & composite

Cast gold

Ceramic

Composite

Post+core build-up with composite (pre-operative)

Post+core build-up with composite (post-operative)

Amalgam

Metal

Ceramic

Composite

Resin-modified glass-ionomer fill-in

Composite fill-in (pre-operative)

Composite fill-in (post-operative)

Core fill-ins

Prosthodontics at a Glance, Second Edition. Irfan Ahmad.

The purpose of a **core build-up** is to provide retention and resistance for the definitive extracoronal restorations. The final restoration can be partial or full coverage, depending on the amount of residual tooth substrate. Cores can be built up on either **vital** or **non-vital teeth**, which have previously received a post to gain additional **intraradicular support** from the endodontically treated root.

Ideal properties of a core build-up material

At present, **a single restorative material does not fulfil all the ideal properties of a core build-up material**, which are:

- **Adequate physical properties** (flexural and compressive strength) to resist intra-oral forces
- **Non-allergenic**
- **Biocompatible**
- **Prevent microleakage** of oral fluids at core-tooth interface
- **Chemical adhesion** or bonding to tooth substrate, both enamel and dentine
- **Similar thermal properties to natural teeth** (coefficient of thermal expansion and contraction)
- **Minimum water absorption**
- **Dimensionally stable**
- **Cariostatic**
- **Ease of manipulation**

Materials for core build-up

The essential factor for a successful and long-lasting core, irrespective of the material used, is ensuring that at least **2 mm of dentine width and height is present for the ferrule effect.** The most popular **materials for core build-ups** are **amalgam**, **resin-based composite**, **glass ionome**r, **ceramics** and **cast alloys**. **Amalgam** has traditionally been used as a build-up material, offering excellent strength, low solubility and bonding by micromechanical retention to dentine using dental adhesives. The disadvantages are poor aesthetics, a protracted setting time requiring a second visit for preparation of the core and patient concerns regarding its possible toxicity, a doubt refuted by scientific research. **Resin-based composites** offer superior aesthetics and the ability to bond to dentine with dental adhesives, and the flowable varieties allow ease of manipulation, especially for cementing posts into root canals. However, their drawbacks are polymerisation shrinkage, hygroscopic expansion, incompatibility with eugenol-based root-filling materials and technique-sensitive protocols. **Glass ionomers (GIs) or resin-modified glass ionomers (RMGI)** have the advantage of chemical adhesion with dentine, but their poor physical properties (low tensile and compressive strengths) are incapable of withstanding intra-oral forces. Therefore, their use is limited to filling in small defects **(fill-in)**, but are unsuitable for bulk build-ups. **Ceramics and cast alloys** require an indirect technique and are reserved for cores with intraradicular posts, offering a unified post and core complex. Cast gold is resilient but has poor aesthetics beneath highly translucent all-ceramic restorations. Also, certain types of ceramics can be fused onto zirconia posts with excellent aesthetics. However, zirconia posts are stiff and difficult to retrieve if there are endodontic complications requiring re-root canal therapy.

Core build-up for vital teeth

Various methods are available for building a foundation for teeth that have lost enamel and dentine due to trauma, caries or previously failed fillings. The two crucial factors for cores on vital teeth are, first, to **preserve the maximum amount of healthy tooth** and, second, to **prevent pulpal involvement**. The importance of retaining as much of the remaining tooth substrate is ensuring tooth stiffness, which depends on preservation of the marginal ridges. If the latter are lost, tooth stiffness is severely compromised, requiring either cuspal coverage (onlay), or a full coverage crown. The techniques for retaining cores on vital teeth include:

- **Pins** – questionable due to dentine crazing, and the possibility of inadvertent perforation into the pulp and periodontium
- **Cavity modification** – judicious and strategic creation of undercuts, slots and grooves to retain the build-up material
- **Dental adhesives** – for enhancing adhesion of amalgam and resin-based composites to coronal dentine
- **Luting agents** – bonding to dentine, e.g. amalgam with wet zinc phosphate or glass ionomers

Core build-up for non-vital teeth

Materials for core build-up on non-vital teeth are similar to that for vital teeth. The **ferrule effect** is also applicable for non-vital teeth. However, since **additional support is gained from intraradicular posts**, the fundamental issue is **minimising material interfaces**. This means that materials of the post/core complex should have similar properties. When **similar materials** are used, there is less stress concentration at the interfaces and **reduced microleakage.** Also, a post/core complex of the same material is structurally better placed to withstand intra-oral forces. This is the rationale for fabricating a unified post/core complex using an indirect technique with either cast alloys or ceramics (powder/liquid or CAD/CAM techniques). With the **direct approach**, a post/core complex is fabricated chair-side during a single visit, but the different material interfaces are often a compromise, with poorer mechanical properties. Therefore, when using a direct approach, precise clinical procedures and appropriate material selection are essential for ensuring longevity of the post/core complex and the subsequent permanent restoration.

Key points

- Core build-ups on vital and non-vital teeth are used to provide retention and resistance for definitive restorations
- It is essential to preserve as much natural tooth substrate as possible, incorporating a ferrule to maintain structural integrity
- Cores on vital teeth should avoid pulpal involvement
- There is no ideal material for a core build-up
- A unified post/core complex is preferred for non-vital teeth, since it avoids different material interfaces

Dental aesthetics

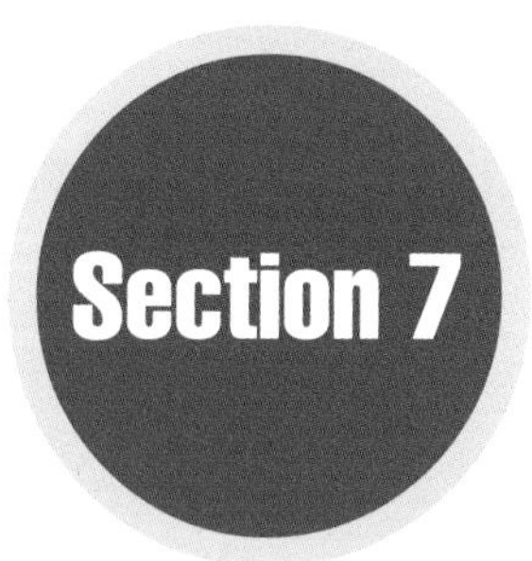

Chapters

Anterior dental aesthetics: basic principles

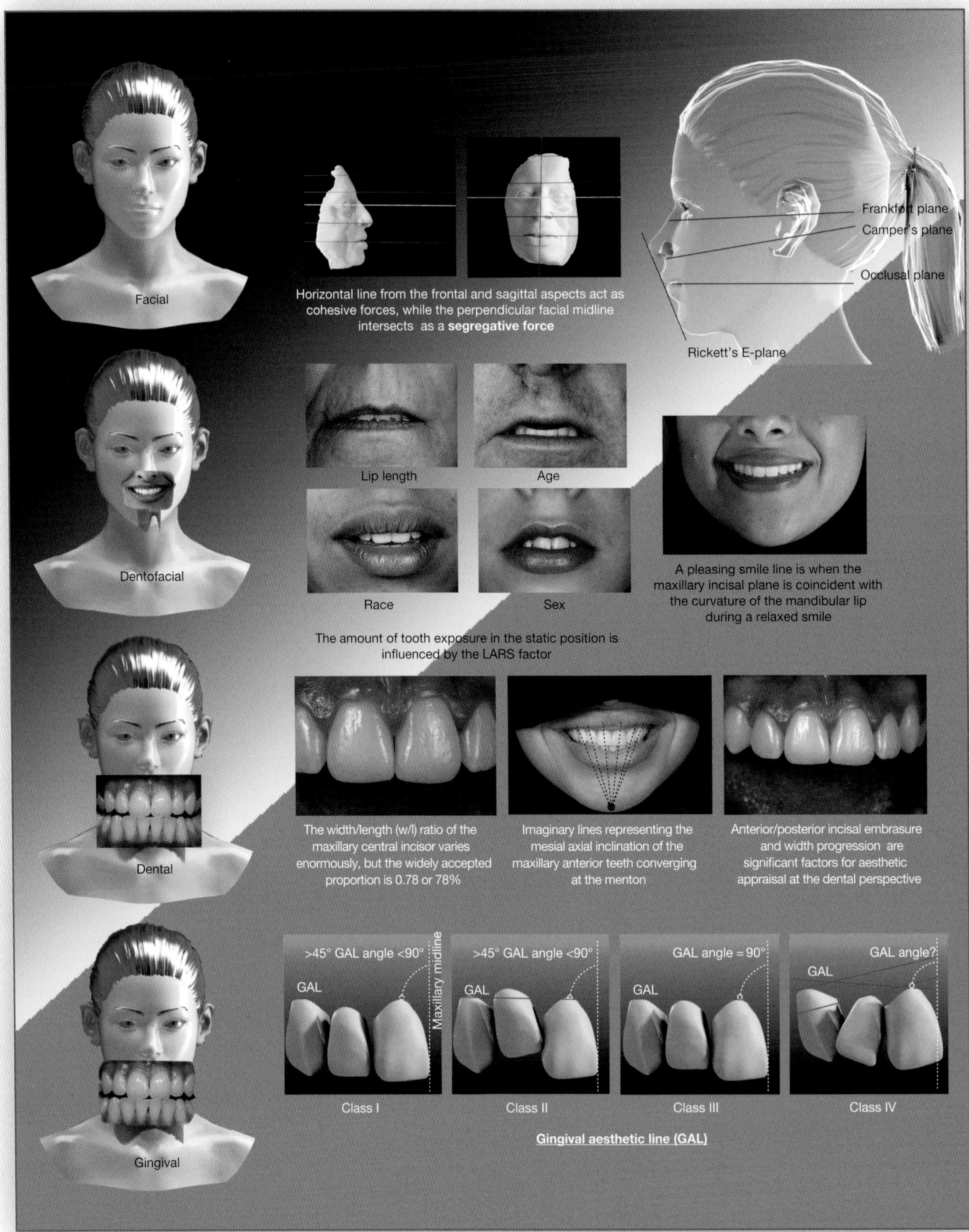

Facial

Horizontal line from the frontal and sagittal aspects act as cohesive forces, while the perpendicular facial midline intersects as a **segregative force**

Frankfort plane
Camper's plane
Occlusal plane
Rickett's E-plane

Dentofacial

Lip length
Age
Race
Sex

The amount of tooth exposure in the static position is influenced by the LARS factor

A pleasing smile line is when the maxillary incisal plane is coincident with the curvature of the mandibular lip during a relaxed smile

Dental

The width/length (w/l) ratio of the maxillary central incisor varies enormously, but the widely accepted proportion is 0.78 or 78%

Imaginary lines representing the mesial axial inclination of the maxillary anterior teeth converging at the menton

Anterior/posterior incisal embrasure and width progression are significant factors for aesthetic appraisal at the dental perspective

Gingival

>45° GAL angle <90°
GAL
Maxillary midline
Class I

>45° GAL angle <90°
GAL
Class II

GAL angle = 90°
GAL
Class III

GAL angle?
GAL
Class IV

Gingival aesthetic line (GAL)

Prosthodontics at a Glance, Second Edition. Irfan Ahmad.

Anterior dental aesthetics is primarily concerned with the appearance of the **maxillary anterior sextant**. The majority of research has been directed towards the size, shape and alignment of the maxillary incisors and canines, their relationship to each other, the antagonist dentition and to the surrounding soft tissues including the gingivae, lips and facial features. Dental aesthetics is best analysed by considering the face and then zooming closer to the dental elements.

Facial perspective

The **facial perceptive** can be divided into frontal and sagittal views. From the **frontal view,** the key features are:

- **Imaginary horizontal parallel lines acting as cohesive forces** for facial symmetry
- **Facial midline, perpendicular to horizontal lines, acting as segregative force** to add interest to the facial composition
- The **interpupillary line** is used as a reference for assessing the inclination of the incisal plane
- From the **sagittal (profile) view**, the analysis consists of:
- **Imaginary horizontal parallel lines acting as cohesive forces**
- **Frankfurt horizontal plane**
- **Ricketts' E-plane**
- **Steiner and Burstone lines**
- **Naso-labial angle**

Dentofacial perspective

Zooming closer, the **dentofacial perspective** (or composition) concentrates on the teeth and their relationship to the surrounding soft tissues in **static and dynamic muscular positions**. The **static position is a habitual** (not relaxed) state, the lips are slightly parted with minimal muscular activity and the teeth are out of occlusion. The **degree of tooth exposure is determined by the LARS factor**:

- **Lip length (maxillary)** – varies from 10 mm to 36 mm. Short lip = greater maxillary tooth exposure. Long lip = greater mandibular tooth exposure
- **Age** – youthfulness equates to greater maxillary tooth display, while reduced muscular tonicity of the maxillary lip musculature in advancing years results in less maxillary and greater mandibular tooth display
- **Race** – increasing maxillary tooth display from Caucasians, Asians to Blacks
- **Sex** – females have shorter maxillary lips and display more of the maxillary teeth compared to men
- The **dynamic positions** are **relaxed and exaggerated smiles**. Some points to consider are:
- **Smile arc (line or curvature)** – imaginary line of the incisal edges of the maxillary teeth, which should be parallel to the concave curvature of the mandibular lip
- **Bilateral negative space** (buccal corridor) – space separating the teeth from the corners of the lips
- **Phonetics** – positions of the teeth relative to the soft tissues (lips and tongue) for proper pronunciation of sounds, for example:

'M' or 'Emma' – habitual muscular position of lips
'F' and 'V' – buccal surface of maxillary incisors contact mucosal (not cutaneous) part of lower lip
'S' – vertical dimension of speech or edge-to-edge position of the upper and lower incisors
'TH' – tongue touches palatal aspect of maxillary teeth.

Dental perspective

The **dental perspective** is concerned with tooth shape, dimensions, alignment and progressive width proportions between the maxillary incisors and canines. Some aspects include:

- **Shape** – genetically determined
- **Size** – the width/length of teeth is referred to as the w/l ratio or its value as a percentage. The w/l ratio for narrow teeth can be as small as 60% and for wide teeth greater than 100% (accepted norm is 78%)
- **Alignment** – intra-arch positioning and axial inclination
- **Incisal embrasures** – angles between the incisal edges or tips of teeth, influenced by the degree of tooth wear. Incisal embrasure angles increase from the anterior to the posterior teeth
- **Width progression** – traversing distally from the centrals to the canines in specified increments or percentage widths of the teeth
- **Anterior overjet** (horizontal: ideal 2.7 mm) and **anterior overbite** (vertical: ideal 4.0 mm)

Gingival perspective

The **gingival architecture** surrounding the teeth is determined by the undulations of the underlying bone and the morphology and size of the teeth. Gingival considerations include:

- **Gingival exposure (maxillary)** – refers to the amount of gingiva visible between the gingival zeniths of the maxillary teeth and the lower border of the maxillary lip during a relaxed smile. The amount of tolerable exposure is around 3 mm
- **Periodontal biotype** – the texture of the attached gingivae, classified as thick, normal or thin
- **Periodontal bioform** – degree of gingival scallop, categorised as highly scalloped, normal or flat
- **Gingival embrasures** – amount of interproximal gingival papilla fill, linked to the distance of the contact points to the interproximal osseous crest. A distance of less than 5 mm ensures complete papilla fill without unsightly 'black triangles'
- **Gingival aesthetic line (GAL)** – gingival contour progression from central incisor to canine:

Class I – GAL angle is 45–90°, lateral incisor is touching or below (1–2 mm) GAL

Class II – GAL angle is 45–90°, lateral incisor is above (1–2 mm) GAL, and its mesial aspect overlaps the distal aspect of the central incisor

Class III – GAL angle is 90° and the canine, lateral and central incisors all lie below GAL

Class IV – the gingival contour cannot be assigned to any of the above three classes

Key points

- Anterior dental aesthetics is primarily concerned with the maxillary anterior sextant.
- Aesthetic analysis is expedited by sequentially analysing the facial, dentofacial, dental and gingival perspectives.

31 Anterior dental aesthetics: theories

Geometric theories

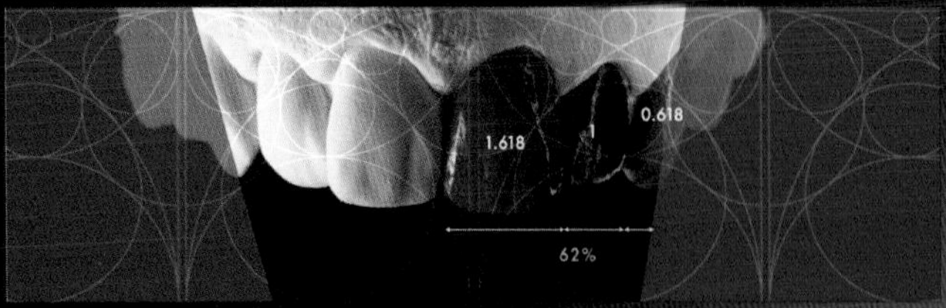

Golden Proportion

Lombardi 1973 — The repeated width proportion of anterior six teeth is in the Golden Proportion viewed from the frontal aspect. Progressing distally, the distal tooth is 62% of the immediate mesial tooth

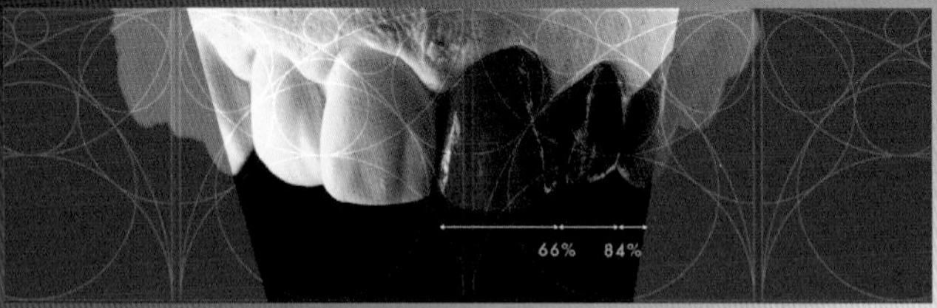

Natural Proportion

Preston 1993 — The repeated width proportion of each tooth is not identical. Progression from central to lateral incisor is 66%. Progression from lateral incisor to canine is 84%

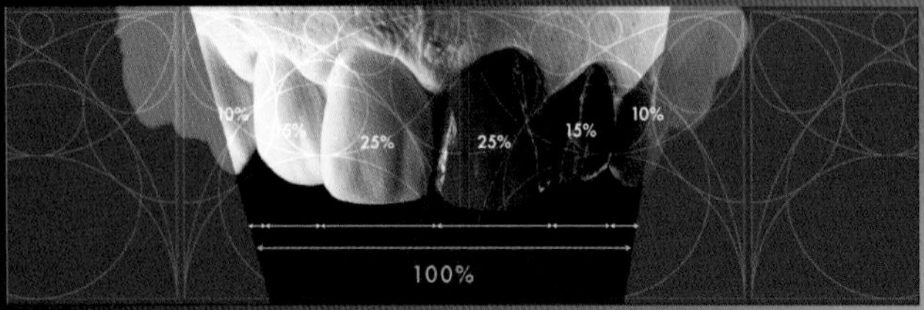

Golden Percentage

Snow 1999 — The width of individual teeth is a percentage of the total width of the anterior six teeth

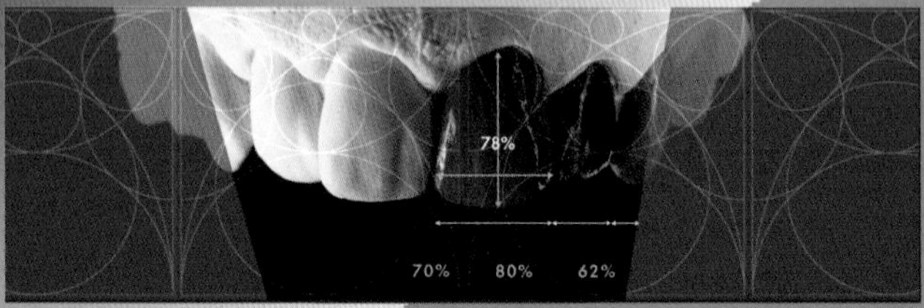

RED Proportion

Ward 2001 — Consistent repeated ratios more important than a specific ratio. For average tooth dimension of 78% (w/l ratio of 0.78), the recommended RED is 70%. For short teeth, 80% RED, and tall teeth a 62% RED (or the Golden Proportion)

Psychological theories

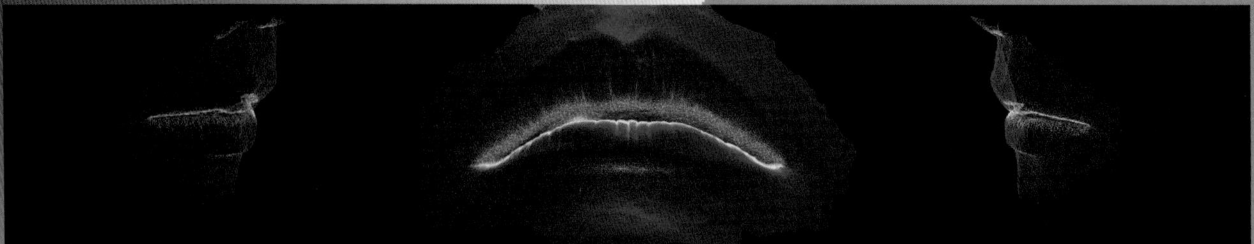

Psychological theories describe 'the way we see ourselves'

Perception theories describe ' the way others see us'

Perception theories

Aesthetic anomaly	Ideal	Tolerance
Smile arc (line/convexity)	2.7 mm	1.2 mm (3 seconds) to 2.7 mm (7 seconds)
Overbite	2.7 mm	5.7 mm
Maxillary central-to-incisal step	1.4 mm	2.9 mm
Bilateral negative space	16% of smile	8 to 22%
Positive canine or molar torque	None	Irrelevant
Maxillary gingival disaply	2.1 mm	+0.4 mm to −3.6 mm

Aesthetic anomaly	Ideal	Tolerance
Central incisor gingival discrepancy	0 mm	2 mm
Lateral incisor-gingival height	− 0.4 mm	+1.2 mm to −2.9 mm
Width of lateral-to-central incisor	78%	45%
Discrepancy dental / facial midline	0 mm	2.9 mm
Discrepancy upper / lower midline	0 mm	2.9 mm
Occlusal plane cant	2.1 mm	3 mm (or 4°)

Degree of tolerance by laypersons for various aesthetic anomalies (afer Ker et al., JADA 2008; 139; 1318-1327)

Prosthodontics at a Glance, Second Edition. Irfan Ahmad.

The search for a **magic formula to quantify beauty** has preoccupied artists, scientist and philosophers for over 5000 years. Yet, to date, there is no formula, law or dictum available that can decisively define the essence of beauty. Many hypotheses, opinions and ideas abound, which can broadly be categorised as **geometric**, **psychological** and **perceptual** theories.

Genesis of beauty

One of the earliest attempts to analyse beauty was by the ancient **Egyptians around 3000 BCE**. The mathematicians of the time realised the importance of proportion for creating aesthetically pleasing objects. The concept of the **Egyptian triangle** was extensively used in arts and crafts, and as an architectural template for building the fabulous sphinxes and pyramids of Egypt. The first person to postulate a mathematical formula for analysing beauty was **Pythagorus in 530 BCE** with the notion of the **golden number, Φ** (1.618), and its reciprocal **(1/1.618 = 0.618)**, the **golden proportion** (**GP**). The significance of the GP is its prevalence in nature as well as inanimate objects. Items perceived as beautiful can be shown to have proportions that are in the GP. **Plato**, **Aristotle**, **Euclid** and others have emphasised the **relevance of proportion in aesthetic appraisal.**

Geometric theories

The concept of proportion and form has been the basis for many **geometric theories** in aesthetic dentistry. Below are some of the authors who have proposed mathematical guidelines for aesthetics of the **maxillary anterior sextant**:

- **Williams** (1914) – classified tooth shape as square, tapering or ovoid
- **Lombardi** (1973) – first person to propose that the width progression of the maxillary anterior six teeth, viewed from the frontal aspect, can be related to the GP
- **Preston** (1993) – disputed the GP and proposed the natural proportion for the width progression from the central to lateral to canine
- **Gillen** (1994) – dispelled the myth of the GP for the maxillary anterior teeth
- **Snow** (1999) – proposed that the anterior six maxillary teeth are in the golden percentage
- **Ward** (2001) – emphasised that a specific ratio is irrelevant, and proposed a fixed recurring aesthetic dimension (RED) for the anterior six teeth
- **Rullinsky** (2009) – coined the golden coefficients for the curvature of the maxillary arch

All the above **theories have been invalidated** by subsequent studies, and none is unequivocally prevalent in the maxillary anterior dentition, particularly the GP, which has been ubiquitously quoted in the dental literature. Nowhere is the saying **'A lie told often enough becomes truth' (Vladimir Lenin)** more pertinent than with the GP. Many researchers have concluded that the **GP is only present in 10% of the population**, yet this pseudo-standard is the cornerstone (and excuse) for many so-called aesthetic '**dental makeovers**'. Furthermore, the **difference** in tooth widths using various theories can be **as little as 0.5 mm**, an amount barely perceptible at close distance, let alone at a social viewing distance.

Psychological theories

Linking psychology with tooth form, contour and colour has also been the subject of numerous studies:

- **White** (1874) – coined the **'temperamental theory'**, correlating tooth differences with an individual's disposition
- **Frush and Fisher** (1958) – **dynesthetic** theory related the sex, age and personality (**SAP**) of a person with tooth form, contour and alignment of the anterior teeth
- **Rufenacht** (1990) – **morphopsychological** concept relating facial and bodily features (morphology) with psychology as the determining factor for the shape and size of teeth
- **Ahmad** (2001) – **synaesthetic perception**; emotional and subconscious decisions and choices take precedence over cognitive or mathematical rationality for aesthetic appraisal

Most of the **psychological theories are opinions**, and cannot be confirmed or refuted by rigid scientific analysis. However, **science cannot explain everything,** and emotional and psychological factors are relevant because they account for patients' **intangible desires** and wishes. For this reason, the **patient's input** should be incorporated into every aesthetic treatment plan.

Perception theories

Perception theories concentrate on what is perceived, both by the providers (dentists, ceramists) and end users (patients). The salient **difference between psychological and perception theories** is that the former concern **'the way we see ourselves'**, while the latter concern **'the way others see us'**. Perceptual theories are currently becoming increasingly popular for aesthetic analysis and assessing the outcome of aesthetic treatment. The seminal perception theory publications include:

- **Kokich** (1999) – first study using photographic image manipulation to assess smile attractiveness, concluding that laypersons are less discriminating than general dentists and orthodontists regarding aesthetic aberrations
- **Pinho** (2007) – concurred that perception between dentists and laypeople vary enormously
- **Ker** (2008) – comprehensive survey of laypersons' perceptions of aesthetic anomalies

Perception theories gauge response from patients (and the dental team) and are extremely valuable for treatment planning, especially for preventing overtreatment. Furthermore, since patients are oblivious to minor aesthetic aberrations, it is the duty of dental professionals **neither to unnecessarily sensitise their patients nor 'manufacture' dental conditions requiring interventional aesthetic therapy.** However, the sample population for many of these surveys is small, specific to particular countries and cultures, and therefore, the findings cannot be applied to all populations or to every individual.

Key points

- There are no magic formulas, no magic numbers, no Holy Grail and no Da Vinci Code for evaluating or creating beauty.
- Geometric theories are a framework, not a formula.
- Psychological theories are pragmatic, not dogmatic.
- Perception theories are subjective, not objective.

32 Anterior dental aesthetics: guidelines

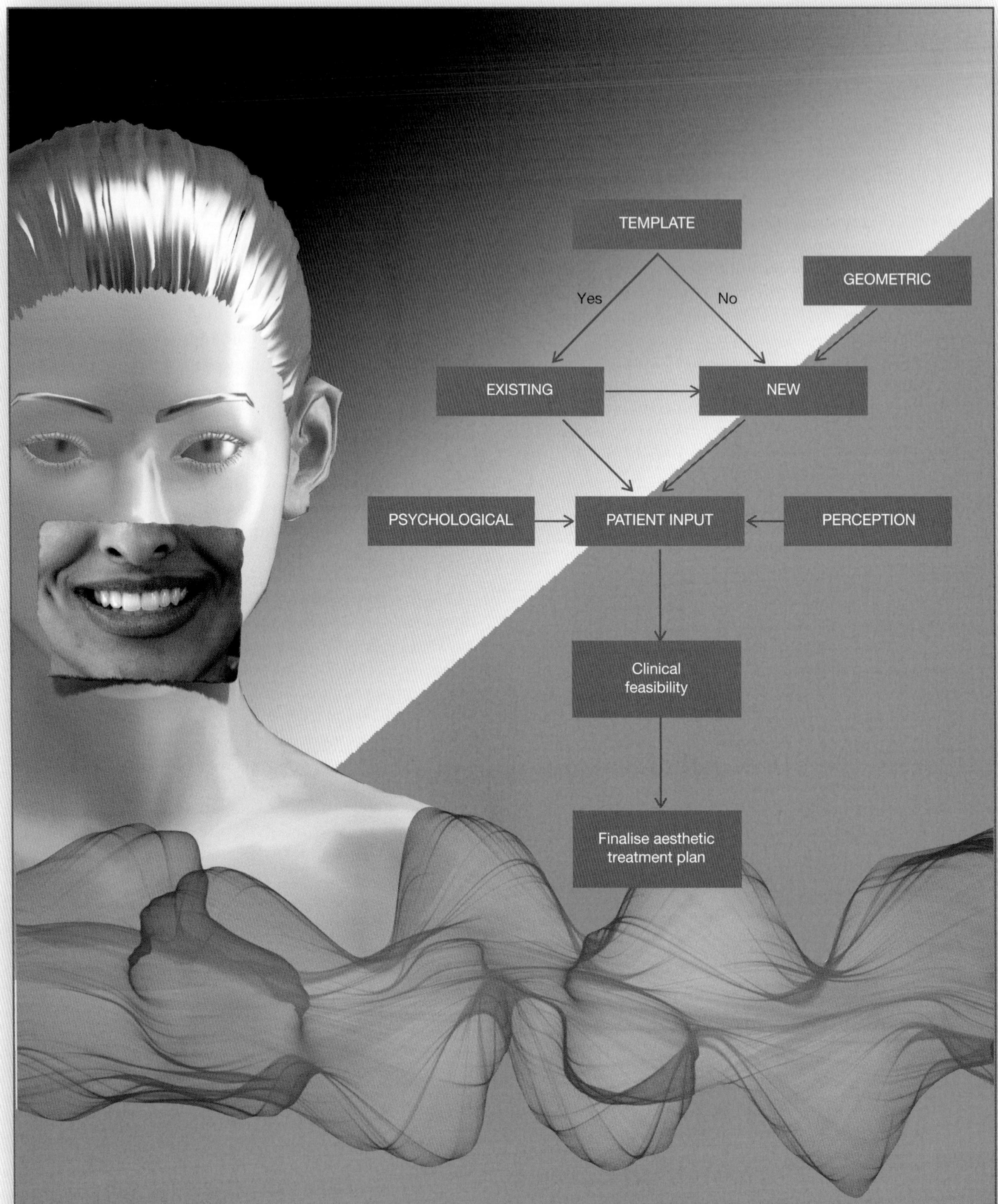

Schematic and sequential guidelines for aesthetic treatment planning

Prosthodontics at a Glance, Second Edition. Irfan Ahmad.

There are numerous theories regarding dental aesthetics, broadly categorised into **geometric**, **psychological** and **perceptual**. No single theory adequately explains the aesthetics of the maxillary anterior six teeth, or can be utilised to prescribe a definitive treatment plan. In reality, **all theories can be synergistically used to analyse and finalise anterior dental aesthetics.**

General guidelines

Before proposing schematic guidelines for dental aesthetics, it is important to **establish principles for treatment planning of aesthetic cases**:

- At present, there are no generally accepted objective standards for designing smiles
- Dental aesthetics cannot be determined or analysed using a single parameter
- Avoid sensitising patients to minor aesthetic anomalies, which they would normally accept or otherwise ignore
- Discourage sensitising patients to minor aesthetic anomalies based on media or peer pressure and social trends
- The culture of **dissatisfaction marketing** for sensitising patients should be discouraged
- Adopt a **minimally invasive approach** for resolving unacceptable dental aesthetics
- **Creating diversity in the maxillary anterior sextant is the key to individuality**

Template

The starting point for a dental aesthetics prescription is establishing a **template**, which can either be existing or new. An existing template is the existing dentition, and the proposed aesthetic changes are designed to integrate within this framework. This ensures a minimally invasive approach, and avoids unnecessary **overtreatment**. If the maxillary anterior sextant is edentulous, or requires extensive alterations, one or more of the geometric theories can be used as a starting point for creating a **new template**. For example, if there is extensive crowding, misalignment or diastemata, a new working template is **designed by simulations**, e.g. diagnostic wax-up or intra-oral mock-ups. The choice of which geometric theory to use is empirical; often the difference in tooth widths between these theories can be as little as 0.5 mm. However, the following aspects should be incorporated into a template:

The **overall** symmetry and balance of the dentofacial perspective is the salient factor for an aesthetically pleasing smile, **rather than individual or localised items**

- **Avoid bilateral symmetry** (mirror symmetry) between the right and left sides of the anterior sextant to ensure individuality and uniqueness
- The average **w/l ratio** of the maxillary teeth is **0.78 or 78%**
- **Dominance of the central incisors**
- The average maxillary **tooth display** during a relaxed smile is 75%
- **No specific ratio for repeated proportions** is applicable to all individuals
- **Smile arc (line)** is parallel to curvature of the mandibular lip during a relaxed smile
- **Acceptable maxillary gingival display** during a relaxed smile is approximately 3 mm, thereby avoiding a 'gummy' smile

Patient input

After defining a working template, either existing or new, the next stage is modification of the template by the patient's input. The **patient's wishes are predominantly related to psychological and perceptual theories**:

- The **patient's input is essential for a successful aesthetic treatment outcome**
- The **patient's persona** is moulded by intellect, culture, social interaction and economic status
- **Women are usually more intuitive and emotional than men,** and therefore make a more critical judgement about beauty and self-appearance

The second aspect regarding the patient's input is **perception**. If an aesthetic aberration is unnoticed or the patient is oblivious to its presence, is it justifiable to correct it? Furthermore, many patients accept gross aesthetic abnormalities, and have little desire to make changes. In both circumstances, **coercive sensitisation** to these irregularities that do not compromise health or function is counterproductive, and at times unethical. In addition, aesthetic anomalies are more apparent to the trained eye of a dentist than that of a layperson, whose **naiveté is often a blessing**. Lastly, most perception theories are based on frontal view assessments but oblique (profile) and dynamic visualisations (video) should also be considered.

Clinical feasibility

The last stage of aesthetic treatment planning is assessing whether the patient's wishes are **clinically feasible,** and if they can be incorporated into the patient's prevailing clinical scenario. For example, if tooth wear has resulted in minimal space for restorative materials due to dentoalveolar compensation, it is futile to provide restorations unless space is created by orthodontic appliances. Another issue is conceding to patients' wishes for irreversible procedures that may compromise dental health in the future, for example, providing elective cosmetic treatment entailing destruction of healthy teeth for the sake of vanity. Many so-called **'cosmetic makeover'** procedures are questionable, ephemeral and possibly unethical.

Finally, **science is dogmatic** with little leeway, while **art is nebulous**, open to interpretation. Since aesthetics is a combination of art and science, the 'aesthetic rules' need to be tailored for an individual. **One size does not fit all.** To date, attempts over the last 5000 years to apply scientific rules and guidelines have failed to determine rigid principles for dental aesthetics. **Aesthetic objectivity is an elusive goal, and perhaps one that should remain enigmatic.**

Key points

- Dental aesthetics is subjective, with no objective rules for analysing or prescribing this treatment modality.
- The best guidelines for aesthetic treatment planning are adopting a minimally invasive approach and combining the available theories, i.e. geometric, psychological and perceptual.
- Patient participation is essential for successful outcome of an aesthetic treatment plan.

33 Anterior dental aesthetics: digital smile design

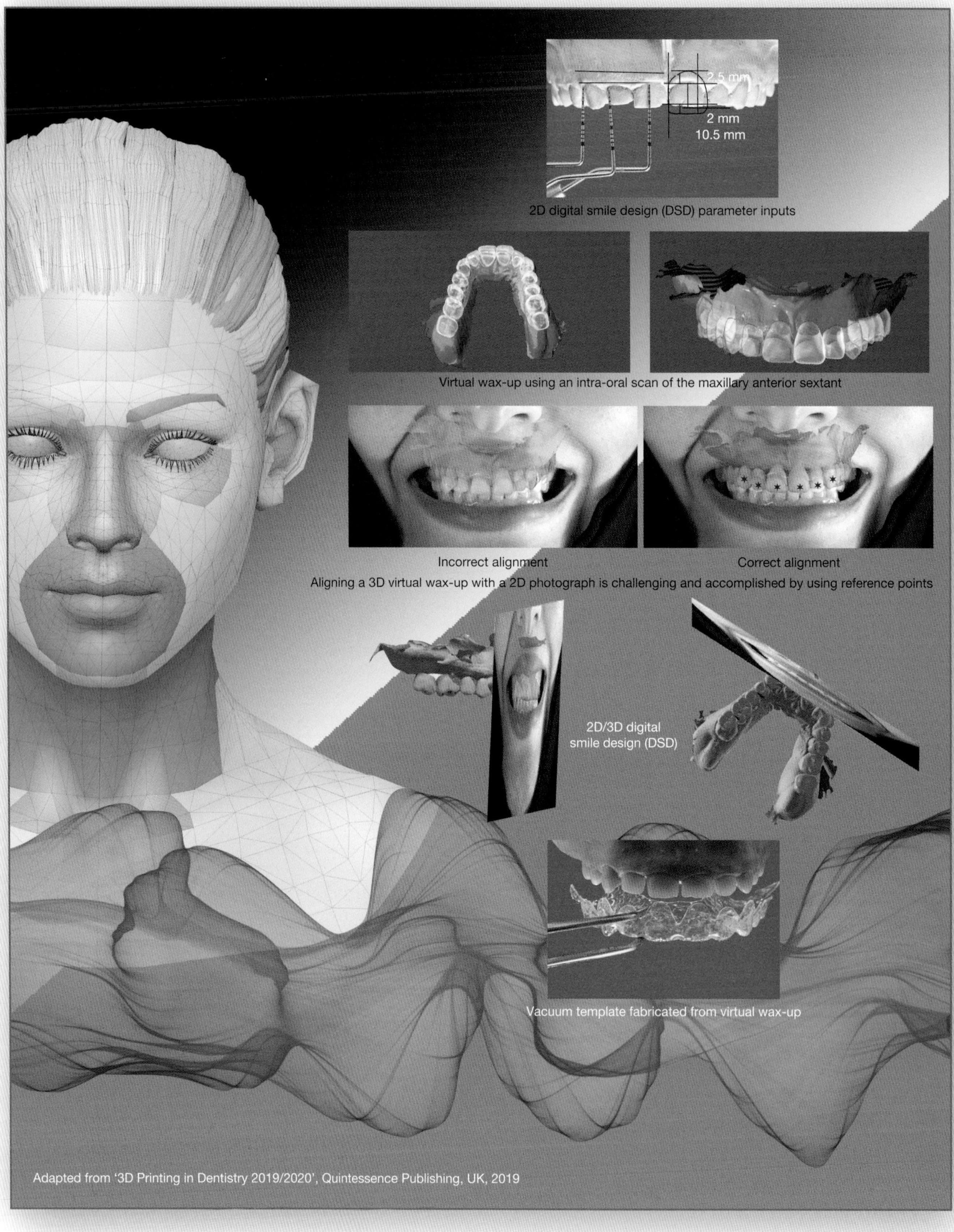

2.5 mm
2 mm
10.5 mm

2D digital smile design (DSD) parameter inputs

Virtual wax-up using an intra-oral scan of the maxillary anterior sextant

Incorrect alignment

Correct alignment

Aligning a 3D virtual wax-up with a 2D photograph is challenging and accomplished by using reference points

2D/3D digital smile design (DSD)

Vacuum template fabricated from virtual wax-up

Adapted from '3D Printing in Dentistry 2019/2020', Quintessence Publishing, UK, 2019

Prosthodontics at a Glance, Second Edition. Irfan Ahmad.

In the last few years, there has been a tremendous fervour about smile design, especially with the addition of the prefix 'digital'. However, the basic concepts for analysing and formulating a treatment plan for restituting anterior aesthetics, usually confined to the maxillary anterior sextant, are based on dental aesthetic principles established decades ago. The bandwagon of the so-called contemporary **digital smile design (DSD)** is simply applying these principles using computer software to facilitate the process. Furthermore, most currently available programmes are capable of essentially 2D simulations, which are ideal for marketing, communication and treatment acceptance, but **translating simulations to harsh clinical reality is challenging and iconoclastic**, often fraught with broken promises and unexpected outcomes. Therefore, a smile design should be considered a guideline rather than a facsimile of what is clinically feasible, and appreciate its limitations of transposing virtual utopia to real-life dystopia.

Virtual smile design

DSD is predominately based on geometric aesthetic theories since computers do not feel and are incapable of expressing an opinion (yet! – see Chapter 20 discussing artificial intelligence). For each perspective, i.e. facial, dentofacial, dental and gingiva, mathematical calculations are used to determine the size, form, alignment and angulations of teeth to intra-oral and extra-oral soft tissue reference points. The principle involves drawing reference lines, shapes and calculating measurements on 2D photographs of the teeth and tissues. The reference markers act as guides to digitally manipulate tooth and soft tissue morphology until **pink and white aesthetics are satisfactorily accomplished**. The information is then utilised for creating either an analogue, or virtual diagnostic wax-up to act as a template for fabricating **intra-oral functional and aesthetic mock-ups**, tooth preparation guides, aesthetic crown lengthening guides, implant surgical guides, provisionals, orthodontic guides for indirect bracket placement and facilitating ceramic layering of definitive prostheses. Furthermore, at the mock-up stage, changes can be made according to patients' wishes **(psychological and perception aesthetic theories)**, and incorporated into the virtual design to finalise an aesthetic treatment plan. **DSD can be 2D, 3D, 4D or a combination of these categories.**

2D smile design

Virtually any imaging, graphics, presentation, designing or drawing software can be used for creating a **virtual smile design**. Some popular software include Adobe® Creative Cloud™ (incorporating Photoshop), Apple® Keynote™, Microsoft® PowerPoint™, Corel Draw®, Autodesk® AutoCAD or innumerable other free download packages. Alternately, specific **smile design programmes** can be utilised such as SmileDesignerPro, SNAP®, Digital Smile Design (DSD) or add-on modules to dedicated dental CAD software. The process involves using a 2D digital image of the patient's teeth as a background, and drawing lines and shapes, which are modified until the desired aesthetic objectives are achieved. Also, preformed **smile design templates** can be imported from 'smile libraries' as a starting point, and altered as necessary for creating the desired simulation. As mentioned in the previous chapter, each tooth should be individual and the composition devoid of bilateral symmetry, which appears contrived and conveys a sense of artificiality.

2D/3D smile design

Whilst a 2D smile design is a useful previsualisation tool, it has several limitations. First, a 2D design lacks the spacial representation of real 3D objects. A 2D photograph of the patient depicts an instance in time and angle, which is static and unalterable. Therefore, the designing process is flawed since it neither accounts for dynamic movements of the lips and teeth, nor different perspectives or angles of view. This presents problems when trying to transpose the 2D design to an actual 3D model of the teeth for producing an analogue or virtual diagnostic wax-up, since the tooth measurements and alignments on the screen monitor fail to match the tangible 3D curved arch models.

One solution that is currently being used is **combining a 2D standardised digital photographs with 3D intra-oral scans** of the arches. This **2D/3D hybrid smile design** is a **step closer to reality** and overcomes some of the limitations of an exclusively 2D design. An intra-oral scan allows the teeth and soft tissues to be represented in three dimensions, which can be manipulated in any angle or plane. However, the extra-oral soft tissue landmarks of the face are still represented in two dimensions. Another drawback of this approach is precisely lining up the 3D intra-oral scan with the 2D digital photograph, which often results in incorrect superimposition.

3D/4D smile design

The **ultimate smile design is an entirely 3D representation** of the intra and extra-oral tissues. This involves **'stitching' 3D facial scans with intra-oral scans** to truly visualise all structures in three dimensions. Additionally, the emerging **4D surface motion techniques** allow facial expressions and movements to be analysed, and complement the unsurpassable diagnostic possibilities with this type of imaging. For example, the teeth and gingiva can be assessed in a visual environment during smiling, speech and laughter. This technology has ongoing developments, but in the coming years will provide extremely sophisticated smile designing capabilities that incorporate **dynamic motions** with **audible phonetic [illegible]**

Key points

- Digital smile design is applying geometric aesthetic theories using computer software.
- A smile design can be 2D, 3D, 4D or a combination of these approaches.
- Future developments will allow dynamic motion and audio to enhance the designing process.

34 Tooth whitening

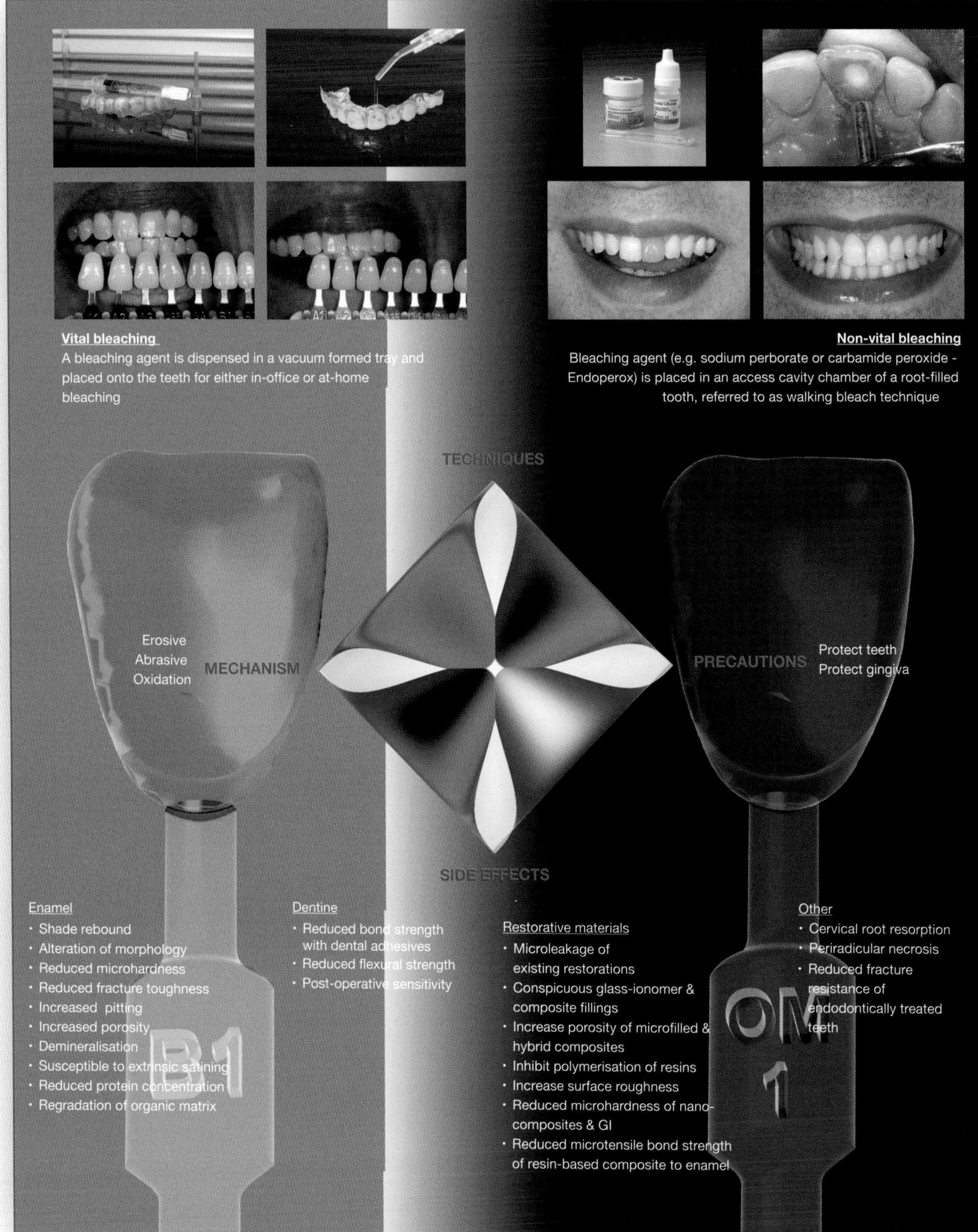

Dental **tooth whitening** or **bleaching** is an effective, economical and **minimally invasive** approach to whitening discoloured teeth. Since its introduction two decades ago by Haywood and Haymann, the at-home technique has proved a successful treatment modality for improving unsightly stained teeth. Bleaching is also therapeutic for periodontal health and favours maintenance of oral hygiene. Furthermore, the transient irritation of soft and hard tissues is innocuous and reversible.

Mechanism

Whitening teeth is achieved by any one of three processes, i.e. **erosive**, **abrasive** and **oxidation**. The most popular method is oxidation since erosion and abrasion potentially damage hard tissues by irreversibly altering tooth morphology. Furthermore, excessive enamel loss is counterproductive for tooth whitening, since it allows visibility of the darker underlying dentine. The **oxidation process** uses bleaching chemicals that penetrate the interprismatic enamel substrate and **convert the pigmented carbon rings to lighter carbon chains**. The higher the concentration of the bleaching agent, the greater and more rapid the effect. This process alters enamel micromorphology, affecting both the organic and inorganic phase of the hard tissue. The negative effect of oxidation is that bleaching chemicals, with a low pH, demineralise enamel. However, the effect is usually transient, since calcium in the saliva and use of fluoride dentifrices reverse the effect by **remineralisation of the enamel** surface layer.

Techniques

The commonly used **bleaching agents** are **carbamide peroxide** (urea peroxide) in concentrations ranging from 1% to 45%, **hydrogen peroxide** (3% to 50%) and **sodium perborate**. These agents are available as gels, varnishes, powder, mouthwashes and toothpastes. The concentration of the bleaching agent determines the duration of treatment. A high concentration results in rapid whitening in a shorter time, while lower concentrations require longer to take effect. There are two main methods for bleaching, either **in-office** or **at-home** (with professional supervision). The latter can be combined with an in-office 'jump start', followed by slower completion at-home.

Vital bleaching is prescribed alone for whitening teeth or be part of a global aesthetic treatment plan, e.g. before veneers, crowns or tooth-coloured 'white' fillings. In isolation, bleaching can be used to alter colour for teeth displaying yellow, brown/grey or tetracycline intrinsic stains. The technique involves fabricating carefully adapted custom made plastic trays using a heat/vacuum tray-forming machine. The trays are filled with the chosen agent and placed over the teeth for specified durations, followed by brushing with a toothpaste containing a high concentration of sodium fluoride (2800 ppm). The duration of treatment depends on the extent of discolouration; the bleaching process can take 2–6 weeks at home if the trays are worn for 2–3 hours per day using 10% carbamide peroxide. The **efficacy is 2–10 shades of colour modification on the Vita Classical shade guide** arranged in order of value. However, there is a **1–2 shade rebound** after 2–4 weeks. Therefore, it is advisable to wait before proceeding with new aesthetic restorations so that the latter can be matched to the stabilised colour of the bleached teeth. For severe stains, e.g. intense tetracycline staining, whitening may take 6–12 months. During the bleaching process, it is essential to provide **professional supervision** throughout treatment, and monitor changes with **photographs** and **reference shade tab guides.**

Non-vital bleaching is a third option used to lighten endodontically treated teeth, often referred to as **intracoronal or walking bleach technique.** Before starting, it is essential to ensure that the existing root filling has a satisfactory apical seal to prevent leaching of the bleaching agents into the periradicular areas, and causing root absorption. The technique involves placing bleaching agents into the pulp chamber and sealing the cavity with either glass ionomer or a resin-based composite filling to prevent microleakage and percolation of bacteria.

Light-activated bleaching involves using bleaching chemicals containing carotene to accelerate the breakdown of the active ingredients when exposed to high-intensity **light or lasers.** However, **light alone has no effect on tooth whitening,** but the heat generated by lights may accelerate the whitening effects of bleaching chemicals. Furthermore, heat can dehydrate teeth, leading to greater postoperative sensitivity.

Precautions

While effective and simple, certain conditions are required before considering bleaching:

- **Tooth protection** – pretreatment of sensitive areas, e.g. cervical or abfraction lesions should be sealed with glass ionomer. Also, bleaching areas of gross tooth wear with exposed dentine may cause further dentine erosion. Finally, for pronounced fluorosis or developmental banding, **microabrasion** may be necessary to avoid uneven bleaching
- **Gingival protection** – rubber dam or other gingival barriers are essential when using in-office high-concentration bleaching gels

Side effects

Although tooth whitening is a **relative safe procedure**, some **side effects** need to be addressed:

- **Reduced enamel microhardness** (outer 25 μm surface) immediately after bleaching, usually reversed by saliva remineralisation in 3–4 weeks
- Excessive bleaching with high concentrations may result in **chemical and morphological changes** in enamel structure leading to **increased porosity,** pitting, reduced fracture strength, erosion or lesions emulating initial caries
- **Sensitivity** (tooth and gingival), particularly with higher concentrations of bleaching agent, but is mitigated by **remineralisation with sodium fluoride, potassium nitrate or sodium [illegible]**
- **Reduced dentine bond strengths** (especially with sodium perborate), but there is little change in enamel bond strength one week post-bleaching
- **Increased microleakage** at the interface between dentine and restorative materials, but margins on enamel remain intact
- Effects of bleaching on **restorative materials**, especially composites and glass ionomer fillings, which may cause existing fillings to become **more conspicuous**
- **Cervical root absorption**

Key points

- Bleaching is a simple, effective and innocuous method for whitening teeth.
- Professional supervision and monitoring are essential to enhance treatment and mitigate side effects.

35 Non-surgical facial aesthetics (NSFA)

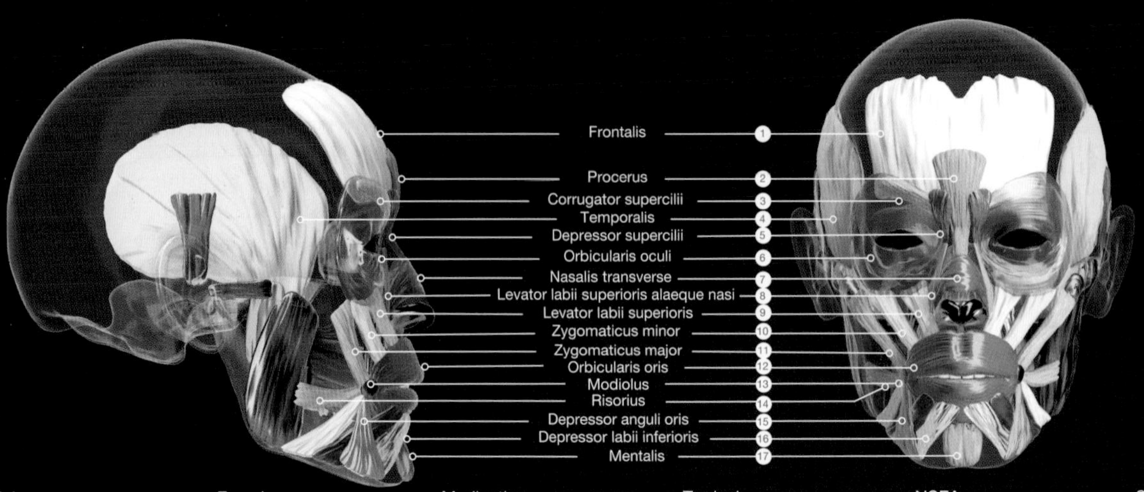

Frontalis 1
Procerus 2
Corrugator supercilii 3
Temporalis 4
Depressor supercilii 5
Orbicularis oculi 6
Nasalis transverse 7
Levator labii superioris alaeque nasi 8
Levator labii superioris 9
Zygomaticus minor 10
Zygomaticus major 11
Orbicularis oris 12
Modiolus 13
Risorius 14
Depressor anguli oris 15
Depressor labii inferioris 16
Mentalis 17

Make-up	Exercises	Medication	Topical	NSFA	Surgery
Cosmetic products	Toning facial muscles	Peptides, vitamins	Creams, chemical/laser peels, dermabrasion	Neurotoxin, fillers	Orthognathic, plastic

Facial beautification continuum

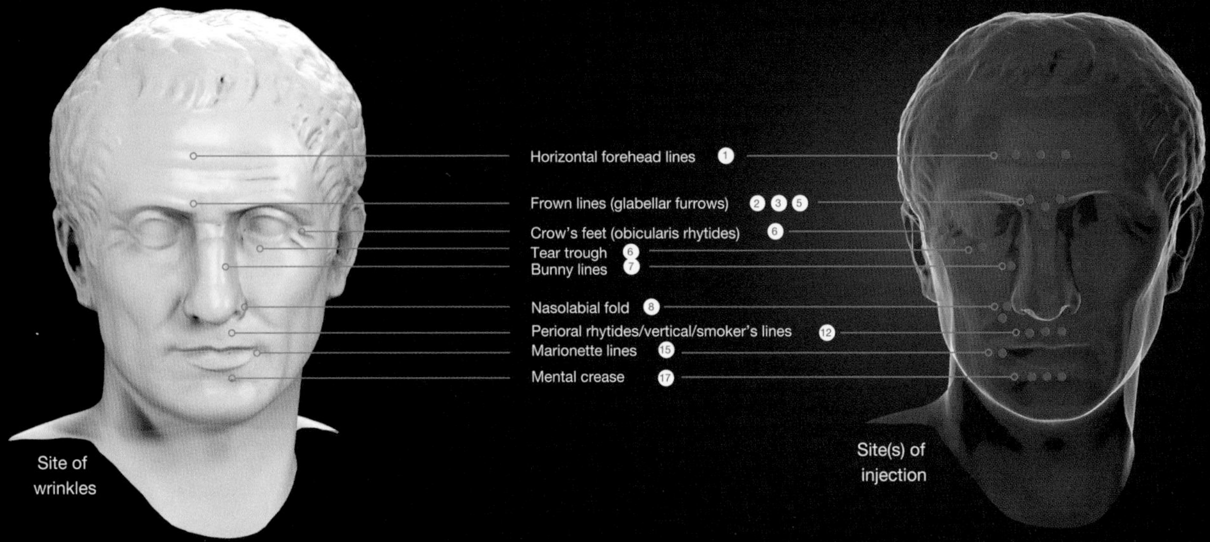

Horizontal forehead lines 1
Frown lines (glabellar furrows) 2 3 5
Crow's feet (obicularis rhytides) 6
Tear trough 6
Bunny lines 7
Nasolabial fold 8
Perioral rhytides/vertical/smoker's lines 12
Marionette lines 15
Mental crease 17
Site of wrinkles
Site(s) of injection

Indications for neurotoxins and fillers

- NSFA
- hyperactive lip
- platysma bands
- reliving suture tension
- dystonias
- strabismus
- migraines
- muscular spasticity
- hyperhidrosis
- lichen simplex
- bilateral masseter hypertrophy
- blepharospasm
- hyperhidrosis
- synkinesis
- Bell's palsy
- pompholyx (dyshidrotic eczema)
- acne vulgaris

Gummy smile

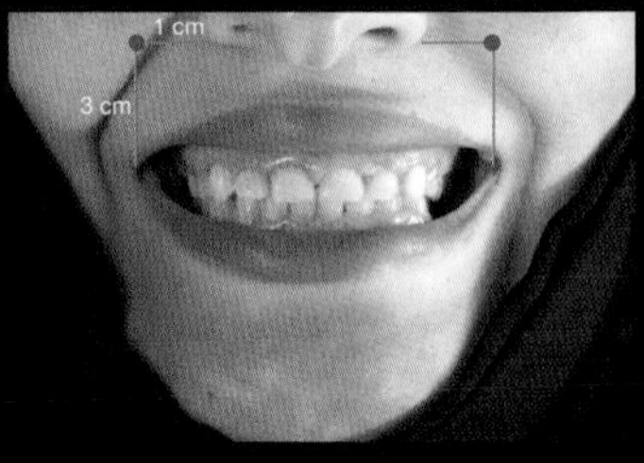

1 cm
3 cm

Yonsei point

NSFA timescale

Time	Effect/Action
Strat of procedure	Burning sensation
24 h	Noticeable changes
2 weeks	Optimal results
2 weeks	Retouch, if necessary
3–6 months	Repeat neurotoxin
6–12 months	Repeat filler

Prosthodontics at a Glance, Second Edition. Irfan Ahmad.

On a facial rejuvenation or beautification continuum, non-surgical facial aesthetics (NSFA) lies just before surgical intervention. NSFA is a **minimally invasive, elective cosmetic procedure** for rectifying rhytides, wrinkles and facial contour disharmonies with intramuscular injections. It is a burgeoning and highly sought after modality, and routinely performed by dentists with predictable results. However, an exhaustive understanding of facial anatomy, aesthetics, specialist training and appreciation of potential pitfalls are prerequisite.

Aetiology of rhytides and wrinkles

Facial muscles are unique since their **attachments are to overlying skin rather than to bones.** As well as **conveying emotions**, facial muscles are responsible for **facial expressions** that are essential for **non-verbal communication**. The formation of **rhytides (lines/creases) and wrinkles (grooves/folds)** is due to dermal atrophy caused by repeated contraction of underlying muscles, ageing, photodamage, scarring or gravitation sagging. The rhytides and wrinkles are **static** or **dynamic**, and may be accompanied by adipose depletion, reduced skin elasticity (flaccidity), thinning, roughness and pigmentation. Several **indices are used for assessing the severity of winkles** and outcome of enhancement procedures, e.g. Wrinkle Severity Rating Scale (WSRS), Wrinkle Assessment Scale (WAS) and Global Aesthetic Improvement Scale (GAIS).

Botulinum toxin

Botulinum toxin is a potent **neurotoxin derived from *Clostridium botulinum* bacterium** that was commercially licensed for cosmetic dermatology in the early noughties. It has **seven serotypes**, but only **A and B have clinical uses**, and botulinum toxin type **A (BTX-A) is predominantly used for cosmetic procedures**. Although **Botox** has become a proverbial appellation for NSFA, there are three **types of BTX-A**: onabotulinumtoxin A (Botox®), abobotulinumtoxin A (Dysport®) and incobotulinumtoxin A (Xeomin®). The formulations vary according to the **complexing proteins**, which can illicit immunogenic reactions (anaphylaxis). The mode of action of the neurotoxin is termed **chemodenervation**, which involves **inhibiting release of acetylcholine** at neuromuscular junctions. This causes the facial muscles to relax giving the appearance of smoothing to the overlying dermal layers. The toxin exerts its effect by cleaving a docking protein (synaptosomal associated protein of 25 kDA [**SNAP-25**]) on the internal surface of neuronal membranes. However, the **effect is ephemeral**, until SNAP-25 reforms to resume muscular contraction. **BTX-A action is more pronounced with dynamic wrinkles compared to static ones,** and is considered safe, and without irreversible damage to targeted nerves or muscles.

After examining and counselling the patient on the benefits and complications of NSFA, a **written content** is obtained, and baseline photographs/videos taken. It is important to set realistic and feasible goals before starting, to avoid disappointments afterwards. The **contraindications for NSFA** are either **somatic** or **psychological**, including allergies to botulinum toxin or its formulation ingredients, acute infection, keloidal scarring, eczema, psoriasis, neuromuscular disorders (e.g. myasthenia gravis and Eaton-Lambert syndrome), drug interactions (e.g. calcium blockers, aminoglycosides cyclosporine and quinidine), pregnancy, lactation, anticoagulant therapy or immunocompromised patients. The other issues are disproportionate **vanity/narcissism,** dysmorphic disorder, histrionic personality disorder (HPD), peer pressure and occupational concerns for individuals relying on facial muscles for non-verbal facial communication (actors, people in public gaze, singers and wind instrument musicians). The **dose** is influenced by the types of product, gender, muscle mass and local anatomy, and is usually around 20–40 units for Botox using a 30-gauge, 1-inch needle. The post-operative instructions are avoiding strenuous exercise, temperance, analgesics, ice packs and not touching the site.

The foremost side effects are diminished facial expressions and non-verbal facial communication, plus **de-personalisation**; so called **plastic aesthetics**. However, is not this the object of the exercise? The **psychometric benefits of NSFA** for improving the quality of life and self-confidence are **subjective**. For some, a dazed expression with ironed out skin appears unnatural, while for other it is a sign of youthfulness and attractiveness. There is no criteria of 'naturalness', but a degree of facial laterality is often acceptable, and even desirable. An assessment of satisfaction is a combination of how a patient looks and feels, and the closer these two entities, the more successful the outcome. The **complications** are categorised as **injection-related events (IRE)** or **treatment-emergent adverse events (TEAE)**, such as vasovagal attack, allergic reactions, oedema, haemorrhage, erythema, ecchymoses, purpura, blepharoptosis, dystonia, paraesthesia, ectropion, facial congestion, dry eyes, facial asymmetries, headaches, nausea, malaise and botulism.

Dermal filers

Dermal filers are indicated and effective for **static wrinkles**, **facial contouring** or **poor response to BTX-A.** The most commonly used dermal fillers are **non-animal stabilised hyaluronic acid (NASHA)**, acidic polysaccharides that are hydrophilic and act as natural moisturisers for making skin more elastic and supple. NASHA are biocompatible and available in **different stiffness gels**. The softer versions, Restylane® Refyne (smaller particles, low density), are for fine lines, while the stiffer, high-density products (Restylane® Defyne) are for facial contouring and volume enhancing. The injections are more painful compared to neurotoxin, and some formulations incorporate lidocaine to mitigate discomfort. Various **injection techniques** are advocated, e.g. anterograde/retrograde linear threading or fanning, depending on whether the wrinkles are diffuse or well defined. Post-procedural precautions and complications are similar to neurotoxin, but massaging the area afterwards is recommended for reducing beading or a lumpy appearance. The severest complication of fillers is **focal tissue necrosis** that can partly be reversed by injecting hyaluronidase.

Smile enhancement

There are various types of smile, and the **type of smile** determines which facial muscles are involved. For example, a **Duchenne smile** signifies ecstatic joy, which is characterised by raised lips and cheeks (zygomaticus major), flaring of the nostrils (nasalis), narrowing of the eyes and appearance of **crow's feet** (obicularis occlui), whereas a **polite or social smile** only involves the zygomaticus major muscles. NSFA is an ideal modality for **fine tuning a smile**, and particularly effective, either alone or as an adjunct with other therapy, for enhancing a smile due to a hypertonic maxillary lip causing **excessive maxillary gingival display** (>3 mm) known as a 'gummy smile'. The usual injection site for reliving a **gummy smile is the Yonsei point.**

Key points

- NSFA is an elective cosmetic procedure using injectable botulinum toxin and/or dermal fillers.
- Meticulous medical and psychological assessment, plus appropriate training are essential.
- NSFA is also effective for soft tissue smile enhancement.

Types of restorations

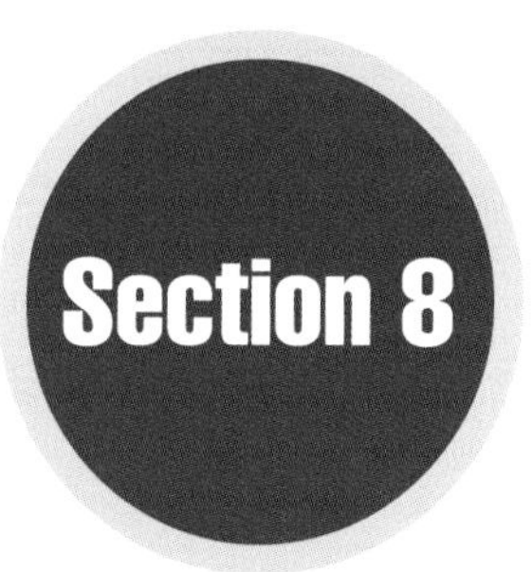

Chapters

36 Choice of intracoronal restorations

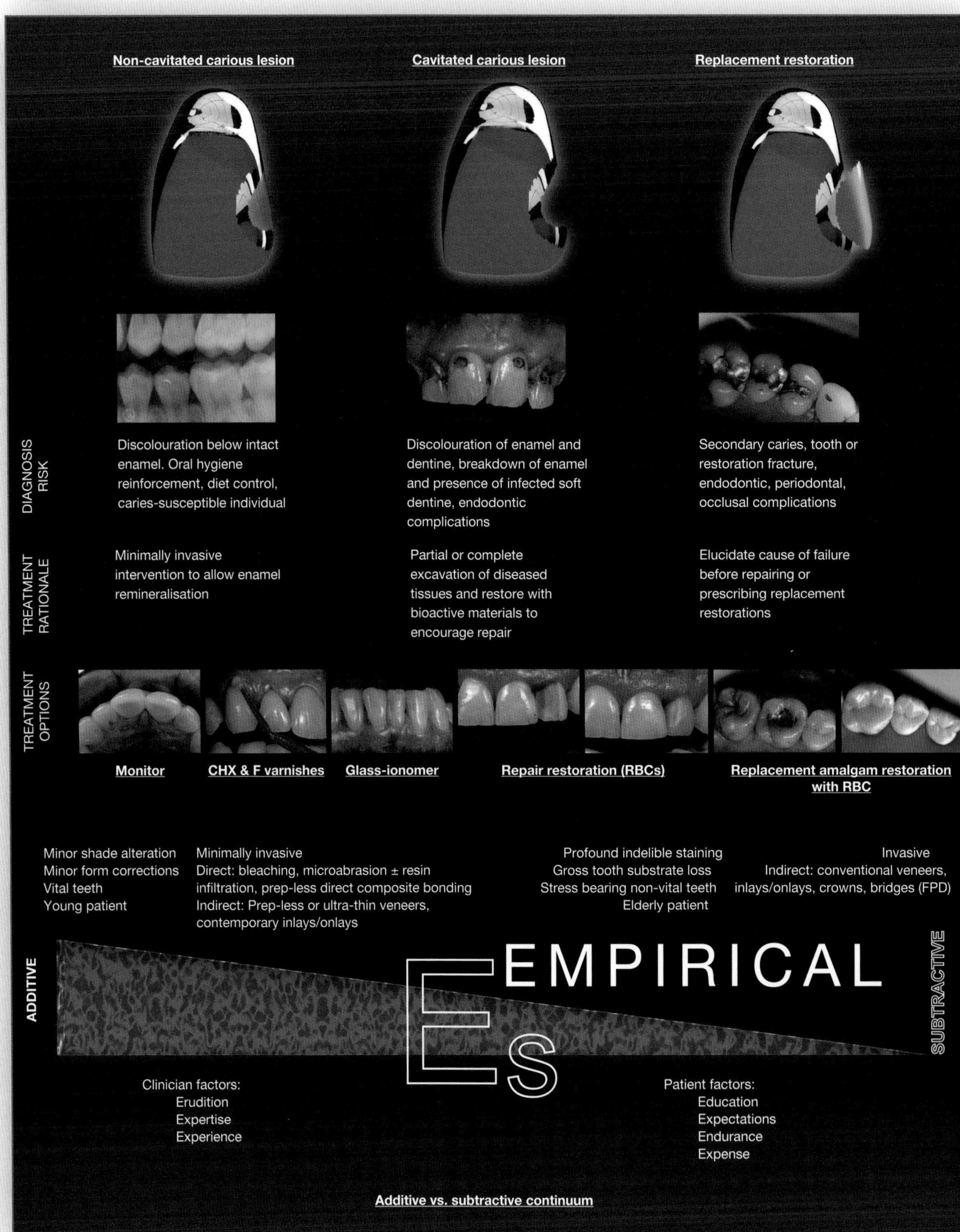

Prosthodontics at a Glance, Second Edition. Irfan Ahmad.

Intracoronal restorations are defined as those **surrounded by one or more natural tooth surface(s)** and can broadly be categorised according to Black's cavity classification; Classes I, II, III, IV and V, and VI. Treatment of intracoronal lesions depends on a variety of factors, and for optimal clinical decision-making, it is necessary to accurately **diagnose** pathology, determine **aetiology**, identify **risk factors** and assess **prognosis** for various treatment options.

Non-cavitated vs. cavitated

A **non-cavitated carious lesion** extending into dentine, with appropriate treatment, has the potential to be arrested by **remineralisation** of the demineralised enamel. However, once cavitation is evident, restorative intervention is necessary to halt progression of the lesion.The factors to consider are:

- **Aetiology** – cariogenic bacteria
- **Clinical presentation** –

Non-cav: discolouration below surface of an unrestored tooth, avoid using sharp probes to prevent piecing the delicate demineralised surface enamel

Cav: fractured and discoloured enamel with underlying carious, discoloured soft dentine, morphology, extent and depth of the lesion depends on the degree of disease progression

- **Symptoms** –

Non-cav: none or sporadic sensitivity

Cav: sensitivity, pain, abscesses

- **Risk assessment** –

Non-cav: patients with poor oral hygiene, inadequate diet control, or individuals with high caries susceptibility requiring restorative intervention

Cav: as above, plus occlusal, endodontic and periodontal complications

- **Treatment options** –

Non-cav: minimally invasive, monitoring for low-risk patients, or restorative intervention for high-risk patients

Cav: minimally invasive (partial or minimal caries excavation and restoration, e.g. atraumatic restorative treatment [ART] technique) or conventional (complete caries excavation and restoration)

- **Type of restoration** –

Non-cav: chlorhexidine (CHX) and fluoride (F) varnishes, fissure sealing (preventive resin restoration – PRR), direct restorations

Cav: direct restorations (using Black's classification to define location of lesions), indirect for larger coronal defects and destruction

- **Choice of restorative materials** –

Non cav: caries infiltration technique, bioactive restorative materials (glass ionomers [GI] or resin-based composite [RBC])

Cav: direct approach using bioactive restorative materials (GI, RBC), amalgam. Indirect approach using ceramics, metal alloys

- **Prognosis/outcome**:

Non-cav:

a. Halted carious lesion with or without remineralisation of enamel – review with periodic application of varnishes and/or fissure sealants

b. Reparative 'healing' with bioactive restorative materials – monitor

c. Progression to cavitated carious lesions – intervention with direct fillings

Cav:

a. As above

d. Tooth or restorative material fractures – cuspal or full coverage

e. Endodontic/periodontal involvement – root canal therapy/periodontal therapy

Replacement restorations

Replacement of failed or defective restorations constitutes about 60% of operative dentistry. Before considering a new restoration, it is essential to elucidate the cause of failure, promote preventive measures and provide an appropriate restoration to prevent future eventualities. The factors to consider for replacement restorations are:

- **Aetiology** – hostile oral conditions such as cariogenic bacteria, occlusal loads, fatigue, temperature changes, aqueous environment, poor clinical technique or incorrect material selection
- **Clinical presentation** – recurrent or secondary caries **(NB, a marginal discrepancy or gap is not necessarily a predictor of secondary caries or disease process)**, fractured tooth or restorative material, poor aesthetics, pulpitis, periapical lesions, periodontal or occlusal complications
- **Symptoms** – pain, abscesses or soft tissue laceration due to sharp edges of fractured teeth/restorations
- **Risk assessment** – assess oral hygiene, diet control, caries susceptibility, endodontic, periodontal and occlusal factors, poor clinical technique
- **Treatment options** – repair vs. replace benefits. For small restorations, a 'like for like' approach may be all that is required, For larger failed restorations, it may be necessary to prescribe an alternative type of restoration, or alternative material, or both
- **Type of restoration** – direct restorations (using Black's classification to define location of lesions), or indirect for large restorations with loss of coronal tissue
- **Choice of restorative material** – bioactive restorative materials (GI and RBC), amalgam, ceramic, metal alloys
- **Prognosis/outcome**:

  a. Reparative 'healing' with bioactive restorative materials – monitor

  b. Tooth or restorative material fractures – indirect inlay

  c. Extensive coronal tissue loss incapable of supporting an intracoronal restoration – extracoronal indirect full coverage

  d. Endodontic/periodontal involvement – root canal therapy/periodontal therapy

Additive vs. subtractive

Before deciding whether to use either a direct or indirect approach, it is also necessary to consider if the procedure is **additive** or **subtractive**. The former involves adding restorative materials to replace diseased or lost dental tissues, while the latter is removing healthy tissues to accommodate artificial restorations. Often the **scientific and clinical rationales are irreconcilable** and decisions based on empirical judgement. However, before resolving this dilemma, it is worth considering the pros and cons of each method and using the **'Es' mnemonic**.

Key points

- The choice of intracoronal restoration depends on accurate diagnosis, aetiology and prognosis.
- Both non-cavitated and cavitated lesions are treated with a minimally invasive approach and periodically monitored.
- It is essential to elucidate the cause of failure before prescribing a replacement restoration.
- Decision making involves either an additive or substrative approach.

37 Choice of extracoronal restorations

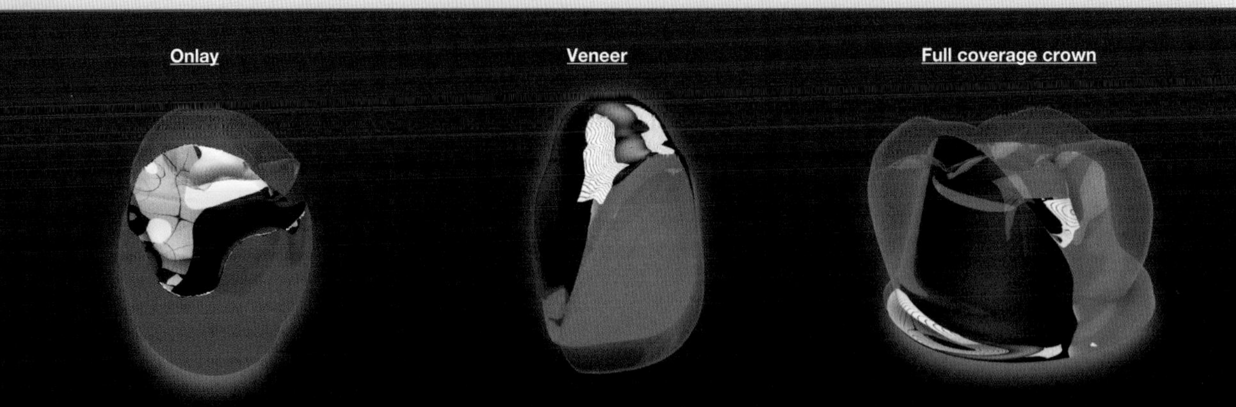

Type of restoration	Survival rate (%)	Period (years)
Inlay and onlays	95	7–10
Porcelain fused to metal (PFM)	> 95	10
Porcelain laminate veneer (PLV)	> 94	12
Leucite-reinforced pressed glass-IPS Empress (anterior single unit)	> 95	11
Leucite-reinforced pressed glass-IPS Empress (posterior single unit)	84	11
Lithium disilicate IPS Empress 2 (anterior and posterior single units)	> 95	5
Glass infiltration - In - Ceram (anterior and posterior single units)	> 98	5
Polycrystalline alumina – Procera (anterior single units)	> 99	7
Polycrystalline alumina – Procera (posterior single units)	> 98	7
Zirconia (multiple unit fixed partial denture [FPD])	74	5

Survival rates of extracoronal restorations

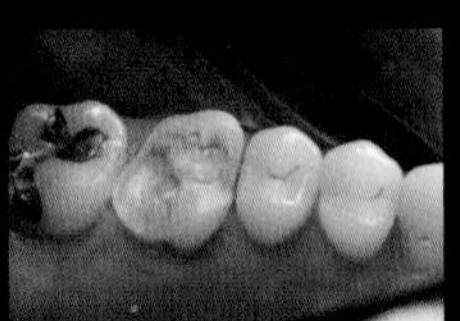

Cavity size

When the width of an intracoronal cavity exceeds 1/2 the distance of the cusp tips, an onlay or crown is advisable

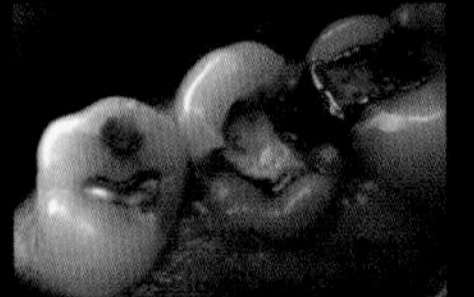

Cracked tooth syndrome

A symptomatic cracked tooth syndrome often required coverage of the offending cracked cusp(s)

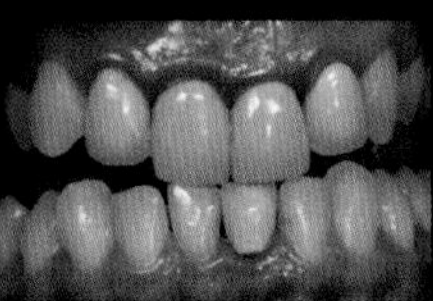

Replacement crown

Defective crowns are a common reason for providing a superior fitting crown to prevent decay and safeguard periodontal health

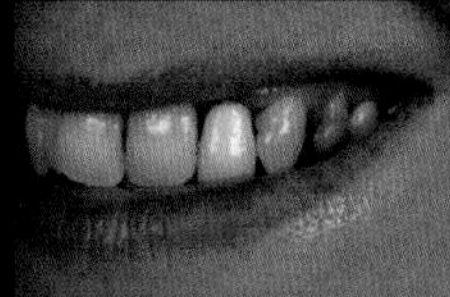

Discoloured cervical margins

Amalgam or metal corrosive byproducts of old restorations can result in unsightly appearance, requiring removal and coverage with an extracoronal restoration

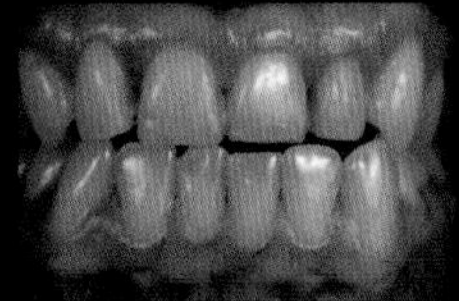

Stained composites

Large, defective, failing, stained composites on anterior teeth are candidates for ceramic PLVs

Prosthodontics at a Glance, Second Edition. Irfan Ahmad.

The **transition between an intracoronal and an extracoronal** restoration is based on the **amount of remaining tooth substrate** following removal of decay and/or existing restorations. If sufficient dentine and enamel are present, an intracoronal restoration (direct or indirect) is the first choice of treatment. With greater tooth loss, reduced retention, coronal destruction and mutilated anatomy, an indirect extracoronal restoration is superior for restoring morphology, function, aesthetics and durability. Essentially, extracoronal restorations are classified as **onlays, veneers** and **full-coverage crowns**. The **distinction between an onlay or veneer and a partial coverage** crown **is nebulous**, and various configurations have been proposed, e.g. ½, ¾, ⅞, etc. depending on the remaining tooth substrate and the type of restorative material used.

Decision-making rationale

Decision-making with informed consent of the patient depends on the following criteria:

- **Minimal intervention** – retaining maximum tooth structure and respecting periodontal, occlusal and pulpal health
- **Tooth integrity** – strength of remaining tooth structure, and performance and durability of the chosen restorative material
- **Clinical feasibility** – access for facilitating preparation, placement, impressions and cementation
- **Prognosis and survival rates** – resistant to wear, occlusal forces, fractures and ease of oral hygiene procedures
- **Aesthetics** – location of tooth in mouth
- **Cost** – dental laboratory fees increases cost compared to a direct approach

Decision making-guidelines

Below are the criteria and indications for indirect restorations:

- **Cavity size** – for posterior teeth with defective restorations, the criteria for replacement depend on the size of the cavity once the restoration and decay are removed. If the occlusal width of the intracoronal preparation is greater than half the distance of the buccal and lingual cusp tips, an extracoronal restoration should be considered. In these circumstances, an onlay or full-coverage crown is necessary to protect the thin cross-section and fragile cusps, and to increase the tooth's resistance to fracture
- **Cracked tooth syndrome** – tooth fracture associated with pain on biting and sensitivity to sugary foods. Diagnosis is by trans-illumination from the buccal or lingual aspects to ascertain the location and depth of the fracture lines(s). Horizontal fracture lines usually result in breakage of the involved cusp. If pain persists, following tooth preparation and temporisation beyond the visible fracture line, endodontic therapy or extraction may be indicated
- **Fractured cusps** – deep apical or subgingival fractures may necessitate endodontic treatment, and/or crown lengthening before crowning
- **Unsupported cusps** – if decay or existing restoration necessitates removal of all supporting dentine, the remaining unsupported enamel should be removed and incorporated into an onlay preparation
- **Endodontically treated teeth** – more susceptible to fractures than vital teeth, since the former **lack proprioceptive response**. The treatment options depend on the size of the access cavity and existing restoration(s). If the access cavity and existing restoration are small, a direct composite is an ideal choice. However, for larger restorations, an onlay, reduced crown, conventional crown or possibly an endocrown (gaining macromechanical retention from the pulp chamber of root-filled posterior teeth) should be considered
- **Parafunctional habits or hard diet** – patients with bruxism or who eat hard food are candidates for cuspal coverage
- **Discoloured cusps** – usually resulting from amalgam leakage byproducts, which are unsightly if visible during a smile may require replacement with an onlay
- **Hemisectioned teeth** – full coverage for splinting to adjacent teeth for stability
- Existing crown requiring replacement due to **fractured porcelain, colour mismatch, defective margins** or **gingival recession**
- **Short clinical crowns** – if the remaining tooth substrate is insufficient for an onlay, full coverage offers better retention
- **Splinting teeth** – mobile teeth can be splinted using crowns, but this is a highly destructive and questionable modality. A less invasive option for symptomatic mobile teeth is splinting with orthodontic wire luted with a resin-based composites (RBCs)
- **Fixed partial denture (FPD)** – either to close a space (questionable for virgin abutment teeth) or to replace a failing FPD
- **Implant-supported crowns** – single and multiple splinted units
- **Elective crowns** – if the patient declines orthodontic treatment to realign teeth, or to mask discolouration for improving aesthetics or to raise the vertical dimension of occlusion (VDO). However, to provide crowns on vital teeth solely for aesthetics is contentious

Survival rates

Inlays and **onlays** can be fabricated from RBCs, ceramics and cast metals. The current trend is to use tooth-coloured restorations, which limits the restorative materials to composites or ceramics. **Unilayered** silica-based ceramics include feldspathic, leucite-reinforced pressed glass or lithium disilicate. Furthermore, the use of CAD/CAM technology has increased the popularity of these indirect restorations. Both inlays and onlays have a **success rate of greater than 95% over 7–10 years,** and bulk fracture of the restoration is cited as the predominant reason for failure. **Porcelain laminate veneers (PLVs)** are usually prescribed for anterior teeth, which require superior aesthetic, but have low structural demands. The most popular materials for PLVs are high glass content silica ceramics that can be adhesively bonded to the underlying tooth structure (preferably enamel). PLVs are extremely successful, with some studies reporting **survival rates after 12 years of greater than 94%**. **Full coverage crown**s can be fabricated using metal, **porcelain fused to metal (PFM)** or all-ceramic (monolithic or porcelain fused to ceramic). The all-ceramic units are usually **bilayered** with a dense ceramic core for strength (e.g. glass infiltrated and polycrystalline alumina or transformation toughened polycrystalline zirconia) and a weaker veneering porcelain (e.g. silica ceramics) for aesthetics. Also, **polychromatic translucent monolithic zirconia** is another option. All-ceramic units on anterior teeth have a higher success rate than on posterior teeth, and the **overall survival rate is comparable to that of PFM crowns.** Once again, the main reason for failure is catastrophic fracture or chipping of the veneering porcelain.

Key points

- Extracoronal indirect restorations are indicated for compromised teeth with reduced tooth substrate.
- Choosing the type of extracoronal restoration depends on the clinical scenario and survival rates.
- The survival rate for indirect ceramic restorations is about 90% over 10 years and is comparable to that of PFM units.

Dental materials

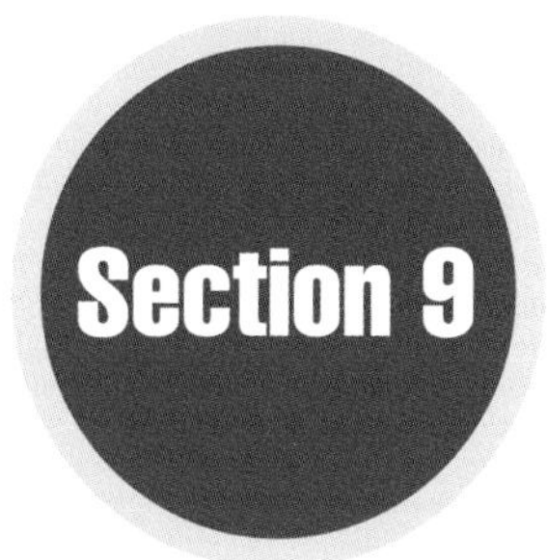

Chapters

38 Materials for direct restorations

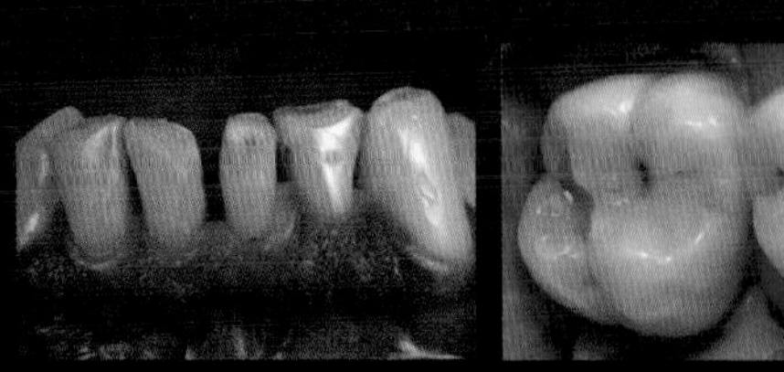

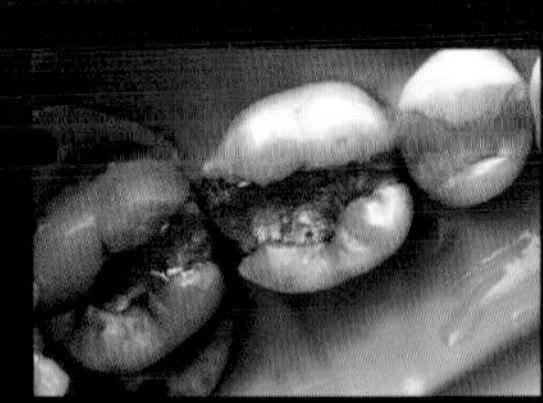

Glass-ionomer: Class V & minimally invasive fillings

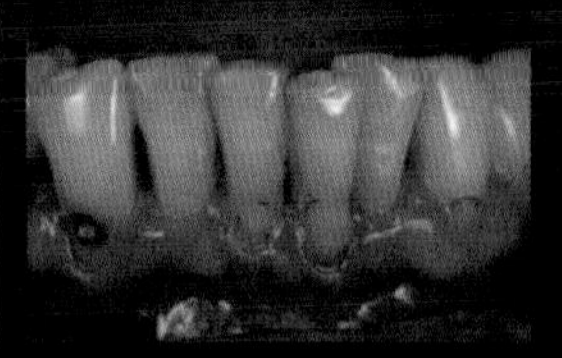

RBCs restorations: defective, stained margins

GLASS IONOMER

Advantages
Indications: pulp capping, linings, fissure sealing, luting cements, Class I and V cavities, fixing orthodontic brackets, atraumatic restorative treatment (ART), fillings in deciduous teeth
Chemical adhesion to enamel & dentine
Bioactivity/anti-cariogenic
Alleviates post-op sensitivity
Several combination materials
Moisture tolerant

Disadvantages
Poor mechanical properties
Unsuitable for load-bearing areas
Water adsorption/crack formation
Inferior aesthetics compared to RBCs

COMPOSITE

Advantages
Indications: pit & fissure sealing, Class I, II, III, IV, V, VI, tunnel cavities, ART, aesthetic masking of discoloured teeth, core build-up, indirect inlays and veneers
Highly aesthetic
Large varieties for varying clinical situations
Minimally invasive cavity preparations
Bond to tooth structure with dental adhesives
Thermal insulators
Acceptable physical and mechanical properties
Reinforce tooth/restoration complex
Light, chemical, dual-cured varieties
Bioactivity

Disadvantages
Polymerisation shrinkage (1–5%) and stresses
Technique sensitive
Microleakage/discolouration/wear/bulk fracture/2° caries/post-op sensitivity/toxicity
Water adsorption/porosity/staining
Increased material costs/longer treatment time

AMALGAM

Advantages
Indications: load bearing areas, core build-up
Established clinical protocols
Long survival rate/durability
Forgiving clinical technique
Micromechanical adhesion with dental adhesives

Disadvantages
Poor aesthetics
Corrosive by-products/galvanic effect
Mercury exposure
Invasive cavities
2° caries

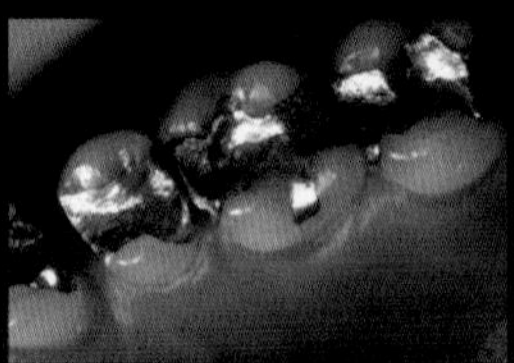

10-year old amalgam fillings

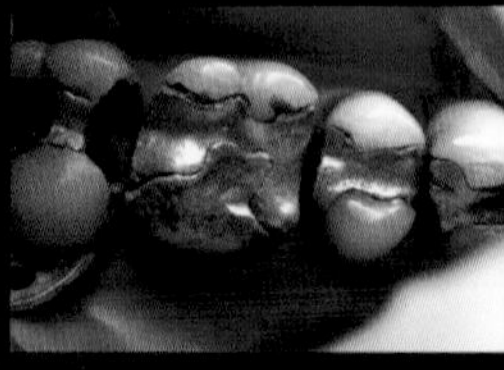

Defective amalgam fillings

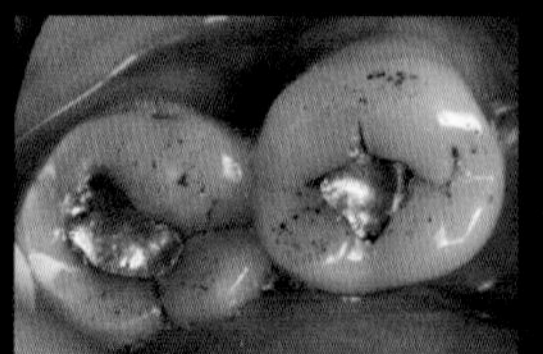

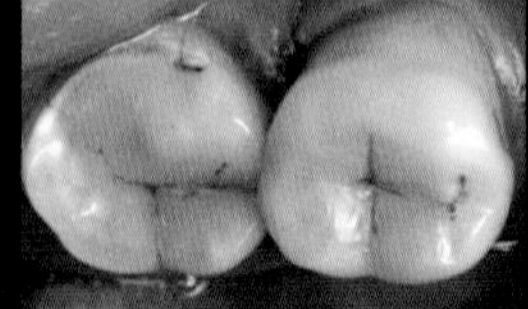

Replacement amalgam fillings with RBCs

Prosthodontics at a Glance, Second Edition. Irfan Ahmad.

Material selection for **intracoronal direct restorations** is a daunting task. At present, there is no material on the market that is a true substitute for dentine and enamel, and a compromise is usually necessary depending on the prevailing clinical situation. **Most intracoronal cavities are restored using a direct technique.** However, inlays are also possible using an indirect technique. The performance and **survival of any direct restoration is multifactorial**, depending on the location of the tooth, type of tooth, restoration design and size, number of surfaces involved, choice of material, operator factors (experience, dexterity and technique) and patient factors (age, attitude to dental care and oral hygiene). Without doubt, **resin-based composite (RBC) fillings** are rapidly becoming the **first choice for direct restorations** and are covered in a dedicated separate chapter.

Palliative dressings

The most popular temporary **palliative dressing** is **zinc oxide eugenol**. Zinc oxide powder is mixed with eugenol liquid to form a condenwsable putty. Care is necessary if the definitive filling is resin-based since **eugenol retards the setting reaction of most RBCs**.

Silver mercury amalgam

The use of **silver mercury amalgam** dates back to the beginning of the last century when **Black** first described his classification of dental cavities. **Dental amalgam** is a mixture of **silver, tin and copper alloy powder** mixed with **mercury**, creating a condensible slurry that solidifies at intra-oral temperature. Amalgam, unlike composites, is a relatively forgiving material, not dependent on stringent clinical protocols. Its use is still widespread, with long survival rates for large direct restorations in posterior, load-bearing teeth. However, recent concerns about **low-level mercury exposure** is scientifically unfounded, but remains contentious for many patients. **Many countries have banned amalgam** use altogether, while others have contraindicated its use in susceptible patients, e.g. females of child-bearing age, immunologically compromised, impaired kidney function, high mercury exposure due to diet (e.g. seafood) or occupation, or suffering from neurological disorders. Other disadvantages include the need to remove excess tooth substrate when creating undercuts (but micromechanical adhesion is possible using dental adhesives), trauma and decay to neighbouring teeth, leaching into enamel/dentine with subsequent tooth discolouration, amalgam tattoos of the oral mucosa and environmental waste concerns. Finally, the **risk/benefit ratio should be assessed before electively replacing amalgam fillings** for more aesthetic alternatives.

Glass ionomers

Glass ionomer (GI) is another popular restorative material. Although the appellation 'glass-ionomer' is predominately used, the **correct terminology** of these acid-based cements is **'glass polyalkenoate cements'.** The ingredients of GIs are a polymeric acid, glasses (alumino-silicate), water, often with fluoride and phosphate additives. The basic reaction is between polymeric acids and powdered glasses, which remain afterwards to reinforce the set material. The physical properties of GIs are influenced by the type of polymer (e.g. homopolymer or copolymer of acrylic acid), concentration of the polyacid, glass particle size, mixing procedure (spatula or auto-mix) and age of the material. For example, high molecular weights increase strength, but also increase viscosity that makes handling difficult for **luting**, but is better suited for **restorative purposes**. Hence, the various formulations of GI display varying degree of initial and delayed compressive strength. The minimum vales of **compressive strength of luting GI cements and restorative GI cements are 70 MPa and 100 MPa, respectively.**

The distinguishing feature of glass ionomers is their **ability to chemically bond to tooth surfaces by chelation of the calcium ions within the hydroxyapatite** with the poly(acrylic)acid in the material. The adhesion is **both micromechanical interlocking and chemical bonding,** with tensile bond strength to enamel higher (2.6–9.6 MPa) than dentine (1.1–4.1 MPa). The failure of GIs is usually **cohesive**, indicating that the bond between the cement and tooth is clinically viable for preventing microleakage.

Other benefits are lowering **post-operative sensitivity, hydrophilic and protection from caries due to F release**, which is accelerated in an acidic environment and **increases pH to buffer the immediate vicinity for neutralising acid from cariogenic bacteria.** The initial F release, or **early burst**, subsides and is followed by lower levels over time. However, the suggested **F recharge is contentious**, since there is a decline in F uptake by GIs as the material matures. In addition, GIs release and take up biologically active ions (fluoride, sodium, phosphate and silicate) that **promote remineralisation.** The high viscosity GI has finer glass particles with anhydrous polyacrylic acids and is intended for use as restorative materials. The **addition of titanium dioxide nanoparticles has shown to have strong antibacterial activity against *Streptococcus mutants*** compared to conventional GIs.

GI combination materials

Several combination materials are available, exploiting the beneficial properties of glass ionomers with other materials. For example, **resin-modified glass ionomers (RMGI)** most closely resemble conventional glass ionomers, while **compomers** (polyacid-modified composite resins) have a closer relationship to composites. **RMGIs contain the HEMA monomer and camphorquinone initiator,** and the setting reaction is both acid–base and photo-polymerisation. HEMA increases strength but has increased hydroscopic expansion, and is less biocompatible due to possible leaching of the monomer. Nano-ionomers, containing nanofillers offer improved aesthetics and polishability. Fibre-reinforced glass ionomer cements have alumina, silica and carbon fibres in an attempt to increase flexural strength and fracture toughness. **Giomers** are resin-based GIs, with enhanced fluoride releasing properties by incorporation of a pre-reacted glass (PRG). **Glass carbomers** were introduced with the potential of enhanced bioactivity by the addition of a hydroxyapatite filler, but tend to be more brittle than GIs.

Key points

- Irrespective of the concerns, amalgam still has good survival rates for large cavities in posterior teeth.
- Although technique sensitive, RBCs are becoming the first choice for direct restorations.
- Glass ionomers offer chemical adhesion to tooth, and are used as luting agents and restorative materials.
- Numerous combination materials are available, exploiting the benefits of GI with other dental restoratives.

Resin-based composites

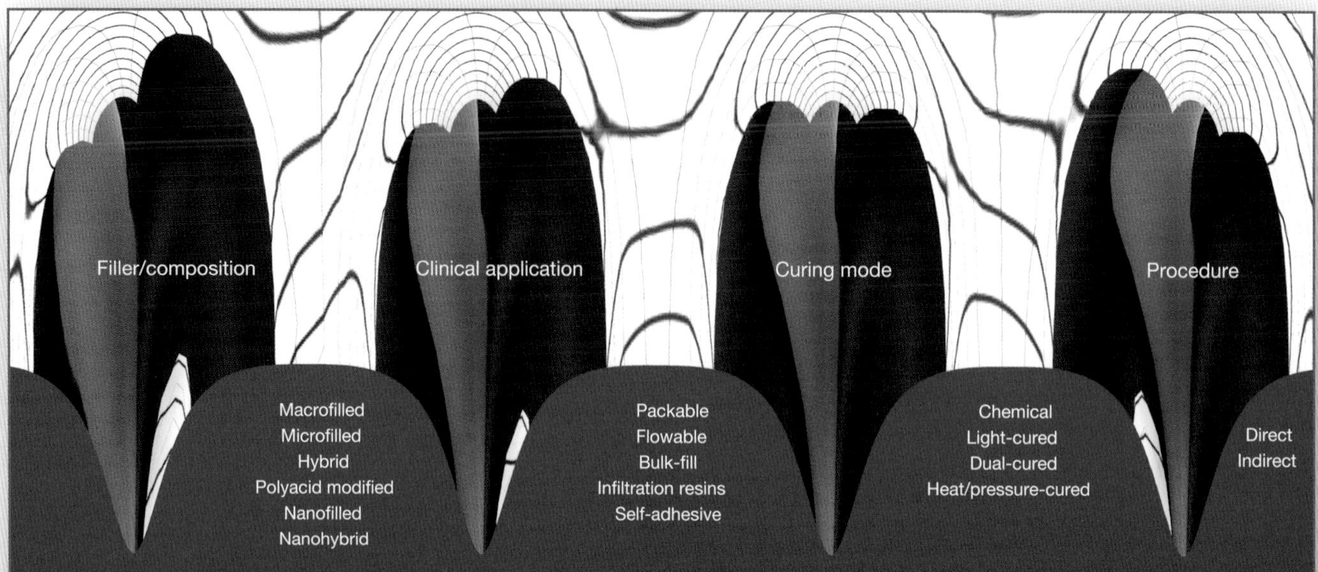

Filler/composition

Macrofilled
Microfilled
Hybrid
Polyacid modified
Nanofilled
Nanohybrid

Clinical application

Packable
Flowable
Bulk-fill
Infiltration resins
Self-adhesive

Curing mode

Chemical
Light-cured
Dual-cured
Heat/pressure-cured

Procedure

Direct
Indirect

Resin-based composite classification

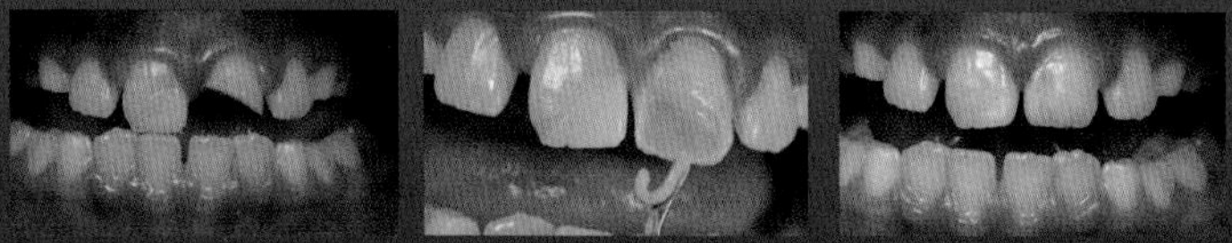

Microfilled composite: incremental layering

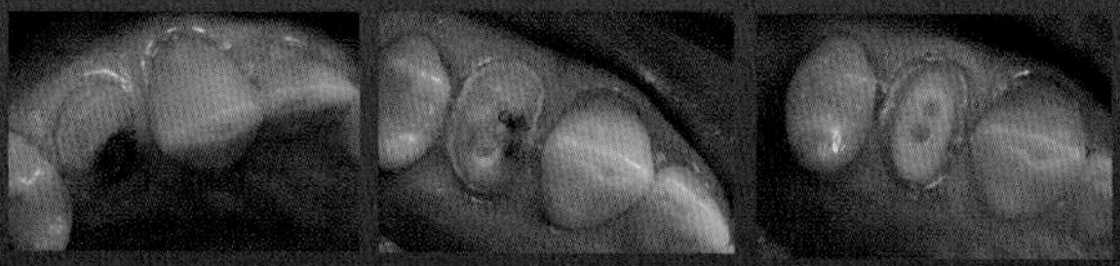

Hybrid composite: core build-up

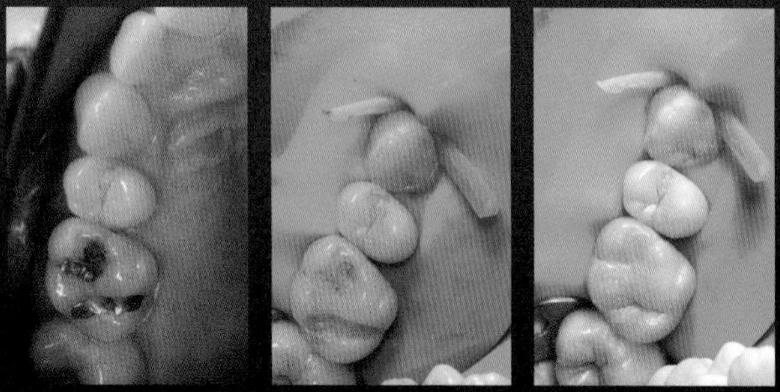

Nanohybrid composite: incremental layering

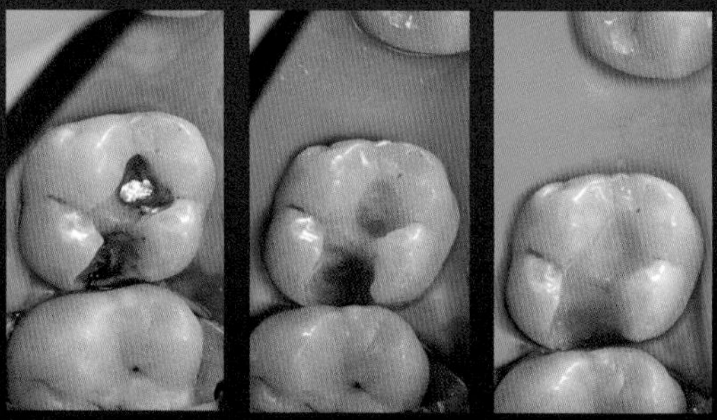

Flowable composite: cavity liner

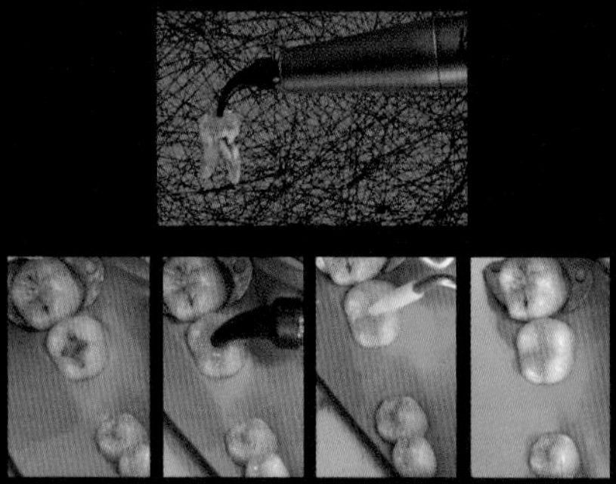

Bulk-fill composite: posterior occlusal filling

Composite	Filler particle size
Macrofilled	10 – 50 μm
Microfilled	40 – 50 nm
Hybrid	10 – 50 μm + 40 – 50 nm
Microhybrid	0.6 – 1 μm + 40 nm
Nanofilled	5 – 100nm
Nanohybrid	5 – 100 nm + 0.6 – 1 μm + 40 nm

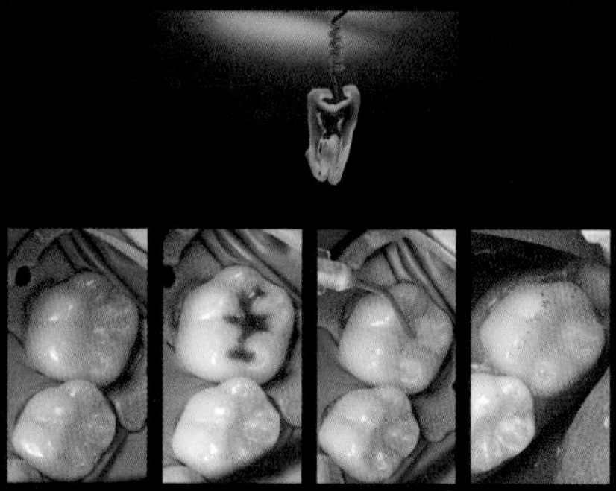

Self-adhesive flowable composite: fissure sealing

RBC according to filler particle size

Prosthodontics at a Glance, Second Edition. Irfan Ahmad.

Resin-based campsites (RBCs) have revolutionised restorative dentistry, and in conjunction with dental adhesives (Chapter 62) represent state-of-the-art materials for direct restorations. Although the indications have expanded, including indirect restorations, RBCs are not flawless. While many deficiencies have been addressed by advances in material science and technology, composites are inherently **bioinert**, **not bioactive** and **replace rather than regenerate** dental hard tissues.

Evolving RBCs

The **main advantages of RBCs are aesthetic appearance** and **preservation of sound tooth** substrate. Since Bowen introduced the **bis-GMA resin** doped with **inorganic fillers** in the 1960s, composites continue to evolve at a rapid pace. The basic constituents of RBCs are an **organic resin oligomer matrix** (bis-GMA, hydroxyethylmethacrylate [HEMA], triethylene glycol dimethacrylate [TEGDM] and urethane dimethacrylate [UDMA]), **inorganic ceramic filler particles**, **coupling agent** (silane, 10-methacryloyloxydecyl dihydrogen phosphate [10-MDP]), visible light **photoinitiators** (camphorquinone/amine system), **stabilisers**, and **pigments** for **shade, fluorescence and opalescence**. Generally, a higher filler content (around 80 wt%) affords superior, mechanical, physical and optical properties, i.e. translucency and opacity for ensuring a correct **translucency parameter** so that filling 'blend' with the surrounding tooth. A recent suggestion is substituting silane with a catecholic coupling agent that provides 10 times greater adhesion, and 50% increase in toughness. The evolution and varieties of RBC are as follows:

- **Packable composites** were introduced to emulate the tactile sensation of placing amalgam, but their durability is questionable.
- **Flowable composites** have a reduced filler content (37–70%), which decreases viscosity and increases flowability, offering superior adaptability to cavity crevices and niches. The improvement in mechanical and optical properties have expanded the applications of flowables to include fit and fissure sealing, stress absorbing liners, relocating deep cervical margins, Class V fillings, injectable resin composite technique, and minimally invasive or preventative resin restorations (atraumatic restorative treatment [ART]).
- **Compomers** (polyacid-modified RBC), a combination of glass ionomer and composites (polyalkenoate acid and glass component), have favourable handling and fluoride release. The drawbacks are long curing times, brittleness, water sorption and poor strength. The main indications are fillings in primary teeth or as liners below stronger overlaying composite.
- **Self-adhesive composites** (compobonds) incorporate a dental adhesive, which is self-etching and/or self-adhesive monomers (10-MDP) to simultaneously condition enamel and dentine. However, the efficacy of adhesion compared to using a separate adhesive is in doubt.
- **Caries infiltration technique** is an approach for remineralising enamel by capillary action for early stage proximal caries and white spot lesions.
- **Bulk-fill composites** provide an alternative method for posterior composite fillings with a single increment rather than successive layers. These flowable materials show excellent adaptation, reduced polymerisation shrinkage, and contain highly light sensitive initiators to cure to a depth of 4–6 mm (e.g. SDR, SonicFill), but the high translucency makes the filling conspicuous.
- **Organically modified ceramics** uses Ormocer® technology with excellent wear resistance, but poor polishability.

Overcoming challenges

The **factors compromising long-term durability** of composites are **material properties, inadequate clinical techniques** and **patient factors. Polymerisation shrinkage** is associated with conversation of the monomer to a polymer and ranges from 1% to 5%. Methods to limit this deleterious effect, including incremental layering to reduce the C-factor, different light curing modes, modifying filler loading, flowable shock absorbing liners or silorane-based composites. Also, the associated stresses are probably more detrimental than volume shrinkage, leading to marginal opening, discolouration, caries, post-operative sensitivity and bulk fractures. **Wear** of the surface of the filling is attributed to abrasion, adhesive affects, and corrosion by acids and fatigue. The **wear resistance** is primarily linked to the resin/filler composition, and to increase wear resistance, several strategies are employed, e.g. spherical fillers and limiting nanofiller loading to 25 wt%, porous and fibrous nanofillers, improving binding of resin to fillers by enhanced silanisation technology or improving polymerisation conversion rates with alternative resins such as bisphenol-S-bis (3-methacrylato-2-hydroxypropyl) ether (bis-SGMA). **Bulk fracture** is influenced by the fracture toughness (K_{IC}), flexural strength and shear bond strength (SBS), i.e. the ability to withstand masticatory shear forces to prevent **adhesive or cohesive fracture**. The K_{IC} is improved by increasing filler loading or reinforcing with silica-fused ceramic whiskers. In general, nanofilled and hybrid varieties have greater K_{IC} compared to microfilled composites. A recent development is the **self-healing composite** that is capable of restitution following fractures.

Recurrent (secondary) caries is major cause of failure, and one approach to overcome this issue is modulating the biofilm with antibacterial and remineralising dental composites. The first option is **incorporating antibacterial agents** for sustained release (releasing composites), e.g. fluoride, chlorhexidine, silver nanoparticles, ZnO nanoparticles or bacteriostatic calcium fluoride nanoparticles against *Streptococcus mutans*. However, the effect is ephemeral and results in porosity and subsequent deterioration of the composite. The second option is incorporating **non-releasing antibacterial, antiviral and antifungal agents** into the resin, e.g. polymerisable quaternary ammonium monomers (QAMs), which act by contact inhibition and are longer lasting than releasing composites. The last option are the **remineralising composites** containing nanoparticles of dicalcium phosphate anhydrous (DCPA) to promote mineralisation. A recently introduced bulk-fill RBC, is alkasite (Cention N – Ivoclar Vivadent, Schaan, Liechtenstein), is anticariogenic (elevates pH to prevent demineralisation), and a shrinkage stress reliever (PEG-400 DMA) to reduce polymerisation stresses. **Post-operative sensitivity** results from **microleakage** caused by polymerisation shrinkage and/or acidic dissolution of the resin matrix. Some solutions to alleviate this unwanted sequelae are placing appropriate linings or using specific bonding agents. The **potential toxicity of composites** is linked to monomer release from uncured resin that is cytotoxic to pulp cells, fibrobalsts and keratinocytes, with possible genotoxicity, tumorigenesis and proliferation of cariogenic bacteria. Furthermore, hypersensitivity to the monomer can elicit anaphylaxis. These issues are counteracted by minimising leaching of uncured monomer, and ensuring its maximum degree of conversion.

Key points

- RBCs are the first choice materials for direct restorations, and development of new varieties has expanded their applications.
- Composites have several issues that require addressing.
- Future RBCs will be bioactive for regeneration rather than repair.

40 Bioactive materials

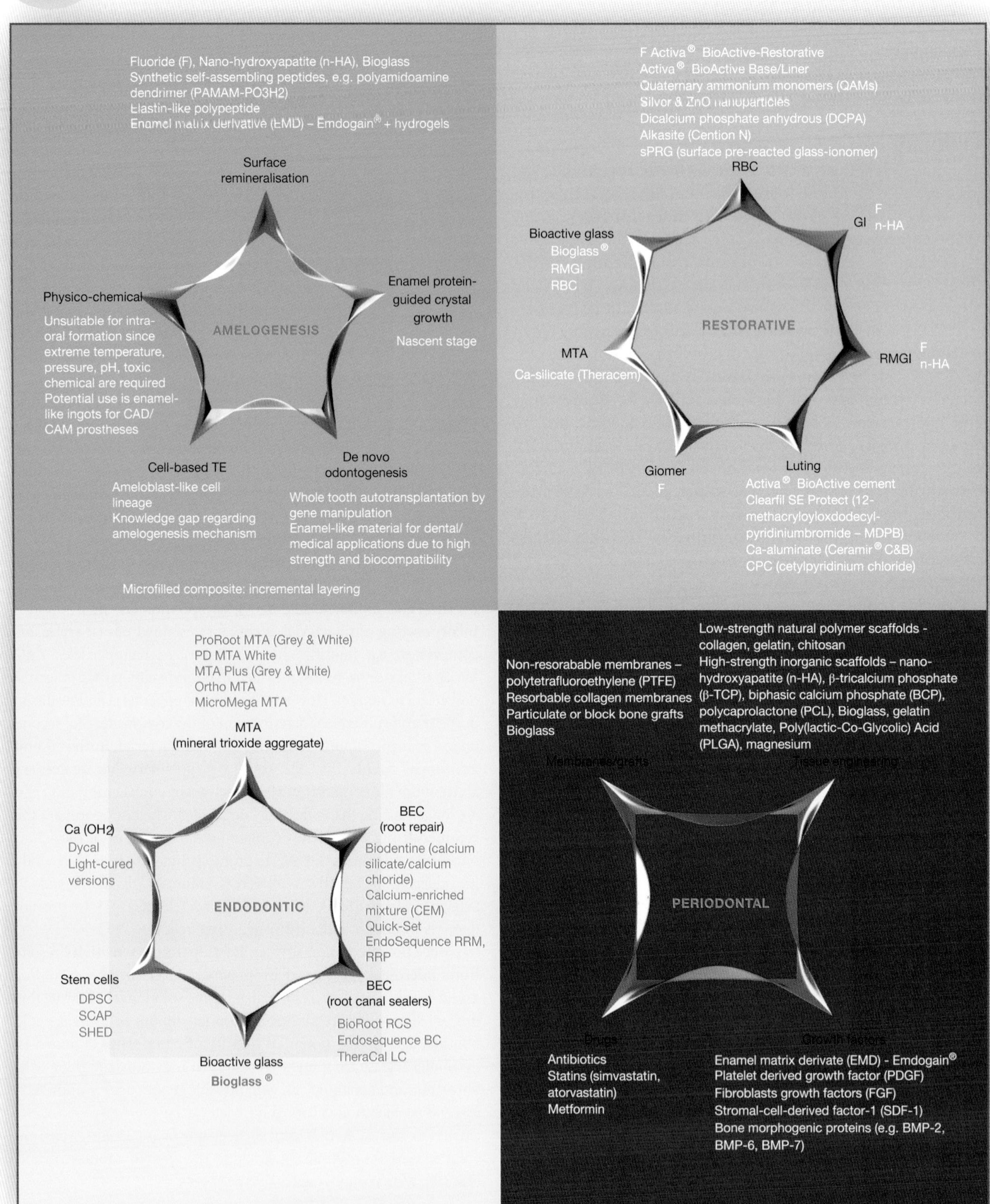

Conventional dental materials are **bioinert**, but the next generation of emerging materials has bioactive properties. A broad definition of **bioactivity** is the ability of a material to interact with or initiate a specific reaction within living tissues. However, in orthopaedics, a bioactive material is one that forms a layer of calcium phosphate apatite. **Bioactive materials regenerate by harnessing and stimulating the innate healing potential of the body**.

Amelogeneis

Amelogenesis is the process by which **ameloblasts secrete enamel proteins** (amelogenin, ameloblastin, enamelin), followed by **apatite biomineralisation** with calcium and phosphate to form parallel, **hydroxyapatite crystals** organised into **enamel prisms.** Several methods are proposed for amelogenesis, but to date, have failed to faithfully reproduce the intricate structure or the physical, mechanical and optical properties of enamel. This is because enamel morphogenesis presents a unique challenge since after its formation, the ameloblasts die to leave an acellular tissue, with little reparative capacity. **Surface remineralisation is a type of in situ tissue engineering (TE)** that has attracted the most attention. Fluoride (F) delivered via drinking water, toothpaste, mouthwashes and restorative materials interacts with enamel to form **fluorapatite** or fluorhydroxyapatites and resists acidic attack from cariogenic bacteria, gastric reflux or dietary products. However, excess amounts of F cause **fluorosis** or mottled enamel. Another material is **nanohydroxyapatite (n-HA)**, composed of 50–1000 nm crystals, is a better source of free Ca, and has the ability to adhere to bacteria, and therefore, modulate the biofilm. Whereas **F acts by combining with enamel to harden its surface, n-HA forms an outer synthetic enamel layer** to protect the surface. Recent formulations of n-HA include zinc carbonate n-HA ($ZnCO_3$/n-HAP) with superior remineralisation compared to F, and provide relief from **dentine hypersensitivity**, especially after bleaching procedures. n-HA (0.25%) added to sport or energising drinks (Powerade®) reduces the rate of erosion and increases **enamel surface microhardness.**

Restorative

A **bioactive restorative material** should interact with the tooth substrate to form a chemical bond and promote remineralisation. Bioactive materials are based organic polymers, metals and ceramics. For example, bioceramics (Ca-phosphates, Ca-aluminates and Ca-silicates) **bond to dental hard tissues** have several applications including cements, fillings, endodontic fillings, sealants, implant surface coatings or bone augmentation constituents. F is the prevalent ion added to restorative materials. **Nanobioceramic-modified cements and luting agents** promote remineralisation by precipitating calcium and phosphate to seal the gap between the tooth and prosthesis for minimising microleakage, e.g. nanostructured Ca-aluminate or MTA-modified Ca-silicate resin cement. Also, n-HA combined with fluorapatite added to glass ionomer cements significantly improves compressive strength and hardness. The **antibacterial monomer MDPB** has been added to dental adhesives (Clearfil SE Protect) to prevent secondary caries, and a novel bioactive composite (Activa®) claims to release greater amounts of F than GI or RMGI, but both require further validation. Lastly, **bioactive glass additives to adhesives and luting cements** encourage formation of **reactionary dentine** to maintain pulp vitality, and **mitigate post-operative sensitivity.**

Endodontic

Dentine and pulp regeneration depends on the size of the lesion and is accomplished by indigenous odontoblast and stem cells, e.g. dental pulp stem cells (DPSCs). The process involves modulating the Wnt/β-catenin signalling pathways that activate odontoblasts. The first material for direct or indirect pulp capping, pulpotomy and **apexification** was $Ca(OH)_2$, which elevates surrounding pH to 12, stimulates growth factors in dentine collagen to form **reactionary dentine** if the pulp is intact or **reparative dentine** if there is pulpal exposure. Mineral trioxide aggregate (MTA) works in a similar fashion, since its bioactive component is $Ca(OH)_2$, but has the added benefit of sealing dentine, releasing calcium phosphate, with reported less root fractures following apexification compared to $Ca(OH)_2$. MTA is also used for revitalisation procedures with DPSCs and intracanal tri-antibiotic paste. **Bioactive endodontic cements (BECs)** are modified MTA formulations with improved performance to overcome shortcomings of MTA, and have expanded applications of repairing furcation perforations, and resolving root absorption, e.g. Biodentine, which promotes mineralisation on contact with DPSCs, but does not cause proliferation of DPSCs. Bioglass® (calcium sodium phosphosilicate glass) forms a hydroxy-carbonated apatite layer and is ideal for pulp capping. In addition, modified BEC formulations, often with addition of zirconium oxide, are used as root canal sealers. If the diagnosis is irreversible pulpitis, pulpectomy is followed by either a root filling or de **novo regeneration/revitalisation of the pulp.** The latter is using DPSCs, **stem cells from human exfoliated deciduous teeth (SHED)** or **stem cells of the apical papilla (SCAP)** seeded onto a TE scaffold, which are inserted into the cleansed root canal(s) (Chapter 75).

Periodontal

Periodontal regeneration of cementum, periodontal ligament (PDL) and alveolar bone focuses on proliferation of cementoblasts, fibroblasts and osteoblasts. The main strategies are **GTR** (guided tissue regeneration), **GBR** (guided bone regeneration) and **TE** accomplished by barrier membranes and bone grafts to prevent apical migration of epithelium and facilitate growth of the PDL and alveolar bone. The membranes are a composite of natural and synthetic biomaterials, multilayered, and carriers of antibacterial and bioactive molecules. TE uses low-strength natural polymers for PDL regeneration, and high-strength inorganic materials for cementum and alveolar bone regeneration. In addition, **biomimetic nanofibrous multilayer scaffolds** are effective for creating an **extracellular matrix microenvironment**, and combine several biomaterials for synergistic effect for simultaneously growing different tissues of the periodontium. **n-HA** is biocompatible, osteoconductive, anti-inflammatory, **chemically bond to bone** and used for **periodontal and cranio-maxillofacial surgery and enhancing osseointegration**. The function of **drugs** and **growth factors** is antimicrobial, altering the disease process, and initiating signalling pathways for **stimulating innate regenerative capacity of the tissues.** The key challenges for periodontium regeneration are a knowledge gap of the formation of these complex structures, the precise concentration/dose and timing of drug/growth factor delivery, regeneration of Sharpey's fibres and incorporating **mechanical cues** in **biomaterial designs**.

Key points

- Bioactive materials interact with, and initiate regeneration of tissues.
- Enamel remineralisation is achieved with F and bioceramics.
- Periodontal regeneration is by membranes, grafts, TE, growth factors and drugs.

Materials for indirect restorations

Ceramic veneer

CERAMICS

Advantages
- Highly aesthetic
- Wide choice of materials with varying properties
- Indicated for substructures (core) and veneering
- Biocompatible
- Low thermal conductivity - less post-op sensitivity

Disadvantages
- Brittle, likely to fracture, depends on type of bond to underlying substructure or tooth
- Minimum thickness necessary for durability
- Opposing tooth wear

TITANIUM

Advantages
- Highly biocompatible
- Corrosion resistance
- High strength and rigidity
- Low density and weight
- Withstands large temperature fluctuations
- Lightweight prostheses
- Laser welding of multiple units
- CAD/CAM technology for milling/3D printing frameworks

Disadvantages
- High casting shrinkage
- Technique-sensitive dental laboratory protocols
- Expensive processing equipment

Cast gold inlay

CAD/CAM Ti framework

CAST ALLOYS

Advantages
- Long-term successful clinical history
- Established clinical and laboratory protocols
- High strength and resistance to fracture
- Versatility for fabricating a variety of indirect restorations
- Ability to fuse porcelain on metal substructure
- Choice of strengths for varying occlusal demands
- Ideal for long-span FPD on both natural and implant-supported abutments
- Ability to solder units, e.g. post-ceramic soldering
- Enhanced micromechanical adhesion with resin cements
- Reduced opposing tooth wear

Disadvantages
- Poorer aesthetics compared to all-ceramic units
- Corrosion by-products
- Allergic reactions to base metals
- Poor insulators, resulting in transient sensitivity to temperature
- Greater plaque accumulation compared to glazed porcelain margins

RBCs

Advantages
- Improved aesthetic and mechanical properties compared to directly placed composites
- Tight interproximal contacts
- Excellent anatomical form
- Precise marginal integrity
- Improved surface texture
- Reduced opposing tooth wear
- Similar thermal expansion as natural tooth
- Fibre reinforcement for increased strength
- Good insulators
- Reduced cost compared to cast metals and titanium

Disadvantages
- Increased cost compared to direct restorations
- Technique-sensitive, adhesive luting protocol
- Weaker materials compared to cast metals and titanium

Indirect RBC inlays

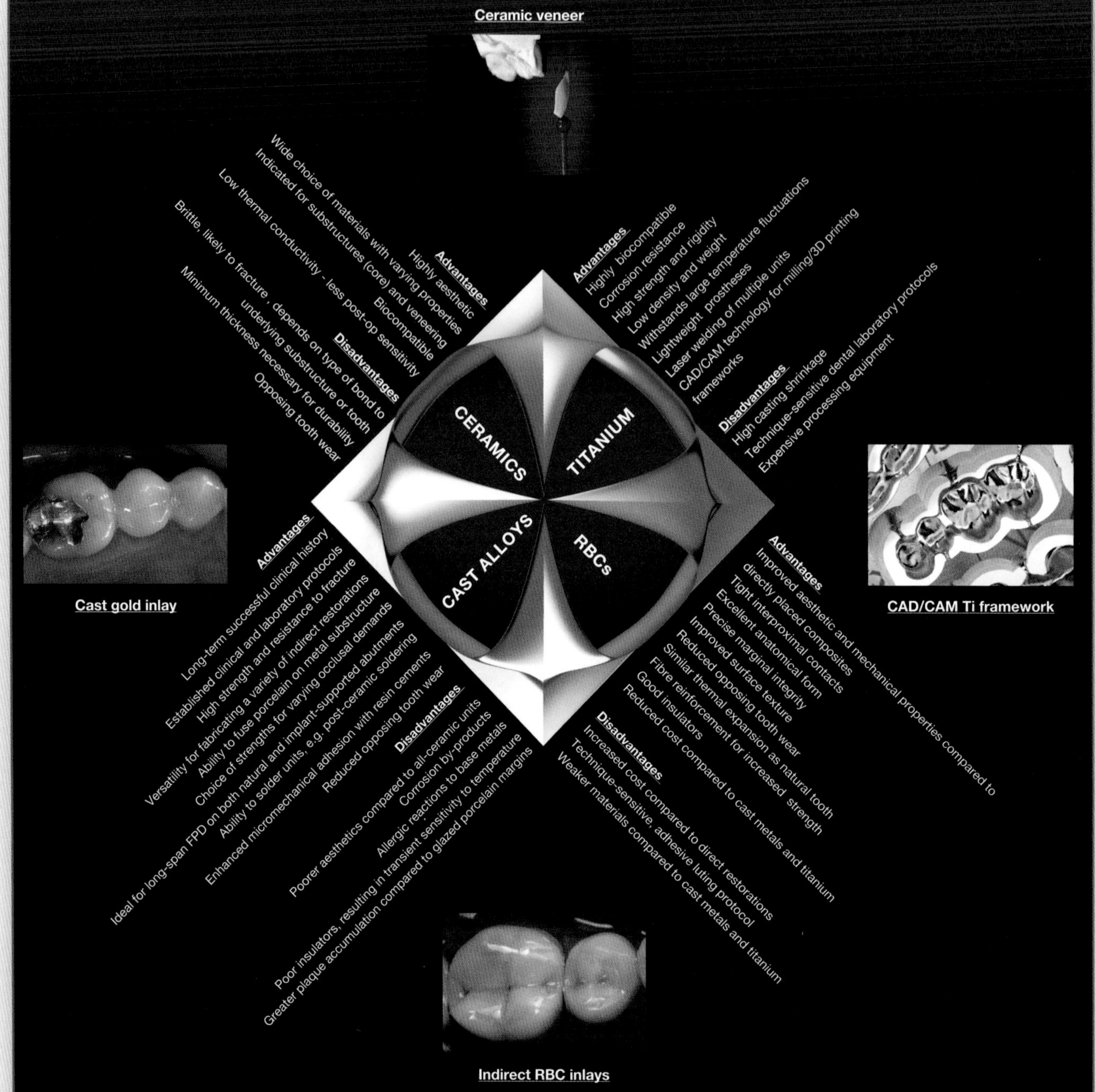

Substrate	Enamel	Dentine	Alveolar cortical bone	Alveolar trabecular bone	RBC filling material	Resin-based cement	Veneering fluorapetite porcelain	Lithium disilicate core	Al_2O_3 (Procera)	Zirconia core	Ti-6Al-4V (Grade 5)	Cast gold alloys
MOE–E (GPa)	73	19	14	1.4	20	9	67	102	300	210	120	80–100

Compassion of modulus of elasticity (MOE)

The **materials for definitive indirect restorations** include **ceramics, titanium, resin-based composites (RBCs)** and **cast alloys.** Traditionally, metal alloys were the ideal choice for indirect restorations, but recent material advances are rapidly changing this paradigm, making composites and ceramics (discussed in the next chapter) formidable contenders for clinical suitability and durability. The **success and longevity of any restorative materials** depends on:

- **Patient factors** – oral hygiene, patient constitution and medical history
- **Material properties** – strength, wear, biocompatibility, marginal integrity, physical and chromatic stability, resilience for resisting occlusal forces and retaining anatomical form and prevention of secondary caries
- **Clinical technique** – material manipulation, placement and maintenance

Strength of restorative materials

Ideally, a restorative material should mimic the physical, mechanical and optical properties of the tissue it is replacing. The **modulus of elasticity (MOE)**, or Young's modulus, plays a pivotal role in determining the success or failure of a material, and the surrounding or underlying natural tooth substrate. Restorative materials with **similar MOE to dentine,** such as RBCs, absorb stresses, allowing dissipation by dentine, the periodontal ligament and surrounding alveolar bone. Conversely, **rigid materials with an MOE similar to enamel,** such as ceramics, are more stress-resistant and transfer forces to the weaker material, i.e. dentine, making the tooth more susceptible to root fracture.

Titanium

Titanium (Ti) and **titanium alloys** are well established in the aerospace industry due to their favourable mechanical and physical properties. Titanium is mined as an oxide, but is refined to a metallic state using the **Kroll process.** Ti is available in **four grades** of pure titanium and three grades of titanium alloys containing traces of aluminium, copper, niobium vanadium, iron and gold (20–30%). Its strength, rigidity and ductility are similar to that of other casting alloys used in dentistry. Pure titanium lacks strength for dental prostheses, and is difficult to machine and polish, especially with CAD/CAM processes. The most popular type for manufacturing dental implants and **implant**-retained superstructures is **Ti-6Al-4V.** Ti is a highly reactive material that readily forms a **passive oxide (TiO_2) film (layer) on its surface when exposed to oxygen.** The bioinert TiO_2 passivation film protects the metal surface and confers **anticorrosive** properties, and **allows bonding of fused porcelain or polymers** for tooth-coloured restorations. In addition, the **implant surface** can be sprayed with apatite coatings for enhancing osseointegration. The passivating oxide layer is also advantageous for forming a soft tissue attachment around Ti abutments. However, in an aerobic environment, due to peri-implantitis, the passive film is degraded leading to Ti corrosion.

Developments in processing methods, such as lost-wax casting, **CAD/CAM milling, 3D printing and electric discharge machining,** have expanded its application in dentistry for crowns and partial denture frameworks for implant-supported prostheses. This is a promising development for the future, and titanium could challenge or replace conventional noble and base metal alloys for indirect restorations, especially using CAD/CAM fabrication.

Resin-based composites

The drawbacks of direct composite restorations include poor wear resistance, chromatic instability, water adsorption and marginal discrepancies. Most of these problems are due to **polymerisation shrinkage, stresses** within the materials and techniques for placement and polishing. To overcome these deficiencies and improve clinical performance, **indirect composite restorations** have been developed. The main difference between direct and indirect composites is the method of polymerisation. With the former, photoactivation is used intra-orally to initiate the setting reaction. In the latter, special ovens are used to **set the material by light, heat (>100°C) and pressure (>150 MPa) in a vacuum,** which **increases the degree of conversion to 98% (compared to 50–70% for direct composites),** hardness and reduces porosity. Indirect processing **improves colour stability and mechanical properties** of the composite such as hardness, tensile strength and flexural strength, and reduces the stresses of polymerisation shrinkage. Furthermore, extra-oral shaping of the restoration allows better proximal contacts and occlusal morphology. Indications for indirect RBC restorations include inlays, onlays, veneers, crowns and fibre-reinforced FPDs, especially for patients who refuse intra-oral metal or have **parafunctional activity**. In addition, **composite ingots** are available for milling a variety of **CAD/CAM restorations.** However, due to the relative low strength of composites, careful occlusal assessment is essential.

Cast metal alloys

The most frequently used cast metals in dentistry are high noble content gold alloys, which are classified as follows:

- Type I – low strength, for small inlays and intraradicular posts
- Type II – medium strength, for large inlays and onlays
- Type III – high strength, for full-coverage crowns and fixed partial dentures (FPDs)
- Type IV – extra high strength, for full-coverage crowns, FPDs and removable denture frameworks

The nobility of dental casting alloys usually depends on the **gold content**, which ranges from **60% to 75%.** For increasing strength, the amount of gold decreases and is replaced by other metals such as silver, copper, platinum, palladium and zinc. **While hardness, MOE and tensile strength increase with decreasing gold content, resistance to corrosion also decreases.** Recent concern about palladium allergy, especially among nickel allergy sufferers, has led to doubts about the use of palladium in dental prostheses. Base metal alloys containing non-noble metals such as nickel, cobalt and chromium exhibit high strength (especially in thin cross-sections), lighter in weight and are indicated for crowns, FPDs and RPD frameworks. The disadvantages include allergy to nickel, greater rigidity compared to noble alloys and therefore, possible fracture of the veneering porcelain in long-span bridges. Furthermore, adjustments to the metal substructure are more difficult.

Key points

- The success of indirect restorations depends on patient, material and operator factors.
- The choice of material depends on specific clinical needs and patient preferences.
- Popular materials include ceramics, titanium, RBCs and cast alloys.

42 Ceramics

Ceramic	Proprietary product	Fabrication	Indication	Etchable
Feldspathic	IPS Empress Esthetic, IPS Empress CAD, Vitadur, Vita VMK 68, Vitablocs Mark II	Platinum oil, refractory die, press, CAD/CAM, layering	PLV, inlay, onlay, layering metal & ceramic substructures	Yes
Fluorapatite leucite	IPS d.sign, Noritake EX-3, Vita VM7, IPS e.max Ceram	Refractory die, press, layering	PLV, inlay, onlay, ant. full crown layering ceramic substructures (e.g. IPS e-max LS_2 or IPS e-max ZirCAD)	Yes
Lithium disilicate (LS_2)	IPS e.max (LS_2), IPS e.am Press, Suprinity, Celtra Duo, Obsidian	Press, CAD/CAM	Ceramic substructure, PLV, inlay, onlay, ant. & post. full crowns, ant. FPD, resin bonded bridges, implant abutment	Yes
Glass-infiltarted	In-Ceram, In-Ceram Spinell, In-Ceram Zirconia	Slip-cast, CAD/CAM	Ceramic substructure, ant. & post. crowns, ant. & post. 3-unit FPD	No
Alumina	Procera AllCeram	Sintering	Ceramic substructure, PLV ant. & post. crown, ant. 3-unit FPD	No
Stabilised zirconia	NobelProcera Zirconia, Cerec Zirconia, Zirkon, Lava, In-Ceram YZ, Cercon, IPS e.max ZirCAD, Zenostar, Katana Zirconia ML, BruxZir Now, Prettau Zirconia, Zirlux FC2, Lava Esthetic	CAD/CAM	Ceramic substructure, ant. & post. crown, FPDs, implant abutments and superstructures	No
ZTA & ATZ	Densilox implants	CAD/CAM	Ceramic substructure, ant. & post. crown, FPDs, implant abutments and superstructures, ceramic implant fixtures	No
Resin ceramics (PICN)	Lava Ultimate, Shofu Block HC, MZ100 Block, CAMouflage Now, Cerasmart, Enamic	CAD/CAM	PLV, inlay, onlay, ant. & post. full crowns, implant abutments	Yes (glass ceramic variety)

PLV – porcelain laminate veneer, ant. – anterior, post. – posterior, FPD – fixed partial denture, CAD/CAM – computer-aided design/computer-assisted manufacture

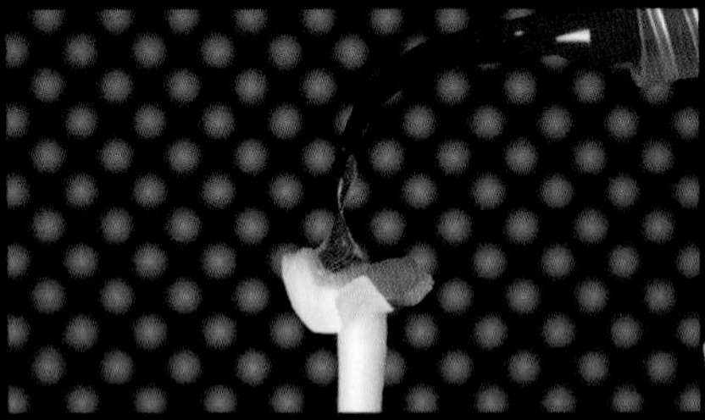

Etching intaglio surface of ceramic inlay with HF acid

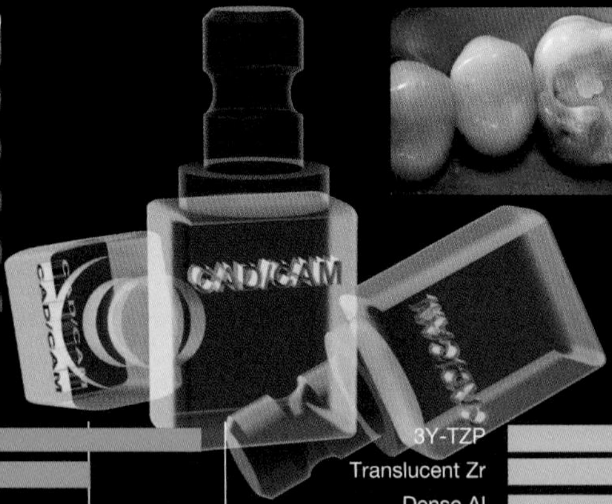

CAD/CAM

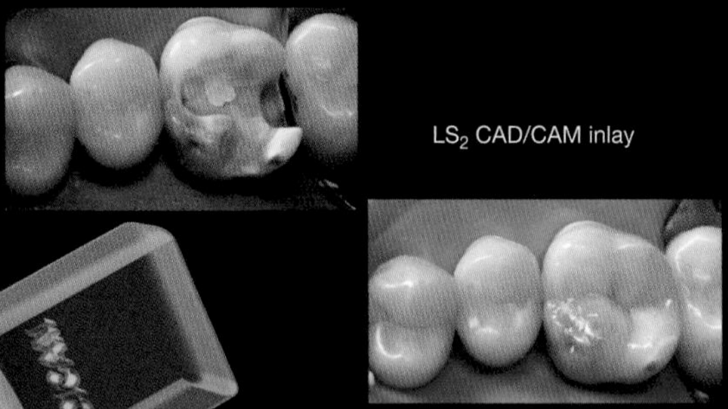

LS_2 CAD/CAM inlay

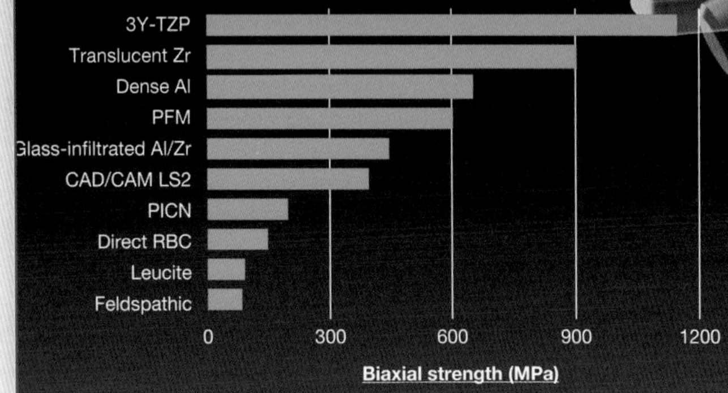

Biaxial strength (MPa): 3Y-TZP, Translucent Zr, Dense Al, PFM, Glass-infiltrated Al/Zr, CAD/CAM LS2, PICN, Direct RBC, Leucite, Feldspathic (axis 0, 300, 600, 900, 1200)

Fracture toughness (KIC) – $MPa.m^{-½}$: 3Y-TZP, Translucent Zr, Dense Al, PFM (veneer), Glass-infiltrated Al/Zr, CAD/CAM LS2, PICN, Direct RBC, Leucite, Feldspathic (axis 0, 1.75, 3.5, 5.25, 7)

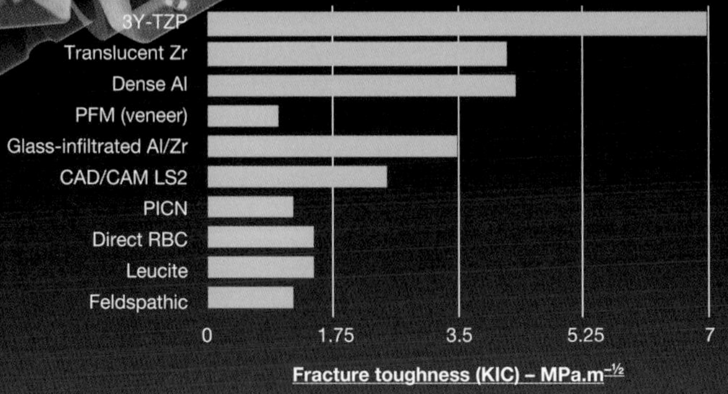

Prosthodontics at a Glance, Second Edition. Irfan Ahmad.

Ceramics are a significant class of indirect restorative materials that are revolutionising contemporary dentistry due to their life-like appearance, and integration into the evolving **dental digital workflow**.

Overview

There are two types of ceramic restorations: first, a **unilayer (monolithic or full-contour)** restoration that is entirely composed of ceramic and gain support from the underlying tooth substrate or is inherently strong. The second, **bilayer** restorations with a high-strength substructure (metal or ceramic) to support a weaker veneering (or layering) porcelain. The recent developments in digital dentistry of **intra-oral scanners** and **CAD/CAM systems** are replacing many traditional methods using labside or chairside milling machines.

Ceramics are inherently brittle materials and susceptible to fracture. Microscopic imperfections within the material are termed **Griffith flaws**, which grow into cracks, and if unimpeded, lead to **catastrophic fracture** of the ceramic. The cracks are propagated by the hostile oral environment: **dynamic (occlusal forces), humid (stress corrosion)** and time-dependent **static fatigue**. Many strengthening mechanisms are used for halting fracture propagation including reinforcement and **infiltration with glasses** as well as **phase transformation toughening**. Preventing fractures not only depends on material properties but also adopting proper laboratory and clinical procedures. Most types of ceramics are available as **cuboid blocks (ingots)** or **blank discs** for use in **milling CAD/CAM** devices. The advantage of using premanufactured ingots is that the industrial process is controlled and repeatable, thus avoiding manual processing errors of **powder/liquid** build-up or hot-**pressing methods**. This improves the properties of the ceramic, e.g. a feldspathic ceramic ingot has a flexural strength of 130 MPa, twice that of conventional layered feldspathic porcelain. As a general comment, ceramics with **high glass phases have superior aesthetics (more translucent) but poor strength**, while those composed of **high crystal phases offer better mechanical properties but poorer aesthetics (more opaque).** Also, some ceramics cause pronounced antagonists tooth wear that is circumvented by selecting the appropriate ceramic, and careful occlusal assessment.

Several **classifications** are proposed to categorise ceramics depending on material composition (type of matrix and filler), aesthetics, strengthening process, method of fabrication (manual or CAD/CAM) manufacturing process (powder/liquid or ingots), etc. The classification below is based on the one proposed by Gracis et al.

Glass–matrix ceramics

The three sub-divisions of **glass ceramics** are **feldspathic, synthetic** and **glass infiltrated**. The feldspathic variety are particle reinforced glasses and used for monolithic, highly aesthetic restorations or layering metal or ceramic substructures. The synthetics are divided into **leucite based** and **lithium dilsilicates (LS_2)**. The composition includes silicon, potassium, sodium and aluminum oxides combined with leucite and other metals to increase strength, especially for substructures. LS_2 ingots are available as a **blue state** to expedite machining, and sintered afterwards to increase strength. The last category is glass-infiltrated materials with **alumina** (In-Ceram), **alumina plus magnesium** (In-Ceram Spinell) and **alumina with zirconia** (In-Ceram Zirconia). However, their use has declined due to the dominance of LS_2 ceramics.

Polycrystalline ceramics

The defining feature of **polycrystalline ceramics** is fine particles that endow strength, but reduced translucency due to limited amounts or absence of glass. The **highly sintered alumina** (Procera AllCeram) has no glass and high strength, but the high MOE (>300 GPa) predisposes to fracture and has made its applications less attractive. **Zirconia is available in three phases** (monoclinic, tetragonal and cubic). Its properties are determined by the amount of fillers, e.g. calcia, magnesia, **yttria** (Y_2O_3) and ceria. The weaker cubic version (<600 MPa) has >5 mol% yttria and is fully stable at room temperature, while the stronger tetragonal phase has 3 mol% yttria (3Y-TZP), >900 MPa, but is partially stable. Increasing the amount of yttria and reducing the alumina content to 0.05%, makes the cubic phase more translucent and is ideal for monolithic aesthetic restorations. However, the drawbacks are lower flexural strength and increased brittleness. An infiltrated variety is also available, In-Ceram® Zirconia. **Zirconia restorations are exclusively fabricated using CAD/CAM ingots** either in the **fully sintered state** or the **green state** that is sintering after milling. Another development is adding alumina to the partially stabilised tetragonal zirconia phase. Two varieties are available, **zirconia-toughened alumina (ZTA)** and **alumina-toughened zirconia (ATZ)**, the difference being the amount of the two constituents. Besides CAD/CAM fabrication, the possibilities of this type of zirconia are manufacturing all-ceramic dental implant fixtures.

Resin–matrix ceramics

These classes of materials contain a resin–matrix polymer that is infiltrated with inorganic glasses or ceramics (greater than 50% by weight), and often referred to as **polymer-infiltrated ceramic networks (PICN).** These materials are exclusively available as ingots for fabricating monolithic CAD/CAM restorations. The advantage of resin–matrix ceramics is that the **MOE is similar to dentine**, the ingots are easily machinable, little or no post-processing is necessary, and intra-oral repair is straightforward using direct RBCs. The ceramic phase can be a combination of silica and zirconia (Lava Ultimate, Shofu Block HC, MZ100 Block), or feldspathic (Enamic®), with a polymer matrix of bis-GMA, urethane dimethacrylate (UDMA) or triethylene glycol dimethacrylate (TEGDMA).

Metal ceramics

Although ceramics are rapidly superseding porcelain fused to metal (PFM) restorations, the latter still have a place in prosthodontics. PFM restorations have over 70 years history of clinical success, and [illegible] versatility for fabricating single and multiple units on both natural teeth and implant abutments. In addition, they have established clinical and laboratory protocols, with survival rates greater than 95% over a 10-year period, and are often used as a benchmark for assessing newer types of all-ceramic restorations. The major disadvantage is poor aesthetics, particularly greying at the cervical margins due to visibility of the metal substructure or 'shine' through thin periodontal biotypes.

Key points

- Dental ceramics are driven by aesthetics and integration into a digital workflow.
- Ceramics are classified as glass-matrix, polycrystalline or resin-matrix.
- Ceramics are indicted for all types of indirect restorations, including implant supported abutments and superstructures.

Lasers

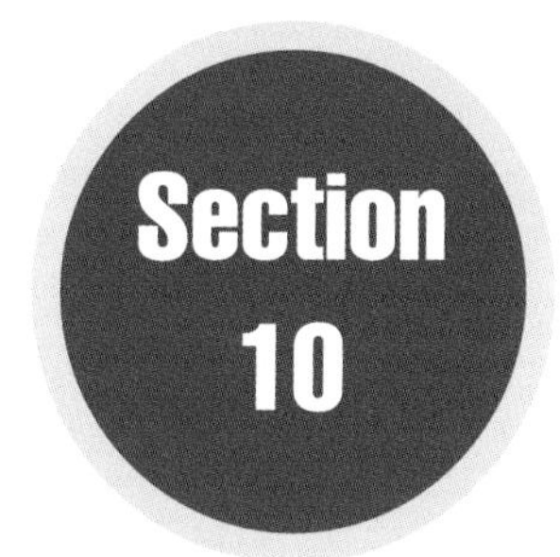

Chapters

43 Lasers 1

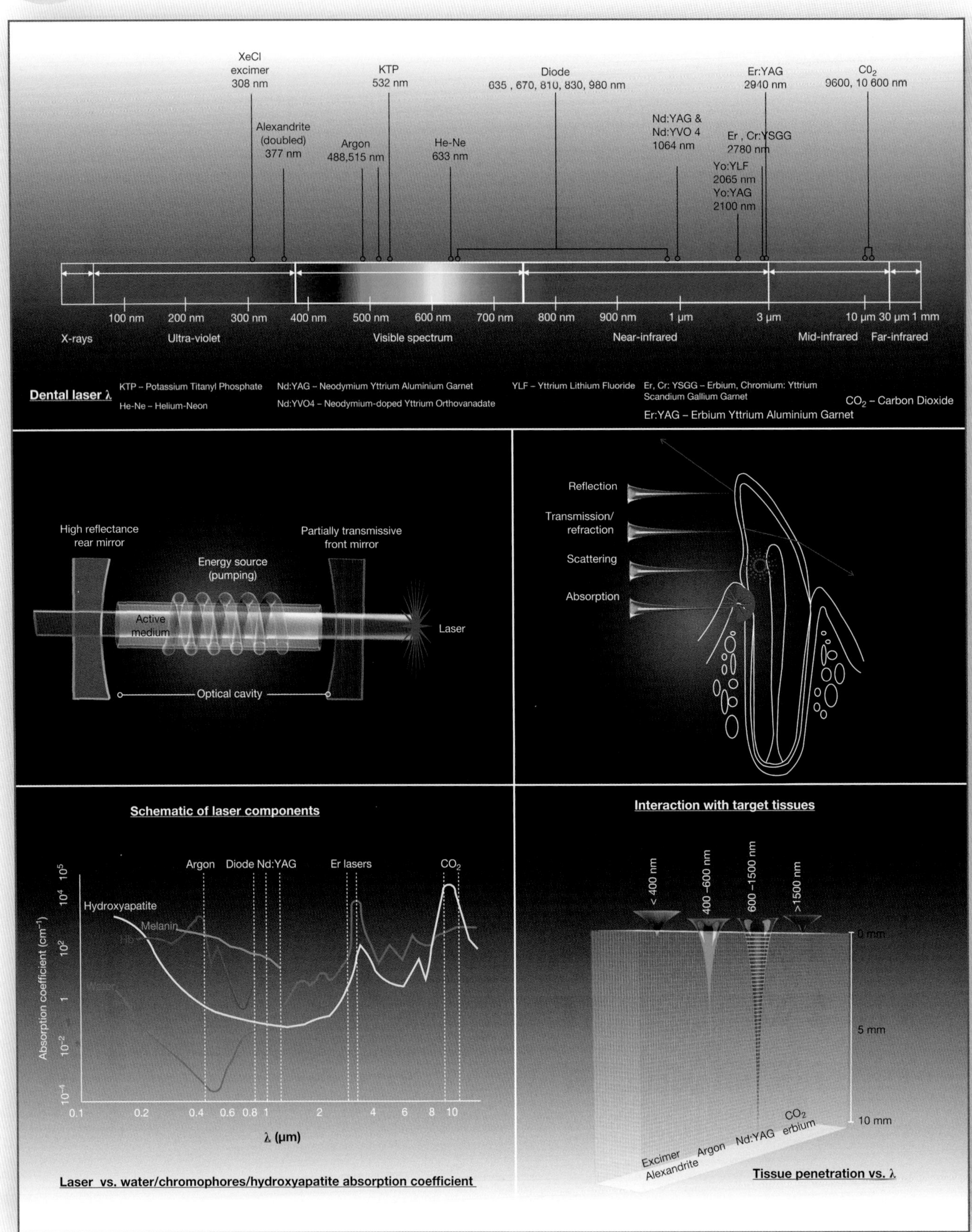

Prosthodontics at a Glance, Second Edition. Irfan Ahmad.

Lasers (Light Amplification by Stimulated Emission of Radiation) were introduced by Theodore Miaman in 1960, and represent cutting edge technology for replacing many conventional protocols. This chapter discusses the basic technology of lasers, while the next chapter concentres on clinical applications of lasers for a variety of dental disciplines.

Laser technology

The components of a laser consist of a **rear highly reflective mirror**, **active medium**, **energy source** and a **front partially transmissive mirror**. To generate a laser, an energy source is supplied to the active medium, a process termed **pumping**. The **active medium** can be a **solid** (e.g. yttrium scandium gallium garnet crystal doped with erbium and chromium for Er, Cr: YSGG), **gas** or **liquid** (dyes) corresponding to various **wavelengths (λs)** of the **nonionizing section of the electromagnetic spectrum.** The energy source is a flash-lamp strobe device, an electrical current or an electrical coil. The energy supplied in the **optical cavity (resonance cavity)** produces stimulated emission of photons that are amplified by mirrors and eventually exit as a concentrated, highly **directional beam**. An ideal laser is coherent, single λ, monochromatic, and without phase delay or retardation. Lasers are classified according to λ, type of active medium, tissue application (hard or soft) or safety classes.

The high intensity light is delivered by a **fibreoptic cable, hollow waveguide** or **articulated arm**, with in-built cooling systems to dissipate heat. The beam is either **focused with micro-lenses' arrays for excisions and incisions** or **unfocused for coagulation**. Lasers operate in either a **continuous wave (CW)** or **pulsed wave (PW)** mode. The PW is preferred to avoid damage to adjacent tissues, termed **selective thermolysis**. Lasers are used with both **contact** (e.g. incising) and **non-contact** (e.g. desensitising) techniques.

Laser/tissue interaction

Lasers **interact with a target tissue in four ways**; reflection, transmission (refraction), scattering and absorption. Reflection from a smooth surface is termed **specular reflection,** while an irregular surface produces a **diffuse reflection**, commonly observed with biological tissues. On the other hand, refraction is 'bending' an incident ray due to the different refractive indices of two disparate media. Absorption occurs when the frequency of the incident beam is equal to natural frequency of vibration of the irradiated tissues. During absorption, with water or macro molecules (proteins or chromophores), light is covered into **kinetic energy** and **heat**. For **dental lasers,** the **'therapeutic λ' range is approximately between 400 nm (argon) and 10,600 (CO_2)**. Finally, scattering occurs when the frequencies of the incident beam and tissue are different.

Mode of action

The **mode of action** of lasers with biological tissues is **non-thermal** (optical) and **thermal**. The extent of interaction with hard and soft tissues is influenced by **irradiation parameters**, i.e. λ, beam characteristics, beam spot size, pulse energy, repetition rate and the properties of the target tissue, i.e. refractive index, scattering coefficient (μs), absorption coefficient (μa), thermal coefficient and anisotropy factor. It is important to note that the **depth of penetration** into tissues is **inversely proportional to the degree of absorption.**

The optical effect relies on reflection and transmission/refraction at low intensifies (<1 mW/cm^2) for **photobiological effects** including photophysical, photochemical and photostimulation (biophotonics), e.g. **photobiomodulation (PBM), also known as low-level laser therapy (LLLT).** The main uses of these types of lasers are **disinfection** and **regeneration**.

The **thermal effect** relies on scattering and absorption, and the degree of temperature elevation of the target tissue is influenced by the irradiation parameters mentioned above. The process of **absorption requires chromophores, water or hydroxyapatite** which have an attraction to a given λ of light. In **soft tissues,** the chromophores are **melanin, haemoglobin, haemosiderin or water,** and in **hard tissues, hydroxyapatite or water.** The thermal effect is necessary for **incising soft tissue and ablation of dental hard tissues.** Since lasers have different absorption coefficient for a specific tissue, different lasers are required for specific tissues. High-power lasers interact directly with the target tissue, whereas soft tissues lasers act indirectly by warming tissue or increasing blood circulation for therapeutic effect. When a laser is absorbed by water, the temperature increase is termed **photopyrolysis** (below boiling point of 100°C), e.g. proteins begin to denature above 40°C. Above boiling point, water vaporises and the process is called **photovaporolysis**. **Photoplasmolysis** is when tissues expand and explode, and is used for soft tissue surgery. Finally, beyond 200°C tissues become dehydrated and burn, termed **carbonisation.**

Soft and hard tissue effects

For soft tissues, the thermal effect is responsible for **healing, coagulation** and **incising.** A temperature increase of 5°C above body temperature is sufficient for **decontamination**, but may cause localised necrosis. **Nd:YAG and diode lasers** have affinity with **haemoglobin** but not for hydroxyapatite, and therefore, are ideal for **cutting soft tissue, coagulation and homeostasis. CO_2 lasers** have **high absorbance with water, but shallower penetration,** and are destructive to dentine and pulp if cooing is not carefully monitored. A temperature rise of 5°C within the pulp can cause irreversible pulpal damage. The temperature needed for rapid incisions is 400°C, but adequate cooling is necessary to avoid carbonisation.

Hard tissue cutting is achieved by photothermal and photomechanical effects. The candidates for **hard tissue cutting (enamel, bone) are CO_2 (9600 nm), Er:YAG (2940 nm) and Er,Cr:YSGG (2780 nm). Erbium lasers cut by thermal ablation**, e.g. Er:YAG interacts with water and elevates temperature to 300°C, the threshold for enamel ablation, while Er,Cr:YSGG interacts with both water and hydroxyapatite to increase temperature to 800°C. The most **promising lasers for enamel ablation are ultra-short pulsed lasers (USPLs)** that operate at very a shorter pulse of one millionth of one billionth of a second (**femtoseconds, fs**) and are currently used in ophthalmology. Compared with lasers of a longer pulse rate, **USPLs offer greater precision in cavity preparation,** minimum damage to adjacent tissue, reduce thermal damage to dentine and can also be used for **selectively removing defective composite, glass ionomer and amalgam restorations.**

Key points

- Laser (Light Amplification by Stimulated Emission of Radiation).
- Different types of lasers are required for a specific type of tissue.
- The λ, depth of penetration and absorption are key factors for selecting a laser for a particular application.
- Interaction with biological tissues is either optical and/or thermal.
- Lasers are used for decontamination and ablation of both soft and hard tissues.

44 Lasers 2

Laser	λ (nm)	Active medium	Emission/ power	Pulse width	Interaction	Clinical application (not exhaustive)
Argon	488,515	Gas	CW, PW/ 600–2000 mW	50–500 ms	Melanin, haemoglobin, haemosiderin	Soft tissue surgery, composite polymerisation, bleaching, caries diagnosis
Diode	810, 980	Semi conductor	CW, PW/ <1 mW	Continuous (50 ms)	Melanin, haemoglobin	Soft tissue surgery, endodontics, decontamination, haemostasis, apthus ulcer & dentine hypersensitivity amelioration, fibroblast proliferation
Nd:YAG	1064	Solid state	CW, PW/ 4050 mW	100 μs	Melanin, haemoglobin	Soft tissue surgery, coagulation, haemostasis, caries diagnosis, endodontics, decontamination, scaling/root planing, hypersensitivity, etching cavities
Er,Cr:YSGG	2780	Solid state	PW/5000 mW	140 μs	Water, hydroxyapatite	Hard tissue ablation (cavity preparation, prevention/inhibition, bone), soft tissue surgery, endodontics, decontamination, CAD/CAM, etching, sleep apnea
Er:YAG	2940	Solid state	PW/ 500–1000J	100–150 μs	Water	Hard tissue ablation (cavity preparation, prevention/inhibition, bone), soft tissue surgery, endodontics, decontamination, CAD/CAM, etching, coagulation
CO_2	10600	Gas	CW, PW/ 25–320–J	Continuous (50 ms)	Water, hydroxyapatite	Coagulation, soft tissue surgery, caries prevention/inhibition, etching

Dental lasers specifications & applications

continuous wave (CW), pulsed wave (PW)

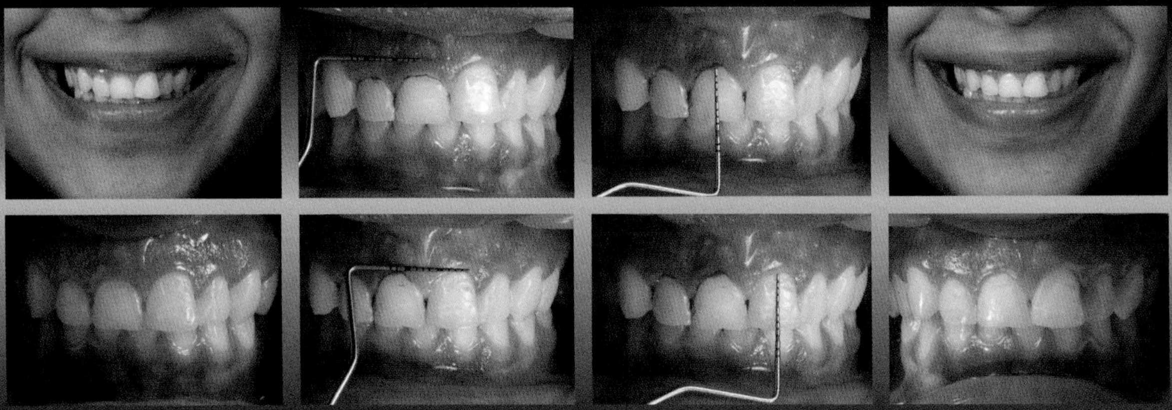

Pre-operative

Asymmetrical gingival contour around central incisors

Aesthetic crown lengthening

Post-operative

Aesthetic crown lengthening to correct gingival asymmetries using a Er,Cr:YSGG soft tissue laser

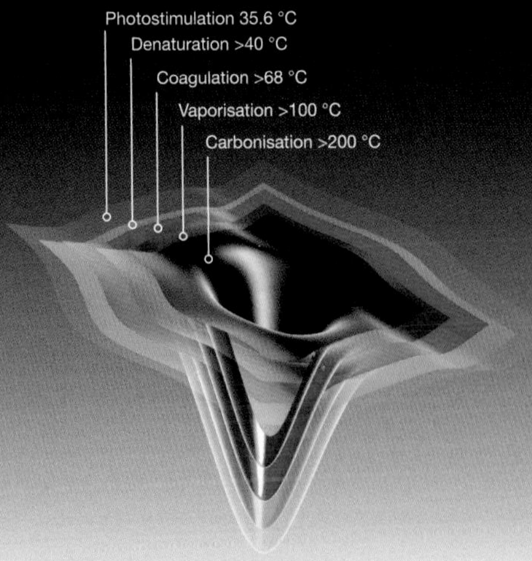

Laser interaction with biological tissues

Class	Wavelength (λ)	AEL (accessible exposure limit)	Risk
1	10 nm–1 mm	Cannot be exceeded	Safe, depends on aperture
1M	302 nm–4 μm	Cannot be exceeded	Safe, if not focused
2	200–700 nm	1 mW*	Safe if exposure time is < 0.25 s
2M	200–700 nm	1 mW*	Safe if exposure time is < 0.25 s, and not focused
3R	302 nm –1 mm	5 mW*	Risk of injury if inappropriately handled
3B	315 nm –1 mm*	500 mW*	Hazardous if directly exposed to eyes and skin
4	10 nm–1 mm	> 500 mW	Direct and indirect risks: eye, skin, fire & explosion

* varies depending on continuous wave (CW) or pulsed wave (PW)

Classes of laser safety according to EN 60825-1

Prosthodontics at a Glance, Second Edition. Irfan Ahmad.

The first dental lasers were introduced in the late 1980s to ablate enamel and dentine, but their use has now expanded to nearly every dental discipline including research. The benefits are **improved patient comfort and clinical efficiency**, but there is a price to pay such as **substantial investment, steep learning curve, stringent adherence to Health and Safety regulations** and **longer healing times**. Furthermore, lasers are **not a panacea, but adjunct tools** for many conventional protocols, and since there is no universal laser, **different types are required for a particular procedure**.

Periodontal/oral surgery

Periodontal therapy and **oral surgery** are the major fields that utilise both soft and hard tissue lasers (e.g. Waterlase® system – **Er,Cr:YSGG**). The main advantages are **painless, avoid anaesthesia, quieter, vibrationless, reduced treatment times, haemostasis, antimicrobial** (sterilising the site), **anti-inflammatory, reduced oedema, no sutures, reduced post-operative pain** and **reduced scarring**. The **shallower penetrating argon** and **CO_2 lasers** are ideal for **tissue soldering/welding** and **epithelial exclusion**, respectively. Conversely, **deeper penetrating diode or Nd:YAG lasers** are efficacious for **pocket de-epithelialisation** and guided tissue regeneration (**GTR**) for periodontal ligament and connective tissue growth with minimum gingival recession, but care is essential to mitigate thermal insult (**laser artefact**) to deeper tissue layers.

The diverse applications of soft tissue lasers include **gingival depigmentation, amalgam tattoo removal, coagulation** of free graft donor sites and **correcting gingival asymmetries (gingival contouring)**. **Photodynamic therapy (PDT)** uses a diode laser (980 nm) in conjunction with a photosensitiser dye (Periowave™) for reducing periodontal pathogens. Also, in non-contact mode, the diode lasers have tactile sensation similar to electrosurgery. Er:YAG and Nd:YAG lasers are best for **prophylactic removal of biofilm and calculus** as well as **biomodification** of the root surface to favour cell attachment and wound healing.

For **implant surgery,** soft lasers can expose implants at second-stage surgery and decontaminate sites of failed implants or peri-implantitis for encouraging re-osseointegration. The concerns about overheating implants and compromising osseointegrated fixtures can be avoided by using CO_2 lasers instead of Nd:YAG or Er:YAG. In addition, **photobiomodulation (PBM)** or low-level laser therapy (LLLT) may facilitate osseoontegration, and ameliorate mucositis and peri-implantitis. Lasers expedite many **oral surgical procedures** such as biopsies, excising hyperplastic gingiva (e.g. operculectomy), **lip repositioning surgery (LPS)**, excising fibromas and oral neoplastic lesions. **PDT (photodynamic therapy)** is another approach for apoptosis of multifocal squamous cell carcinoma and carcinoma in situ. Also, the haemostatic properties of CO_2 are beneficial for removing vascularised tumours with reduced post-operative complications. However, CO_2 lasers are contraindicate for lesions <3 mm since the thermal injury and defragmentation to the excised tissues make histological evaluation impossible. Another indication of LLLT is accelerating the regeneration of inferior dental nerve following surgical damage. Hard tissue lasers perform ostectomy and osteoplasty, as well as surgical reconstructive procedures, e.g. alveolar cleft grafts, or Lefort I osteotomies.

Restorative/endodontic

Restorative indications include **diagnosing occlusal caries** using laser fluorescence (DIAGNOden – 655 nm), **anticariogenic** properties of Nd:YAG (carious dentine absorbs 1064 nm wavelength greater than healthy dentine) and enhances the **antibacterial** and **remineralisation** effect. **Cavity preparation** is frequently executed without anaesthesia, especially minimally invasive removal of occlusal decay prior to pit and fissure sealing. **Etching** with Er, Cr:YSGG or Er:YAG lasers produces surface micro-irregularities without a smear layer, but there are conflicting reports whether laser etching improves the shear bond strength (SBS) of dental adhesives. The symptomatic relief of **dentine hypersensitivity** is due to alteration of electrical activity of pulpal nerves, making them less sensitive to pain stimuli and is also useful for reducing post-operative pain with LLLT following fillings or tooth preparation. Other applications are **polymerisation of composites resins**, and **bleaching** alone or combined with chemical agents for synergistic photo-oxidation (photochemical and photothermal) effect for intrinsic staining.

The main application of lasers for **endodontics** is **decimating pathogens** (e.g. *Escherichia coli, E. faecali, P. gingivalis*) in root canal and periapical areas using Nd:YAG, diode (810 nm and 980 nm) or erbium by the thermal and/or photodamage effect. The advantages of **photo activated dye (PAD)** compared to chemico-mechanical methods are improved penetration into complex root canal morphology and lateral channels, rapid elimination of endotoxins, reducing leakage after obturation, altering the smear layer and sealing dentine tubules. Furthermore, the prisms in enamel and dentine act as optical conduits to irradiate all parts of the root canal(s). **Er,Cr:YSGG offers an effective method for pulpotomy**, and is particularly beneficial for children or anxious adults since local anaesthesia is superfluous. Also, Er:YAG and CO_2 may be used to **sterilise endodontic files**, and as diagnostic tools for **vitality tests** and differential diagnosis of pulpitis.

Orthodontic

LLLT is known to alleviate pain associated with certain orthodontic procedures such as rapid maxillary expansion or rapid tooth movement, while **high-intensity laser therapy (HILT) for correcting soft tissue complications** associated with orthodontic treatment, such as exposing impacted teeth, gingivectomy/gingivoplasty, circumferential supracrestal fiberotomy, and labial or lingual frenectomies to resolve ankyloglossia and tooth movement relapse. Also, **white spot enamel lesions**, after bracket removal, can be remineralised with lasers.

Safety

Lasers are potentially hazardous, and cause deleterious effects to irritated tissues, including severe burns and **irreversible tissue damage**. The **retina and eyes lens** are susceptible to λs from 400 nm to 1400 nm. The safety precautions in a dental practice are appropriate training, correct clinical application, **PPE** including safety glasses to protect against specific laser λs, **high speed aspiration** to avoid **plasma plume** and avoiding reflective surfaces that cause indirect or diffuse irradiation. These include metallic restorations, metal dental instruments, clips, wrist watches, rings, earring and bracelets worn by patients or the dental team. Another concern is ignition of **flammable liquids**, such as alcohol-based surface disinfectants or surgical spirit impregnated swabs.

Key points

- Lasers can be advantageously utilised in nearly every dental discipline but have limitations.
- Main uses include antibacterial, soft and hard tissue ablation.
- Safety is paramount to avoid irreversible damage to target/adjacent tissues or other parts of the body, especially the eyes and skin.

Tooth preparation

Section 11

Chapters

45 Microinvasive and minimally invasive techniques

Caries infiltration concept

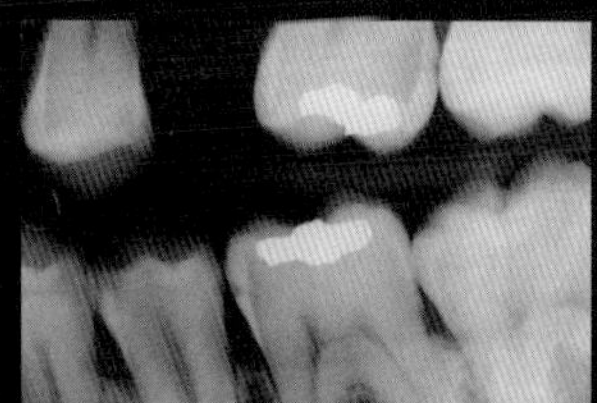

Bitewing radiograph showing early, interproximal, non-cavitated carious lesions

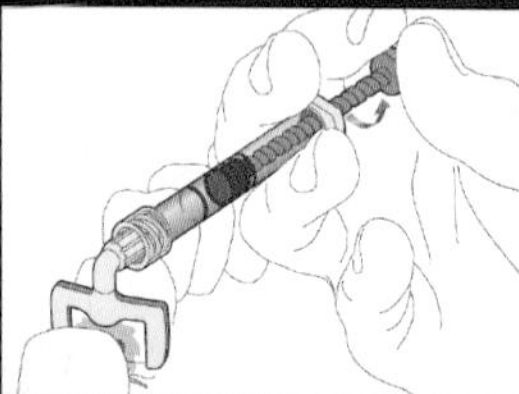

Resin infiltration for sealing interproximal enamel porosity

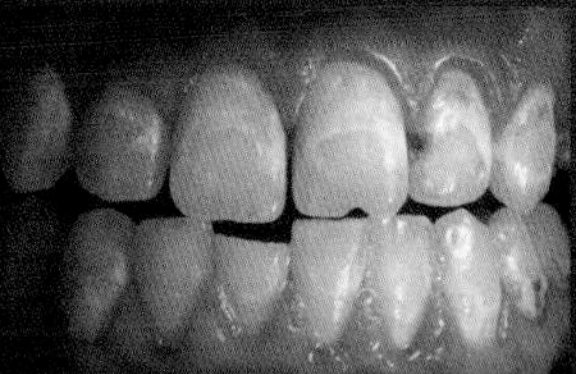

White spot lesions following removal of orthodontic brackets

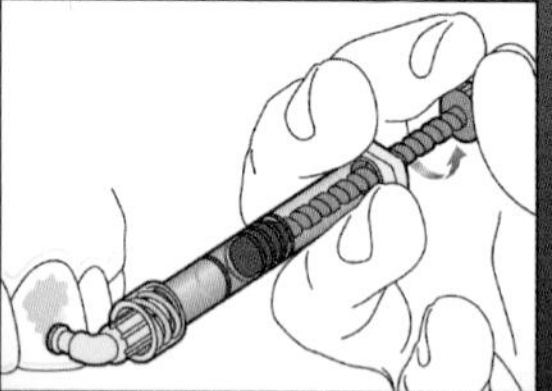

Resin infiltration for aesthetic improvement of facial white spot lesions

Microabrasion

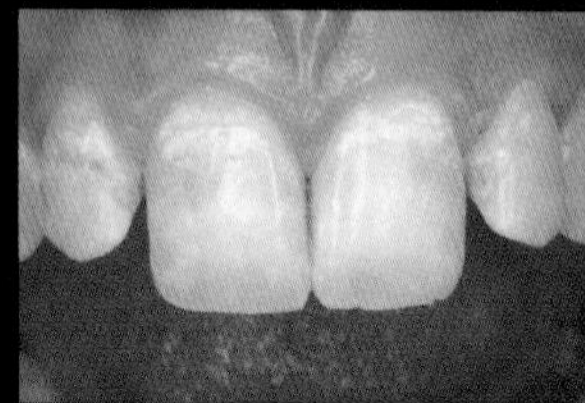

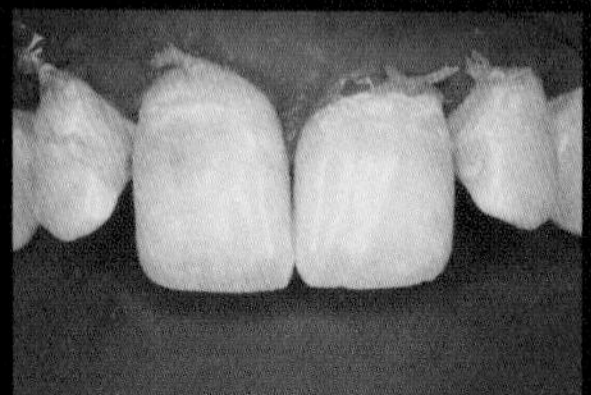

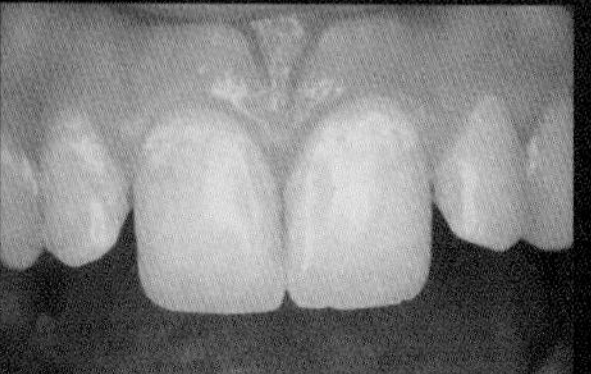

Microabrasion for removing enamel staining

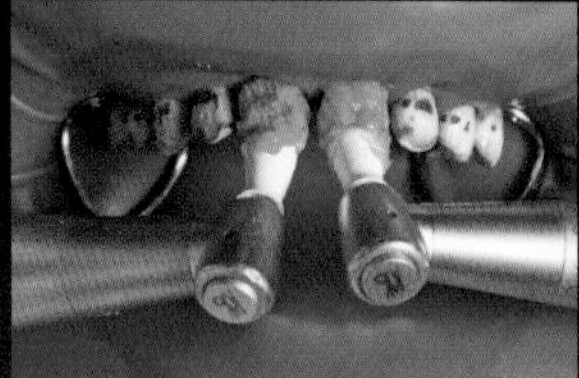

Microabrasion with HCl+pumice or phosphoric acid+pumice slurry

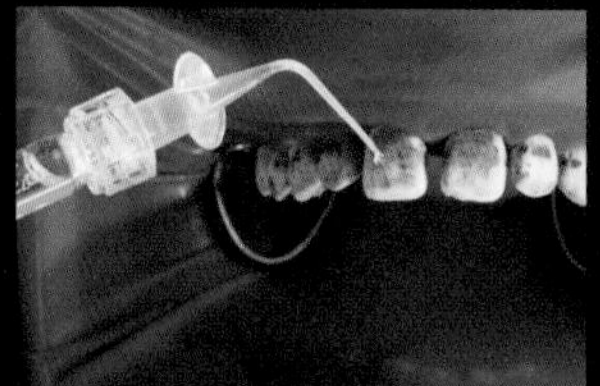

Ethanol for drying enamel surface

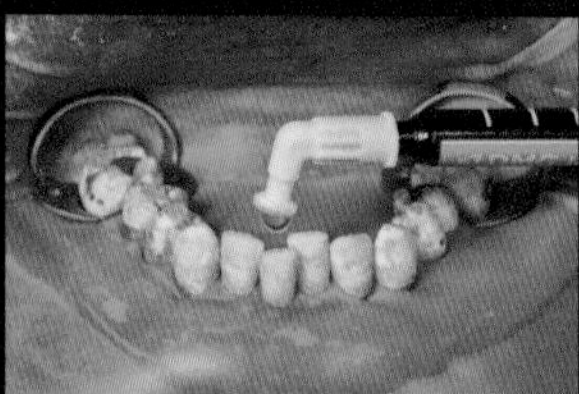

Resin infiltrate for sealing enamel surface

Technique	Constituents	Mechanism	Indications
Caries infiltration concept	10% HCl, ethanol and resininfiltrate	Chemical	Early, non-cavitated interproximal or facial carious lesions
Microabrasion	Various concentrations of HCl and abrasives	Chemo-mechanical	Superficial enamel staining, e.g. dental fluorosis
Air abrasion	Aluminium oxide, silica or bicarbonate soda particles	Mechanical	Cleansing fissures, removing early surface carious lesions, class VI carious and erosive cavities, removing small old composite restorations, removing superficial enamel stains, prophylaxis, and roughening composite cores before luting definitive indirect restorations
Carisolv	Gel combined with hand and rotary instruments	Chemo-mechanical	Caries excavation, especially in deciduous teeth
Lasers	Various types	Photo-thermal	Caries excavation, especially in deciduous teeth
Oscillating tips	Fine grit diamond tips	Mechanical	Shaping cavities following caries or defective restoration removal

Comparison of micro-invasive & minimally invasive techniques for tooth preparation

Prosthodontics at a Glance, Second Edition. Irfan Ahmad.

This first chapter on tooth preparation discusses **microinvasive** and **minimally invasive** techniques. These treatment modalities are minimally invasive, atraumatic, avoiding more traditional and invasive **rotary techniques for tooth preparation.**

Microinvasive techniques

Caries describes the process and lesion of dental decay. Caries is an infectious disease, and the **protagonist bacteria** is ***Streptococcus mutans***, which attacks dental hard tissues. The driving force of caries is not the bacteria per se, but the **biofilm** that contains the bacteria and carbohydrates. If the biofilm is removed or disturbed, caries can be reversed or arrested by **remineralisation** with calcium and fluoride ions present in saliva. The earliest carious lesion is termed a **'white spot'** that can be active or inactive. Microinvasive techniques, such as the **caries infiltration concept** (Icon, DMG, Germany), aim to arrest early caries before cavitation occurs. This is probably the least invasive method of tooth preparation. The first step is isolation with rubber dam or MiniDam, followed by etching with hydrochloric acid (HCl) and applying an infiltrate (low-viscosity resin), which penetrates and seals the lesion by **capillary action**. This treatment is indicated for early **interproximal lesions (smooth surface caries)**, and is also effective for immediate improvement of aesthetics after removal of fixed orthodontic brackets.

Microabrasion

Microabrasion is recommended for removing unaesthetic staining that is limited to the superficial layer of enamel due to **fluorosis**, **prosthodontic demineralisation**, **localised hypoplasia** or other idiopathic brown/white **enamel dysmineralisation**. **Enamel fluorosis**, especially of the maxillary anterior teeth, is due to excessive intake of fluoride (greater than 1 ppm) during the second and third years of life. The source of fluoride is from foodstuffs such as milk, salt, vitamins, infant preprepared food and the indigenous water supply or dental preventive measures such as toothpaste and rinses. Although fluoride is an anticaries measure, excess amounts prevent maturation of the enamel, increasing its **porosity** and presenting as white, yellow or brown striations and staining.

The **microabrasion process** involves **simultaneous acidic erosion and mechanical abrasion.** The technique uses a slurry of HCl, usually mixed with pumice or other abrasive, that is applied to the surface enamel either with a hand applicator or using rubber cups in a slow dental handpiece. A 6% HCl concentration reveals a **micromorphological appearance that is similar to intact, untreated enamel** without an etch pattern, and is less erosive than 37% phosphoric acid, confirming that this type of minimally invasive treatment does not damage the structure of enamel prisms. Also, fluorosed teeth are hypermineralised, with a higher concentration of fluoride in the outer 200 µm layer of enamel that is more resistant to acid etching. The technique involves isolating the teeth beforehand with conventional or light-cured rubber dam to prevent ulceration of the soft tissues. The slurry is applied and repeated until the stains are removed and an acceptable tooth colour is achieved. This is followed by application of **topical sodium fluoride** to encourage remineralisation of the enamel. A possible explanation for the improvement in tooth colour after microabrasion is that the acid penetration into enamel may remove the retained **amelogenin proteins** that are attributed to the lesion of enamel fluorosis. Furthermore, the polished tooth surface results in enhanced **specular reflection** that camouflages underlying enamel imperfections. The drawback of microabrasion is the risk of **caustic burns to the gingiva**, and rubber dam is therefore mandatory. If the slurry is incessantly applied and the dentine exposed, **hypersensitivity** is possible. However, microabrasion should be considered the first line of treatment for removing intrinsic enamel stains before more aggressive restorative options are considered. In severe fluorosis, a variation of the macroabrasion technique is to use **fine diamond burs (60 µm grit) for initial removal of intense fluorotic stains** and to adjust the **macromorphology**. The enamel surface is then polished with aluminium oxide discs and silicone tips before continuing with the HCl slurry. In addition, **office or home bleaching** is prescribed to lighten the teeth. This combination of chemical and mechanical abrasion is often referred to as the **chemomechanical** approach.

Other methods

Other methods of minimally invasive tooth preparation include **air abrasion**, which is a mechanical method for roughening the tooth substrate to increase mechanical retention for resin-based fillings. Particles of silica, **aluminium oxide (50 µm)** or bicarbonate of soda are jetted onto the tooth from a dental handpiece using compressed air. The procedure is painless, rarely requiring anaesthesia. A wide range of clinical applications are possible, ranging from **cleansing fissures, to removing small old composite restorations.** Necessary **precautions** include wearing protective glasses, PPE, isolation of the affected teeth with rubber dam to prevent inhalation and avoiding contact with intact resin-based or glass ionomer fillings. Treatment of small cavitated carious lesions, especially in deciduous teeth, or cleansing fissures of organic debris before sealing, can also be achieved with other minimally invasive protocols. **Carisolv**® is a chemomechanical technique using a gel to dissolve denatured collagen in cavitated carious lesions, followed by hand and rotary instrumentation for debridement of the cavity. **Lasers**, e.g. Er:YAG are also employed for painless carious excavation (Chapter 44). **Oscillating diamond tips that utilise sono-abrasion** are less invasive than burs, and are useful for shaping cavities following caries removal. Finally, the methods mentioned above (air abrasion, femtosecond lasers and sono-abrasion) **all lower the smear layer interference with dental adhesives** compared to rotary tooth preparation with burs.

Key points

- Microinvasive and minimally invasive tooth preparation techniques are aimed at preserving as much natural tooth as possible.
- The caries infiltration concept is the least invasive method for treating early carious 'white spot' lesions.
- Microabrasion is atraumatic and highly effective for restoring aesthetics due to superficial enamel staining.
- Other minimally invasive preparation techniques include air abrasion, Carisolv®, lasers and oscillating diamond tips.

46 Guidelines for rotary tooth preparation

Diamond grit coated bur

Tungsten carbide (TC) bur

EVA tip in reciprocating handpiece to remove unsupported enamel from preparation margins

Soft tissue integrity is maintained by using a flat plastic, Zekrya gingival protector and gingival retraction cords

Hard tissue integrity is maintained by copious irrigation, intermittent preparation, & immediate dentine sealing (IDS) after tooth preparation

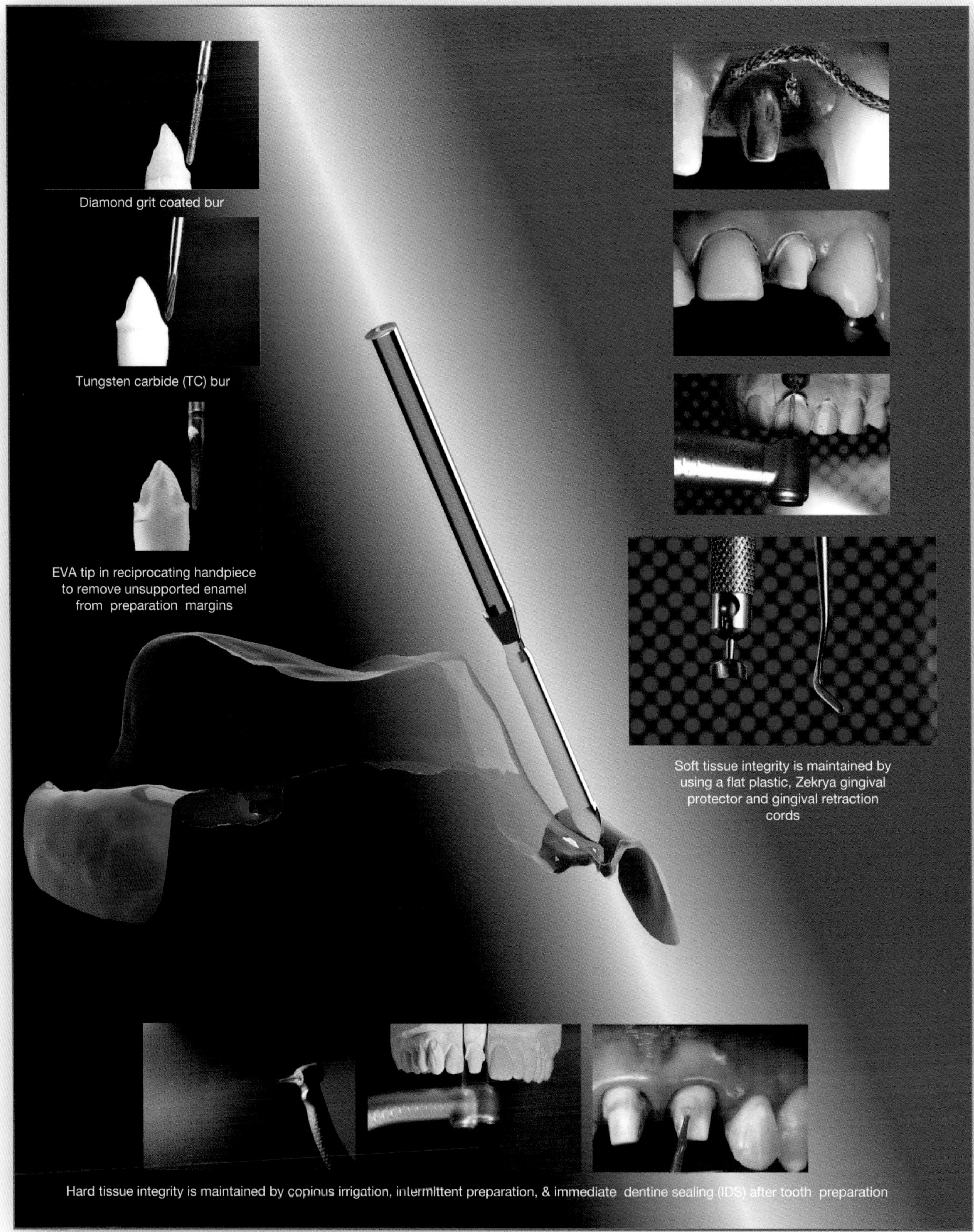

Conventional tooth preparation involves using **rotary instruments** for preparing teeth to receive either direct or indirect restorations, and is currently the most widely used method worldwide. Tooth preparation is potentially destructive to both the hard and soft tissues, and should be carried out efficaciously, expediently and with extreme care **to avoid inadvertent or iatrogenic damage**. The guidelines presented below are applicable to all types of tooth preparation using rotary instruments.

Instrumentation

Rotary instruments refer to **burs** that prepare a tooth by either **grinding** or **cutting.** A **dental bur** has a stainless steel shank with **blades of various geometries and shapes**. Alternatively, the bur shank can be **coated with diamond grits** or **tipped with tungsten carbide (TC) blades or flutes**, for cutting or polishing, respectively. The most popular variety are diamond burs, which are classified according to their shape, size and the **diamond grit particle size** that varies from **10 µm to over 200 µm**. The bur shank fits either a **friction grip (FG) turbine handpiece** or a **latch-type** attachment of a **micro-motor contra-angle (CA) handpiece**. The specifications of handpieces vary according to the manufacturer, but are broadly divided into **turbines** rotating at speeds up to **500,000 revolutions per minute**, while the slower micro-motors' speeds vary from **1,000 to 40,000 revolutions per minute**, depending on torque and gear reduction/increasing ratios.

Soft tissue integrity

The **soft tissues** of the oral mucosa, tongue and lips should be sufficiently retracted to allow a clear field of view and to prevent lacerations by the rotary instruments. The circumferential friable gingival margin requires special attention, to minimise not only transient but also long-term effects of trauma. The **initial trauma** is bleeding, which hinders clinical procedures such as margin visualisation, impressions (analogue or digital) and cementing procedures, while **long-term effects** includes persistent gingival inflammation, periodontal pockets or unwanted gingival recession, **compromising 'pink aesthetics'** in the anterior regions of the mouth. Gingival recession is highly likely with pronounced scalloped gingival contours and/or thin biotypes. Protection of the gingiva is by transient retraction using hand instruments, such as small **flat plastics**, **Zekrya gingival protector** and **gingival retraction cords.** All these methods provide protection against inadvertent violation of the biologic width, and for promoting a haemorrhage free protocol

Hard tissue integrity

Besides soft tissue protection, it is also essential to **protect the dental hard tissues**: enamel, dentine and the alveolar housing of teeth, to avoid morbidity or mortality. The long-term eventualities are endodontic complications, bone resorption and periodontal pockets. Various studies have endeavoured to evaluate the number of teeth undergoing **pulpal pathosis following tooth preparations**. The number of teeth losing vitality following full coverage crowns has varied from as little as **2% to over 13% over a 10-year period.** Therefore, any tooth scheduled for full coverage crowns should have a preoperative endodontic assessment including history of previous symptoms, clinical and radiographic examination, and vitality tests.

The two factors for maintaining hard tissue integrity of teeth are **cutting efficiency (CE) and temperature elevation**. Cutting efficiency is defined as the most expedient method for tooth preparation. The **critical threshold for CE of diamond grit size is 150 µm.** A larger diamond grit size does not increases CE, but leads to microscopic cracks in the enamel and dentine, which weakens the remaining tooth substrate. In addition, the roughened surface created with coarser burs leads to a greater **surface roughness (Ra),** which complicates laboratory procedures such as waxing and casting, and introduces porosity in the luting agent at the cementation stage. Furthermore, the coarser grit generates heat precariously close to the **pulpal necrosis temperature of 41.5°C**. Hence, it is prudent to choose burs with a grit size of <150 µm and progressively reduce the grit size as the preparation approaches dentine, to prevent overheating and to create a smoother surface finish. Other factors to consider during tooth preparation are:

- **Size of pulp chamber**, which should be assessed radiographically and the amount of tooth reduction carried out precisely with silicone or 3D printed indices. In young teeth, the pulp is larger than in older teeth because the pulp chamber in the latter is reduced due to deposition of secondary dentine in response to carious, restorative, occlusal and extra-oral traumas
- **Preservation of natural tooth substrate** is essential to ensure tooth rigidity and insulation from temperature fluctuations, and to prevent impregnation of the dentine tubules with oral pathogens
- **Non-vital teeth** are structurally compromised with **reduced proprioceptive response,** predisposing them to fracture. Care is therefore necessary to design extracoronal restorations that enhance the fracture resistance of the remaining tooth. Teeth with intraradicular support are prone to coronal microleakage that may compromise the root filling as well as the final restoration
- **Cooling with copious irrigation** at water temperatures below 32°C mitigates the frictional heat generated during preparation. However, to minimise airborne micro-organism transmission with any **aerosol-generated procedures (AGP)**, **high-speed HEPA air filtration units**, **FFP3 respirator masks** and **PPE (Level 3 PPE)** are essential
- **Pressure applied during tooth preparation** should be **minimal and intermittent** to reduce temperature elevation, and allow heat dissipation. Excess pressure is usually applied when burs are damaged, degraded or clogged with debris. Ideally, burs should be discarded after a single tooth preparation, or cleaned in an ultrasonic bath before sterilisation. Furthermore, the **trauma to the dental pulp is cumulative.** Heavily or repeatedly restored teeth are especially vulnerable to additional trauma of tooth preparation, which may result in pulpal necrosis
- **Time** taken to prepare a tooth should be an absolute minimum. Relentless and protracted preparation is unproductive, often resulting in endodontic complications
- Preparation should be **accomplished with burs of progressively finer diamond grit (smoother burs) to compact the smear layer** to enhance adhesion of the definitive restoration using dental adhesives
- **Immediate dentine sealing (IDS)** of prepared teeth with a dental adhesive seals patent dentine tubules, halts bacterial ingress, reduces postoperative sensitivity and results in superior bonding of the definitive restoration when using a resin-based cement

Key points

- The use of rotary instruments, or burs, is the most popular method for preparing teeth for direct and indirect restorations.
- Tooth preparation is potentially destructive and caution is necessary to maintain both soft and hard tissue integrity.

47 Resin-bonded fixed partial dentures (RBFPD)

Anterior

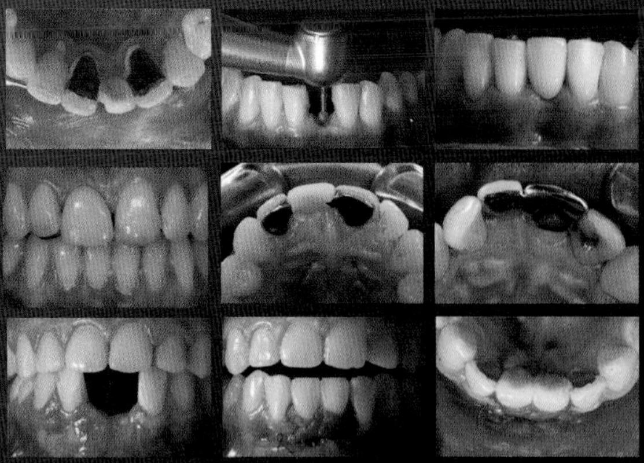

Posterior

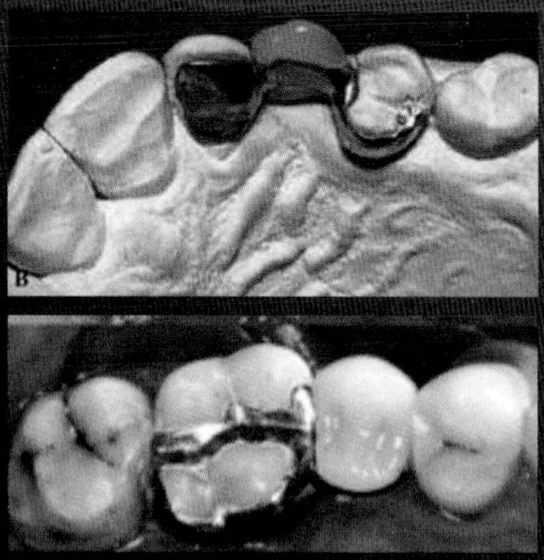

Anterior metal RBFPDs can be two wings or cantilever style and are indicated for permanent prostheses, or temporary measures awaiting a more permanent solution

Posterior RBFPDs have a metal wraparound retainer on the lingual or palatal surfaces. The retainer can be C- or D- shaped, extending onto the occlusal surface

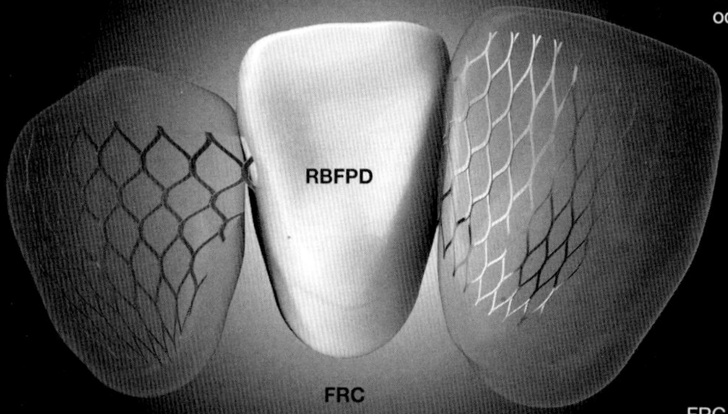

METAL

RBFPD

FRC

FRC FPDs are metal-free, reinforced with fibres, and are more aesthetic, especially for the anterior regions of the mouth

FRC can either be intracoronal ('inlay' retained), or full coverage (extracoronally retained). For posterior teeth, the pontic sites can be further strengthened by incorporating multidirectional fibres, or rods

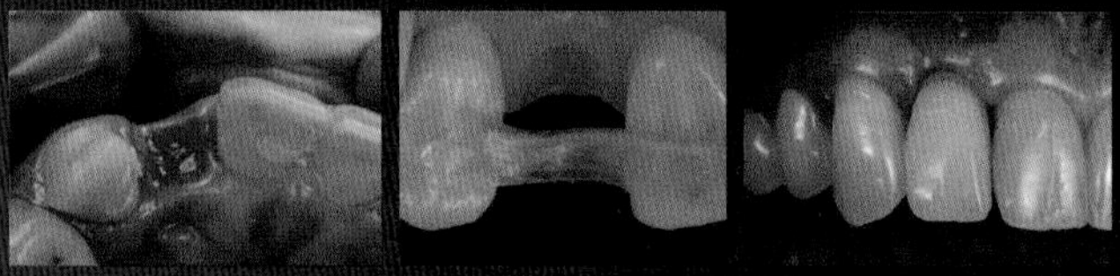

Anterior

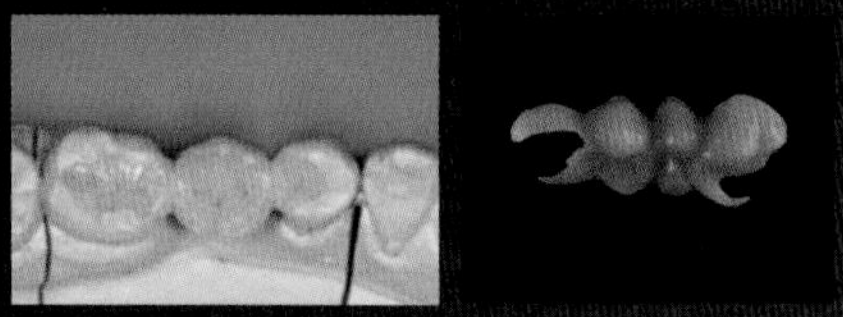

Posterior

Advantages	Disadvantages
Minimal tooth preparation	Survival rate of 5 years
Excellent short-term prostheses for young patients, and while awaiting healing of bone and soft tissue grafts and implants, splint mobile teeth	Debonding likely, especially with parafunctional habits
Choice of metal, composite and ceramic frameworks	Short-span bridges, limited to 2 or 3 units
Economical compared to conventional FPD or implants	Exacting adhesive protocol for cementation

Advantages and disadvantages of RBFPD

Prosthodontics at a Glance, Second Edition. Irfan Ahmad.

Resin-bonded fixed partial dentures (RBFPDs) were introduced by Rochette in 1973 for splinting periodontally compromised mandibular anterior teeth. The indirect prosthesis is made of perforated cast metal retainers or wings, with or without pontics, which are cemented to the lingual or palatal surfaces of abutment teeth with a **resin-based luting agent**. RBFPDs are **minimally invasive,** requiring less tooth preparation compared to conventional FPDs. They are usually indicated for short spans of two or three units. Longer spans are possible if the occlusion is satisfactory without bruxist activity. However, increasing the number of abutments causes **interabutment stresses** leading to a greater chance of **debonding**. RBFPDs are indicated for anterior and posterior regions of the mouth, with the following uses:

- As **minimally invasive fixed prostheses for unrestored, intact adjacent teeth**, teeth in younger patients with large dental pulp chambers, or following acute trauma resulting in avulsion of a tooth
- As **temporary or stop-gap prostheses** while awaiting integration of hard and soft tissue augmentation or during the osseointegration phase of implant therapy
- A **short-span FPD as an alternative** to conventional FPD or implant-supported prostheses
- For **splinting mobile, periodontally compromised teeth**

Several configurations of RBFPD are described. These include retentive **wings** either side of the pontic, or a **cantilever design**, using only one abutment tooth for the retainer, with a suspended pontic. For the latter, the pontic on the opposite side of the retainer can be supported by an intracoronal **rest seat** for correct location and stability. RBFPDs have approximately **90% survival rate over a five-year period**, with greater success reported in the maxilla than the mandible.

Rochette and maryland appliances

Both the **Rochette and Maryland FPDs** are fabricated from cast metals and their fitting surfaces etched in the dental laboratory. The difference between the two is the design of the metal retainers: the **Rochette retainers are perforated** to increase mechanical retention, while **Maryland retainers are non-perforated**. If a pontic is incorporated, its metal sub-structure can be veneered with a resin-based composite or porcelain. The draw backs of metal retainers are the metal shine-through or greying of thin abutment teeth, debonding and overcontoured retainers.

Fibre-reinforced composite (FRC)

To improve aesthetics, gain additional retention and reduce opposing tooth wear, cast metal retainers can be substituted with a reinforced resin composite. **Fibre-reinforced composite (FRC)** FPDs are composed of two types of composite:

- **Substructure** – either pre-impregnated fibres in a resin matrix or non-impregnated polyethylene fibres
- **Superstructure** – a hybrid or micro-filled veneering composite bonded to the substructure composite with heat and light polymerisation. To prevent delamination and create high bond strengths, it is essential to maintain an oxygen inhibition layer between composite increments, or to condition the substructure composite with a silane coupling agent. **FRCFPDs** can either be **full coverage (extracoronal)** or **partial coverage (intracoronal)** 'inlay' retained, depending on the restorative status of the adjacent abutment teeth

The framework design of FRC depends on whether full or partial coverage is planned. Nevertheless, the framework should offer sufficient rigidity to support the veneering composite and resist occlusal forces, which is achieved by incorporating **multi-directional fibres**, adequate **bulk of fibres** and including **bars at pontic sites**.

Tooth preparation

The tooth preparation for an RBFPD depends on the existing restorations in the abutment teeth. Heavily restored teeth with extensive amalgams or composite filling require full coverage type of preparations, while for smaller class I, II and III restorations an intracoronal approach is appropriate. In addition, retentive features, preferably confined within the enamel, such as **proximal/occlusal grooves and lingual steps** are beneficial and avoid overcontoured prostheses and sufficient occlusal clearance. For intact, virgin teeth, **no preparation is usually necessary**, except creation of **guiding planes, occlusal stops and finish lines** for path of insertion and location, respectively.

Prosthesis design

Metal substructures or frameworks can be fabricated from **both noble and base cast metals**, such as nickel chrome alloy. The framework is designed for maximum extension onto the lingual/palatal surfaces to increase the surface area for bonding, without compromising aesthetic, occlusion or periodontal health. For molar abutments, the framework is wraparound to maximise retention and resistance form, and can be either **C-shaped,** confined to the lingual surface, or **D-shaped,** extending onto the occlusal surface. In addition, the retainer thickness should be >0.8 mm for sufficient strength. Other options include fabricating a high-strength **CAD/CAM ceramic framework**, with **pressed or layering veneering porcelain** for the pontic.

Cementation

Luting an RBFPD involves using an **adhesive bonding technique**, which is operator-sensitive and influences the longevity of the prosthesis. A **conventional or self-adhesive resin-based luting agent** is recommended. The intaglio surface of the retainers is pretreated with air abrasion, electrolytic etching or silanation. The fitting surface of the abutment tooth can also be air-abraded and/or etched with 37% phosphoric acid to enhance bonding. Since dentine is rarely exposed, the **bond to enamel is more predictable**, assuming proper isolation to prevent contamination by saliva and blood.

Key points

- Resin-bonded fixed partial dentures are minimally invasive, indirect prostheses.
- They are indicated for a variety of clinical applications, and have a survival rate of approximately 90% over five years.
- The framework can either be cast metal or fibre-reinforced composite that is veneered with either resin-based composite or porcelain.
- An adhesive technique is necessary for luting RBFPDs using resin-based cements.

48 Preparation for inlays and onlays

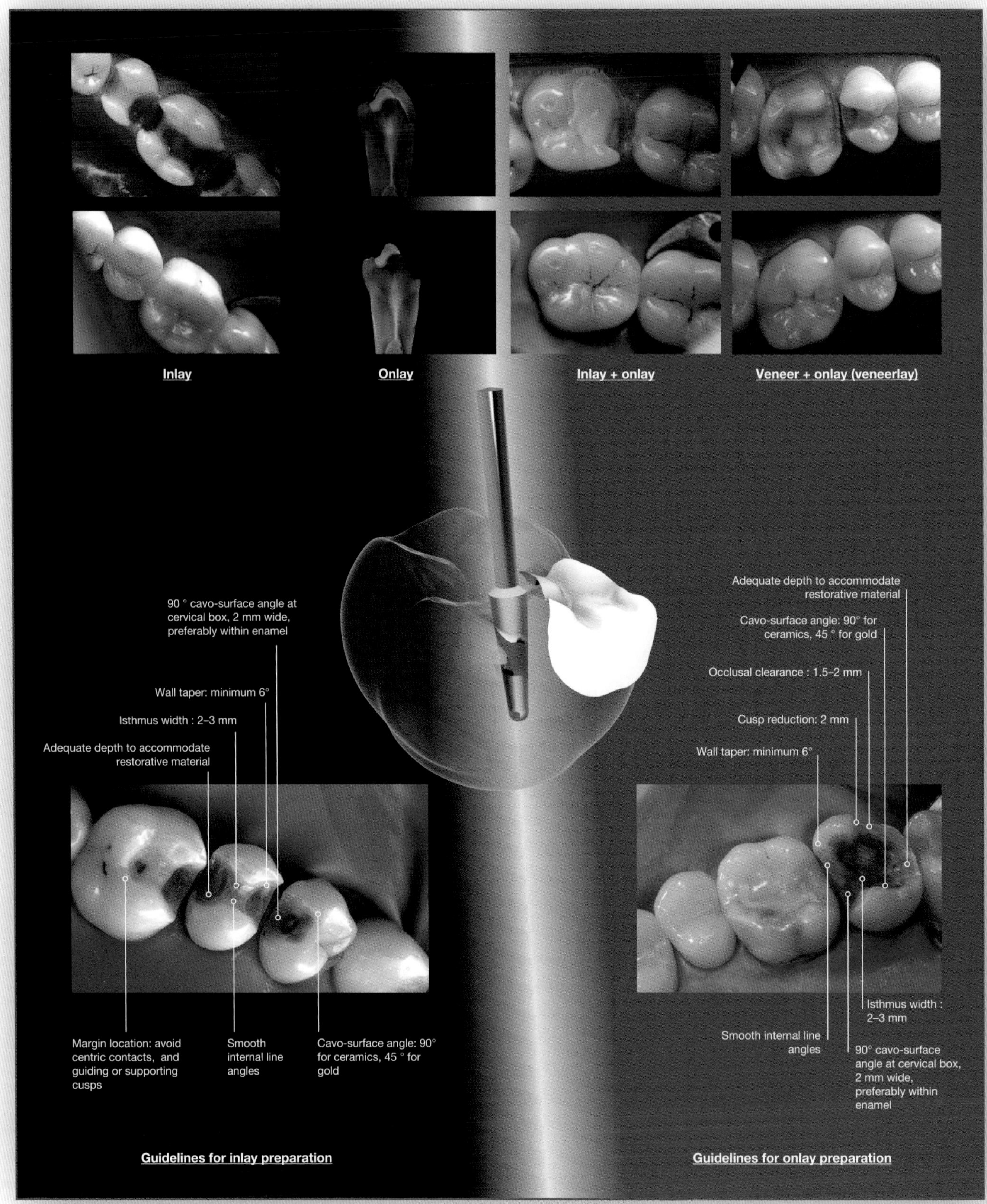

Inlay

Onlay

Inlay + onlay

Veneer + onlay (veneerlay)

90 ° cavo-surface angle at cervical box, 2 mm wide, preferably within enamel

Wall taper: minimum 6°

Isthmus width : 2–3 mm

Adequate depth to accommodate restorative material

Margin location: avoid centric contacts, and guiding or supporting cusps

Smooth internal line angles

Cavo-surface angle: 90° for ceramics, 45 ° for gold

Guidelines for inlay preparation

Adequate depth to accommodate restorative material

Cavo-surface angle: 90° for ceramics, 45 ° for gold

Occlusal clearance : 1.5–2 mm

Cusp reduction: 2 mm

Wall taper: minimum 6°

Isthmus width : 2–3 mm

Smooth internal line angles

90° cavo-surface angle at cervical box, 2 mm wide, preferably within enamel

Guidelines for onlay preparation

Prosthodontics at a Glance, Second Edition. Irfan Ahmad.

Conventional teaching stipulates that **tooth preparation be material orientated, i.e. geometric,** to accommodate the properties of the restorative material. Conversely, **contemporary techniques** dispel this destructive over-preparation in favour of **disease- or defect-orientated preparations.** Modern restorative materials are capable of restoring teeth that have smaller or **minimally invasive preparations**, and therefore allow a larger amount of natural dental tissues to be retained. Indirect **inlays** and **onlays** are indicated for **extensive cavities in premolars and molars**, due to rampant caries, or to replace defective existing restorations. An inlay or onlay preparation **conserves more of the natural tooth, removing less tooth substance (6–27%) compared to a full-coverage crown (68–76%).**

Definitions

An **inlay is an indirect intracoronal restoration** that does not support or replace cusps of a tooth. Furthermore, all occlusal contacts in centric, protrusive and lateral excursions are guided by cusps of the natural tooth. An **onlay is an indirect restoration that incorporates, supports and replaces one or more tooth cusps.** The functional occlusion is supported by the restorative material that covers the involved cusps. An onlay can incorporate an inlay preparation or be restricted to the occlusal surface to replace an **eroded occlusal table**, or to **raise the vertical dimension of occlusion (VDO).** Various cavity configurations of onlays and veneers are possible; for example, a **veneerlay** restoration that combines an onlay and veneer preparation.

Guidelines for inlay preparation

The conventional guidelines for inlay preparations are:

- **Taper** – the occlusal and cervical boxes should have 6° tapers for adequate path of insertion/withdrawal
- **Isthmus width** – 3 mm at the mesial and/or distal aspects
- **Cavity depth** – 3 mm to accommodate an adequate bulk of restorative material (cast gold, composite or ceramic)
- **Internal line angles** – smooth, devoid of undercuts
- **External line angles** – occlusal and cervical box finish lines should have a **90° cavo-surface angle for ceramics and composites,** and a **45° bevel for cast gold** to allow burnishing
- **Occlusal margin location** – avoiding centric contacts or guiding/supporting cusps
- **Cervical margin location** – finish line within enamel, and if possible, coronal to the cement–enamel junction

However, the ongoing improvement in material properties and refined clinical techniques afford greater latitude, allowing a more defect- or disease-orientated preparation. In the past, it was essential to remove minor undercuts (either due to caries or existing amalgam fillings retained by undercuts) by removing enamel at the occlusal surfaces to expand the cavity. But now, the **undercuts can be filled with relative ease using either glass ionomer or dental adhesives with flowable composites.** This is particularly beneficial for digital impressions with an intra-oral scanner, which cannot faithfully scan deep undercuts. Alternately, minor **undercuts can be left in situ**, since modern impression materials are flexible enough to allow removal of the impression without distortion or tearing, and the undercut subsequently blocked out on the plaster cast in the dental laboratory, and filled in at the luting stage with resin cements.

Guidelines for onlay preparation

Tooth preparation for onlays follows similar guidelines for inlay preparation, but offers greater leeway. An onlay preparation can incorporate an inlay preparation or **cover the entire occlusal table** without an inlay preparation. In the former situation, an inlay preparation is carried out, and if deemed necessary, susceptible cusps are reduced by 2 mm to accommodate the restorative material. The cavo-surface finish line is 90° for ceramics and bevelled 45° for cast gold. An onlay is indicated for severe coronal destruction and ensuing loss of tooth substrate resulting from tooth wear, decay or endodontic complications, and for restoring or **raising the VDO**. In these circumstances, the preparation is minimal, limited to defining finish lines with correct cavo-surface angles. Finally, a minimum of **1.5–2 mm occlusal clearance** or opening (if increasing the VDO) is necessary. Recent research has verified that irrespective of the number of cusps (both functional and non-functional cusps) incorporated into an onlay preparation, the fracture resistance of the indirect restoration is unaffected, and can even restore the fracture strength to the equivalent of an unprepared, intact tooth. Furthermore, compared to inlays, **onlays are more efficacious in protecting tooth structure** because an onlay preparation design is more resistant to tooth fractures.

CAD/CAM inlays and onlays

Inlays and onlays can be fabricated **chairside** in a few hours by **CAD/CAM technology**. The technique involves making an intra-oral digital impression of the preparation or extra-oral scanning of a plaster cast of the cavity. The virtual restoration is designed in CAD software, and subsequently milled using machinable resin-based composite or ceramic ingots (feldspathic, pressed leucite glass, lithium disilicate, alumina and zirconia). The milled restoration is polished, stained, glazed, etched and silanated, ready for adhesive luting. The guidelines for tooth preparation for CAD/CAM restorations are identical to those for conventional fabrication methods. However, for digital impressions, the **margins should be clearly delineated with sinuous line angles, and devoid of undercuts**. In addition, the finish lines, when possible, should preferably be located supragingivally to facilitate digital scanning of the preparation (or a plaster cast of the preparation).

Key points

- Inlays and onlays are indirect restorations for large cavities in or on premolars and molars.
- Inlay and onlay preparations are more conservative than full coverage crowns, and the ensuing restoration can enhance fracture resistance of a tooth.
- CAD/CAM technology offers efficacious fabrication of various indirect restorations using a variety of ceramic and resin-based composite materials.

Preparation for porcelain laminate veneers

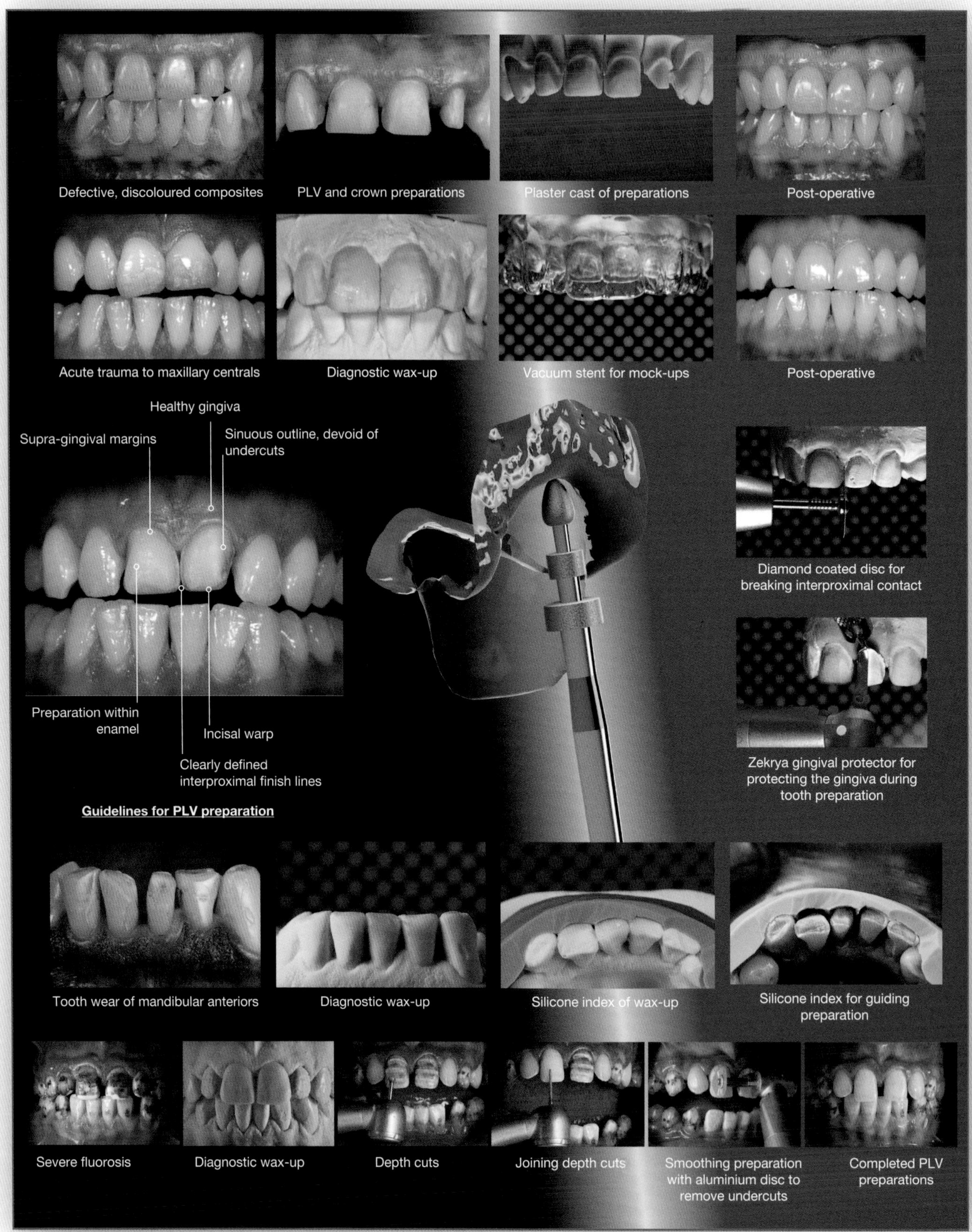

Defective, discoloured composites

PLV and crown preparations

Plaster cast of preparations

Post-operative

Acute trauma to maxillary centrals

Diagnostic wax-up

Vacuum stent for mock-ups

Post-operative

Healthy gingiva

Supra-gingival margins

Sinuous outline, devoid of undercuts

Preparation within enamel

Incisal warp

Clearly defined interproximal finish lines

Guidelines for PLV preparation

Diamond coated disc for breaking interproximal contact

Zekrya gingival protector for protecting the gingiva during tooth preparation

Tooth wear of mandibular anteriors

Diagnostic wax-up

Silicone index of wax-up

Silicone index for guiding preparation

Severe fluorosis

Diagnostic wax-up

Depth cuts

Joining depth cuts

Smoothing preparation with aluminium disc to remove undercuts

Completed PLV preparations

Porcelain laminate veneers (PLVs) have proved to be one of the **most successful and long-lasting indirect aesthetic restorations.** However, PLVs are also one of the **most clinically and technically challenging restorations**, and their success is attributed to careful and meticulous protocols. PLVs are the most frequently used, and abused, restorations in **cosmetic dentistry**, especially in the case of **'extreme dental make-overs'**. In addition, careful **analysis of the patient's psyche** is essential before embarking on irreversible **elective cosmetic procedures**, particularly if expectations are beyond clinical feasibility.

Rationale

The ethos of PLV is based on the principles of preserving as much natural tooth substrate as possible, especially enamel, and utilising this natural hard tissue foundation to support thin veneers of porcelain. Generally, **resin-bonded PLVs require ¼ to ½ tooth reduction compared to complete coverage crowns.** In addition, PLVs conserve natural tooth structure, tooth vitality, rigidity and structural integrity, prevent postoperative sensitivity and therefore, ensure longevity of both the tooth and veneering porcelain. To prevent mutilation of tooth structure for spurious short-term aesthetic gains, it is worth remembering the following dictum before prescribing PLV:

> ***The purpose of PLV is replacing lost enamel and dentine***
> ***NOT***
> ***As a substitute for enamel and dentine***

Indications

PLVs are primarily aesthetic restorations for **improving tooth colour, morphology and alignment.** They are usually placed on buccal surfaces of teeth in the maxillary anterior sextant, but are also indicated for:

- **Space management,** e.g. diastemata closure or correcting imbrications
- **Restitution of vertical dimension of occlusion (VDO)** using the Dahl concept, following bite collapse due to tooth wear
- **Combination restorations**, e.g. veneerlay (combination of a veneer and an inlay or onlay)
- **Palatal veneers** to repair fractures, erosion, GERD (gastroesophageal reflux disease) or breakdown of defective restorations

Preparation designs

Unlike crown preparations that have predefined geometric configurations to provide retention and resistance form, **PLV preparations are non-retentive and entirely dictated by a diagnostic wax-up.** Consequently, there is **no ideal preparation design,** and tooth reduction (if necessary) is influenced by aesthetic objectives, occlusal and functional needs, endodontic and periodontal considerations, amount of remaining tooth substrate, existing fillings, tooth morphology and alignment, choice of ceramic and patients' wishes. There are **four aspects to consider for PLV preparations are**:

- **Buccal (facial)** – retain ²/₃ to ¾ enamel for maintaining enamel rigidity, finish lines within enamel, cervical ¹/₃ reduction (or space) of 0.4 mm and remaining ²/₃ facial reduction (or space) of 0.7 mm
- **Incisal edge**

Window – conservative, poor aesthetics
Feather-edge – conservative, chipping at incisal edges, poor aesthetics
Incisal wrap (with palatal chamfer, bevel or butt joint) – invasive, superior aesthetics, requires 1 mm occlusal clearance, allows tooth lengthening (especially following tooth wear)

- **Cervical** – ideally margins within enamel, supragingival or subgingival to mask discolouration and/or conceal the porcelain/tooth interface
- **Interproximal** – retain or break contact areas depending on clinical situation and treatment objectives

The PLV preparation should feature **clearly defined finish lines, smooth surface roughness**, a **sinuous outline devoid of undercuts**, and **sufficient space to accommodate adequate porcelain thickness for strength** and **to prevent an overcontoured restoration**. If preparation is unnecessary, any **aprismatic enamel should be roughened** using microabrasion techniques to enhance bond strength before bonding the veneers with a dental adhesive and resin-based cement. Pre-existing composite fillings can reduce bond strength and may require replacement beforehand, or during the cementing process. Similarly, definitive cementation of PLVs to bleached teeth should be deferred for one week to ensure viable bonding to the underlying tooth substrate.

Preparation guidelines

A **diagnostic wax-up (analogue or virtual)** is the starting point for PLV preparations (Chapter 17). This allows 3D visualisation of the proposed outcome, and is preferable to 2D image manipulation software simulations. Also, a diagnostic wax-up serves as a template for:

- **Silicone or 3D printed index** for guided tooth preparation
- **Transparent vacuum-formed stent or thermoplastic matrix** for intra-oral mock-ups and temporary coverage
- **Guide for fabricating the definitive porcelain veneers**

Many methods have been proposed for tooth preparation, including **freehand**, **index guides** and **cutting through intra-oral composite or acrylic mock-ups**. The most precise method is using indices in several planes, to guide and minimise inadvertent tooth reduction. Tooth reduction (if necessary) is accomplished by placing depth cuts with **individual round diamond burs** of varying diameters or a **single bur incorporating predefined depth wheels**. The depth cuts are then joined together for the axial reduction using **straight-sided 135° chamfer burs** of **progressively decreasing particle size diamond grit**, and smoothed with **tungsten carbide finishing burs**. The reduction should **mimic the tooth curvature in all planes** (mesiodistal, inciso-gingival) for ensuring an even, predefined thickness of porcelain. If required, **interproximal contacts** are broken with finely coated diamond discs. To prevent laceration of the gingival margin or interproximal papillae, the latter are protected by either **flat plastic instruments or the Zekrya gingival protector**. If dentine is exposed, **immediate dentine sealing (IDS)** using a dental adhesives is advisable before impressions or fabricating provisional restorations.

Key points

- PLVs are highly aesthetic and predictable restorations, but require meticulous attention to detail for long-term success.
- There is no ideal tooth preparation (if necessary) for PLVs, which depends on the clinical scenario and treatment objectives, and is guided by a diagnostic wax-up.
- Preservation of enamel is the key to success.

Preparation for full-coverage crowns and FPDs

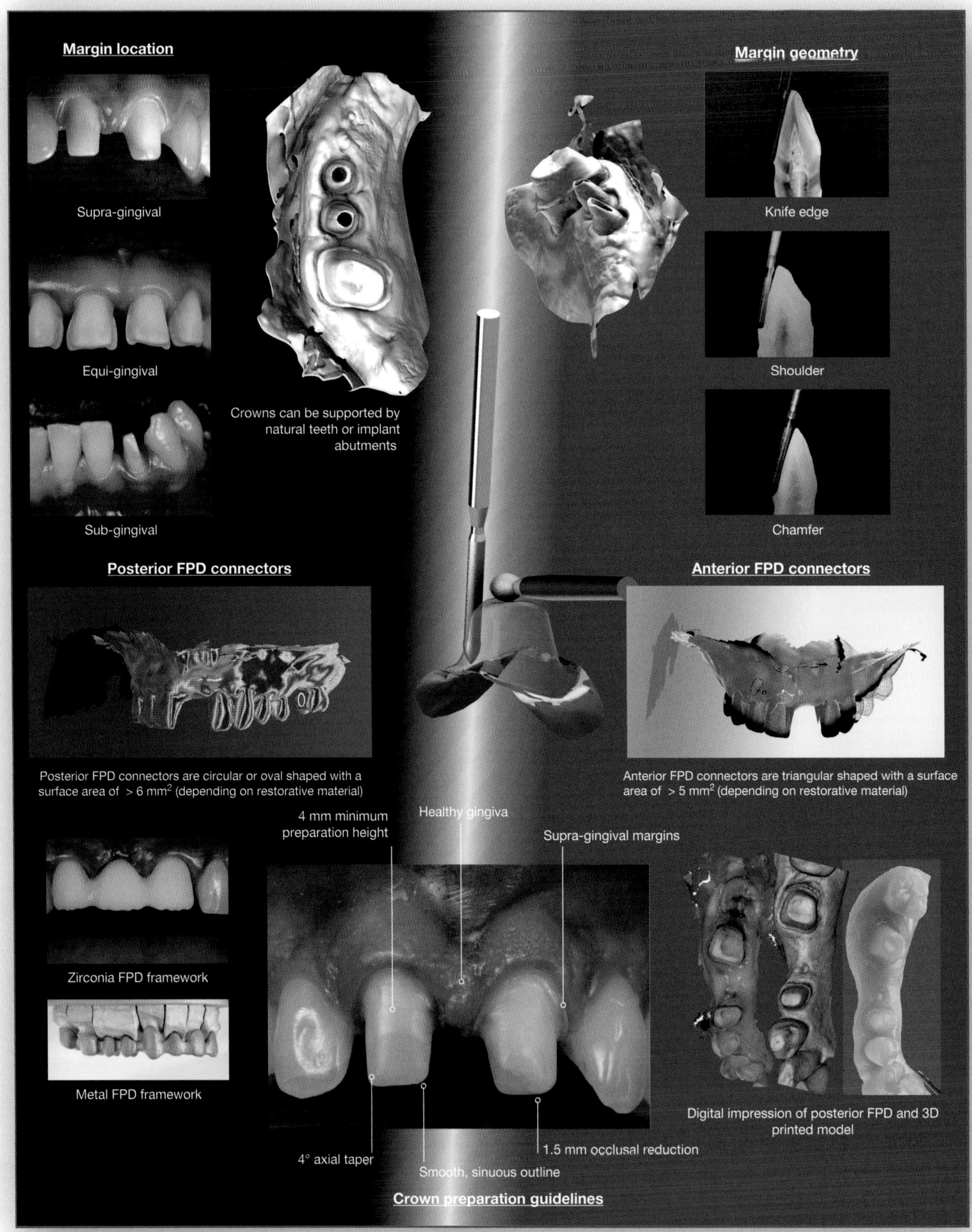

Margin location

Supra-gingival

Equi-gingival

Sub-gingival

Crowns can be supported by natural teeth or implant abutments

Margin geometry

Knife edge

Shoulder

Chamfer

Posterior FPD connectors

Posterior FPD connectors are circular or oval shaped with a surface area of > 6 mm^2 (depending on restorative material)

Anterior FPD connectors

Anterior FPD connectors are triangular shaped with a surface area of > 5 mm^2 (depending on restorative material)

Zirconia FPD framework

Metal FPD framework

4 mm minimum preparation height

Healthy gingiva

Supra-gingival margins

4° axial taper

Smooth, sinuous outline

1.5 mm occlusal reduction

Crown preparation guidelines

Digital impression of posterior FPD and 3D printed model

Prosthodontics at a Glance, Second Edition. Irfan Ahmad.

Full-coverage crowns or **abutments for fixed partial dentures (FPDs)** on natural teeth are probably the penultimate indirect prostheses before contemplating extractions or implants. Furthermore, before embarking on these destructive and irreversible preparations, alternative adhesive restorations such as onlays, PLVs, endo-crowns or RBFPDs should be considered. Full-coverage crowns are also indicated for implant-supported single-unit crowns and FPDs, which minimises the number of implants required for oral rehabilitation. There is an ongoing debate that in view of newer and more predicable restorative materials, and the fact that crown preparation is highly destructive, does this **signal the demise of crowns?** Certainly, decimating virgin teeth for elective cosmetic procedures, or bridge abutments for replacing missing teeth is a travesty and should be avoided at all cost.

Crown preparation is usually for **360° coverage**, but **various configurations** are possible such as **½, ¾, ⅞,** etc. depending on the remaining tooth substrate. Essentially, **tooth preparation for crowns is material-oriented,** i.e. the tooth preparation is geometric to accommodate the properties of specific restorative materials such as gold, resin-based composites or ceramics.

Margin location

The **preparation margins, or finish lines** can be placed in three locations:

- **Supragingival** – indicated for low lip lines, posterior crowns, knife-edge finish lines or thin periodontal biotypes. This is an ideal position since it allows both oral hygiene access, and clinical visibility for monitoring. Furthermore, gingival inflammation is minimal, and biologic width integrity is preserved
- **Equigingival** – ideal when the underlying tooth colour is acceptable and an all-ceramic restoration is utilised
- **Subgingival** – indicated for high lip lines, profound tooth discolouration, masking or altering unsightly tooth colour or for all-ceramic crowns with a dense opaque core (e.g. zirconia) to conceal the crown/tooth interface. However, **subgingival margins should only be considered for thick periodontal biotypes,** which have less propensity for postoperative gingival recession, and **located within the gingival sulcus** to prevent violation of the biologic width. For subgingival carious lesions, **crown lengthening** or **orthodontic extrusion** may be necessary to locate the finish lines in a more favourable position.

Margin geometry

Margin geometry describes the shape of the tooth preparation finish lines. Three basic shapes are possible: **knife or feather-edge, shoulder** (or butt joint) and **chamfer**. The **knife-edge** is minimally invasive and conservative, advocated for full metal crowns, especially in the posterior regions of the mouth. Because the preparation is minimal, the margin must be located supragingivally. The disadvantages include indistinct finish lines and larger margin opening compared to a butt joint, bulbous crowns due to under-preparation, and is therefore contraindicated for all-ceramic crowns. The **shoulder preparation** (90° to 120°) is more aggressive than a knife-edge margin. It is suitable for PFM (porcelain fused to metal) and all-ceramic units. However, the internal line angles should be rounded, devoid of undercut. The **chamfer preparation** has a generally accepted geometry angle of 135° that allows a gradual shade tooth/crown transition, aids scanning with intra-oral scanners and is ubiquitously recommended for most all-ceramic units and electroformed crowns. Furthermore, because **the smallest CAD/CAM millings tips are 1 mm,** they cannot reproduce preparation detail below this threshold.

Preparation design

A crown preparation requires **retention form** to prevent dislodgement and **resistance form** to resist occlusal and masticatory forces. As a general guide, full metal crowns require less tooth reduction compared to PFM or bi-layer all-ceramic units. A preparation design should incorporate the following features:

- **Occlusal/incisal reduction** – 1–1.5 mm in all excursions for clearance, and for enhanced fracture resistance of the restorative material
- **Axial taper** – ideal 4° mesial and distal taper (or 8° convergence angle), acceptable range is 6–15°, i.e. translating to a mesial and distal interproximal reduction of 0.75–1.5 mm
- **Facial and lingual reduction** – 1–1.5 mm depending on the margin geometry, and the facial-lingual thickness of the tooth
- **Incisal-gingival height** – a minimum of 4 mm is desirable for adequate resistance form. It may be necessary to build-up or fill-in deficiencies with resin-modified glass ionomer or resin-based composites or to incorporate retention grooves for added retention
- **Sinuous outline, devoid of undercuts and a smooth surface** is essential for impression making, cementing and facilitating fabrication of the restoration in the dental laboratory. Furthermore, sharp line angles initiate fractures at the fitting or intaglio surface of all-ceramic restorations
- **Follow the contours and anatomy of the natural tooth,** retaining as much enamel and dentine as possible.
- **Trim serrated, unsupported enamel margins** with either hand chisels or preferably with reciprocating EVA diamond tip for delineating a clearly visible finish line

FPD considerations

Tooth preparation for FPD abutments is identical to single units but with the following additional considerations:

- **Parallelism** – all abutment teeth should have the same path of insertion/withdrawal. Various methods are available for achieving parallelism, e.g. intra-oral jigs
- **Connector dimensions** – are the weakest link of FPD frameworks, and their dimensions depend on the type of restorative material and location of the tooth. Cast metal or titanium frameworks require less surface area for connectors than ceramics, e.g. 6.25 mm^2 for porcelain fused to metal, 9–16 mm^2 for alumina and zirconia and 12–20 mm^2 for glass ceramics
- **Pontic design and size** – e.g. ridge-lap, ovate or modified ovate pontics depending on morphology of the alveolar ridge(s)
- **Precision attachments** – are incorporated to relieve stress in long-span FPDs. Precision attachments require additional space at the occlusal and interproximal areas, and can only be used with cast metal frameworks

Key points

- Full-coverage tooth preparation is highly destructive and requires careful consideration.
- Factors to consider for crown preparation are margin location, margin geometry and preparation design.
- Additional features for FPD abutments include parallelism, space for connectors, pontic design and incorporation of precision attachments.

Temporary restorations

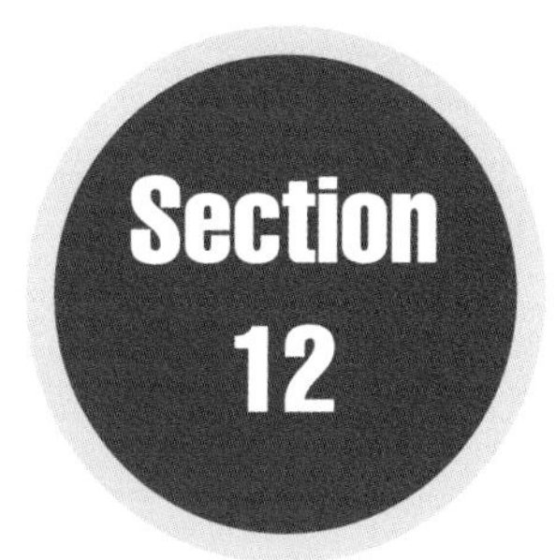

Chapter

51 Provisionals

Material	Advantages	Disadvantages
Metal	Pre-formed morphology, no matrix required, can be relined with self-cured resins	Require extensive adjustment to obtain good marginal fit, contact points and occlusion, poor wear resistance, poor aesthetics
Polycarbonate	Pre-formed morphology, no matrix required, can be relined with self-cured resins, good wear resistance, good aesthetics	Require extensive adjustment to obtain good marginal fit, contact points and occlusion
PMMA	Resilient, good wear resistance and aesthetics, heat and pressure polymerisation improves physical and mechanical properties of material, easy intra-oral relining, repaired with flowable composites, suitable for long-term use and long span multiple units, can be reinforced with metal copings for increased strength for lengthy use, especially for the healing phase of implant-supported prostheses, available as CAD/CAM ingots/3D printing resin	High exotherm, unsuitable for intra-oral fabrication, high shrinkage, unpleasant odour, free monomer causes gingival irritation, requires matrix, higher cost for laboratory-fabricated provisionals
PEMA	Less exotherm than PMMA but higher than bis-acryl, suitable for intra-oral fabrication, selection of shades and stains, easily relined, and repaired with flowable composites, suitable for medium-term use, ideal for relining metal, polycarbonate and PMMA shell crowns	Poorer wear resistance than PMMA, prone to staining, considerable shrinkage, allergies to residual uncreated monomer, unsuitable for long-span multiple units for lengthy period of use, unpleasant odour
Bis-acryl	Most popular of all materials for provisionals due to ease of use and delivery via syringe mix, low exotherm, no objectionable odour, minimal shrinkage, stronger than PEMA, ideal for single and short-span multiple units, and suitable for long-term use, available as CAD/CAM ingots/3D printing resin	High cost and waste, matrix required, brittle, difficult to reline, unsuitable for long-span multiple units
UDMA	Light-cured, good mechanical properties, large selection of shades, good aesthetics, easier relining than bis-acryl, CAD/CAM ingots/3D printing resin	High cost and waste, matrix required, high exotherm due to light-curing polymerisation
Resin-based composite restoratives	Excellent aesthetics, ideal for temporary veneers, can be useds with or without matrix but temporary cement is not necessary, also possible to make laboratory provisional to compensate for polymerisation shrinkage for improved mechanical and optical properties, CAD/CAM ingots/3D printing resin	Expensive, time consuming, difficult to distinguish natural tooth substrate and filling material and may require time-consuming removal and/or damage to tooth preparation
Modified composites	Low viscosity, ideal for intracoronal provisionals for inlays, matrix and temporary cement not necessary	Weak, prone to wear, poor interproximal and occlusal contacts, discolouration with food dyes, difficult to remove if undercuts present

Temporary resin crowns fabricated using a vacuum stent (top 6 images)

Temporary PEMA inlay

Defective crowns on maxillary centrals

Digital impression

CAD

3D printed models

3D printed resin temporary crowns

Prosthodontics at a Glance, Second Edition. Irfan Ahmad.

A **provisional (or temporary restoration)** is used as an interim before fitting the indirect definitive restoration or prosthesis. In essence, **a provisional is disposable**, but should remain for the intervening period while awaiting the permanent analogue.

Function of provisionals

Besides acting as a stopgap, provisionals have numerous useful functions for assuring the ultimate success of the permanent restoration, such as:

- **Health** – of exposed dentine and pulp vitality. In addition, periodontal health requires monitoring, especially if there is prevailing inflammation due to previous defective restorative margins, crown lengthening procedures, implant surgery and bone/soft tissue augmentation. **Healing may be accompanied by gingival recession that may require relocation of the preparation margins**, particularly for restorations in the aesthetic zone. In addition, a provisional is useful for **tissue sculpturing**, either at a pontic site or around tooth or implant abutments to achieve **optimal pink aesthetics**
- **Function** – for planned occlusal changes such as anterior guidance, lateral excursions and vertical dimension alterations. Also, the restorations should be comfortable and not an impede phonetics or embouchure
- **Aesthetics** – when gross morphological changes are planned, e.g. restitution of worn dentition, or for elective cosmetic procedures. Provisionals based on diagnostic wax-ups are ideal for assessing aesthetics and function before carrying out irreversible tooth preparation
- **Tooth preparation** – sufficient tooth removal to accommodate restorative materials using intra-oral guides for precise and calculated tooth reduction, e.g. for adhesively retained PLVs

Choice of materials

The number of materials on the market for provisionals is both impressive and confusing, and the choice is dictated by the intended use and the clinical scenario. Materials for provisionals are broadly divided into metals and resins:

- **Metals** – pre formed single crowns or short-span FPDs without the need for a matrix, e.g. stainless steel, aluminium, nickel and chromium
- **Resins** – polycarbonate (pre-formed single units), PMMA (polymethyl methacrylate), PEMA (polyethyl methacrylate), bis-acryl, UDMA (urethane dimethacrylate), resin-based composites (flowable and non-flowable) and modified composites (for inlays and onlays). Also, many resins are available as ingots for milling long-term temporaries (e.g. Vita CAD-Temp®, Telio® CAD) or 3D printing (e.g. Vita A3 shade Temporis DD-1000-A3, Temporary CB, LuxaPrint, HARZLabs Dental Sand, Raydent Crown & Bridge Resin, NextDent C&B Micro Filled Hybrid)

Techniques for fabrication

Nearly all provisionals (besides pre-formed) require some type of **matrix or template for fabrication. Freehand fabrication** is possible but time-consuming, e.g. temporary composite veneers. The matrix can either be pre-formed or custom-made, which is the most popular method. There are **two techniques** for fabricating provisional: the **direct (intra-oral)** and **indirect (extra-oral)**. The **direct technique** involves using a matrix, for example:

- **Based on existing tooth morphology**, using a rigid and dimensionally stable impression material, e.g. polyvinylsiloxane putty, prior to tooth preparation
- **Based on envisaged tooth morphology** from a diagnostic wax-up using a vacuum-formed thermoplastic matrix
- **Pre-formed metal or plastic shell crowns**

The **indirect technique (extra-oral)** involves using a dental laboratory or in-office casting of models. This technique is ideal for long spans that are intended for lengthy periods of usage, especially for implant-supported prostheses while awaiting osseointegration. Two methods are available:

- **Simulating tooth preparations** on a preoperative or diagnostic wax-up model, and creating PMMA shells in the laboratory that are subsequently relined in the mouth with cold-cured resins after tooth preparation
- **Analogue impression of the prepared abutments**, and then fabricating PMMA provisionals that are cemented with an appropriate temporary cement
- **Digital impression of prepared abutments** and laboratory or chairside **milling or 3D printing provisionals**

Provisionals for PLV present a challenge because little retention is offered from minimal tooth preparation. In these circumstances, if the preparation is within enamel and the contact points are retained, no temporisation is necessary. However, if dentine is exposed or contact areas broken, the options are as follows:

- **Freehand composite build-up with spot etching**, without a bonding agent
- **Composite, bis-acryl or PEMA**, either alone or in combination with a vacuum-formed matrix or silicone impression matrix, and cemented with spot etching and a flowable composite. Also, linking multiple provisional veneers improves retention and prevents dislodgement
- **Chairside or laboratory milling or 3D printing provisionals** from a digital impression

Provisionals for intracoronal restorations such as inlays can be fabricated from a variety of resins, but the most popular materials are light-cured modified composites that are directly dispensed into the cavity preparation and set with a light-curing unit.

Temporary cements

A **temporary cement** should be strong enough to retain the provisional, yet weak enough to remove the restoration. Furthermore, it should be **palliating and therapeutic** to the hard and soft tissues, maintain structural integrity and vitality of the tooth, and promote gingival health. The most popular temporary cements are **zinc oxide/eugenol formulations,** available as **non-eugenol and transparent varieties.** Other cements include zinc phosphate, polycarboxylate and flowable composites. To minimise the marginal gap between the provisional and tooth preparation margins, the provisional should not be overfilled; the temporary cement should be judiciously applied to the cervical margins and axial walls, but not to the occlusal intaglio surface.

Key points

- Provisionals are interim restorations used while awaiting the definitive restoration or prostheses.
- Properly constructed and accurately fitting provisionals are essential for the long-term success of the permanent restoration.
- A selection of materials is available for fabricating provisionals, using either the direct or indirect techniques.

Impressions

Section 13

Chapters

Soft tissue management

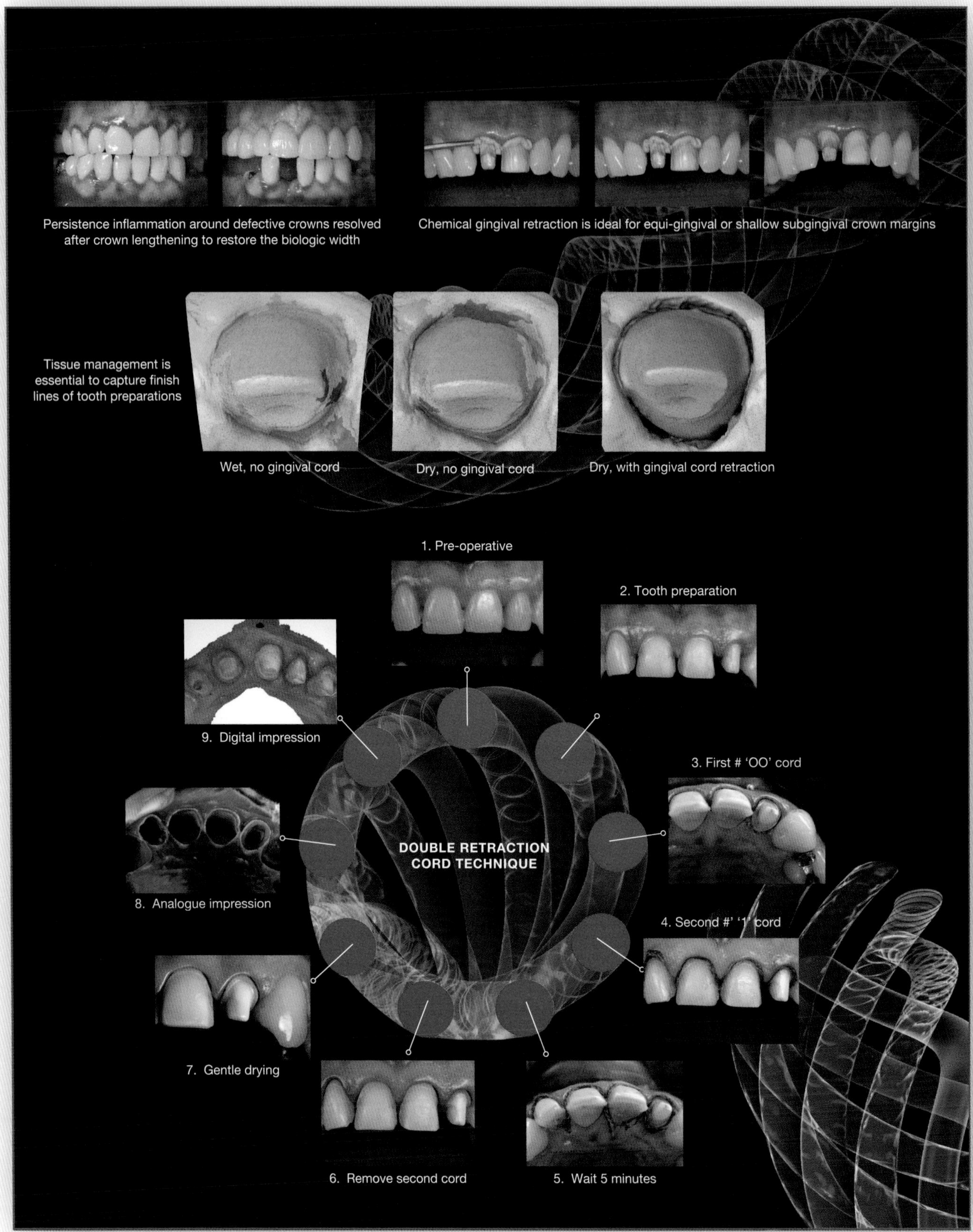

Persistence inflammation around defective crowns resolved after crown lengthening to restore the biologic width

Chemical gingival retraction is ideal for equi-gingival or shallow subgingival crown margins

Tissue management is essential to capture finish lines of tooth preparations

Wet, no gingival cord

Dry, no gingival cord

Dry, with gingival cord retraction

DOUBLE RETRACTION CORD TECHNIQUE

1. Pre-operative
2. Tooth preparation
3. First # 'OO' cord
4. Second #' '1' cord
5. Wait 5 minutes
6. Remove second cord
7. Gentle drying
8. Analogue impression
9. Digital impression

Prosthodontics at a Glance, Second Edition. Irfan Ahmad.

The first factor determining the accuracy of an impression is **efficacious soft tissue management**. The definitive restoration is only as good as the impression. Adequate soft tissue management is **essential for both analogue and digital impressions.** Apart from the need to choose the appropriate impression material and to use a correct impression technique, most defective impressions are attributed to ineffective soft tissue control. Soft tissue management can be categorised as, first, **achieving and maintaining periodontal health,** and second, manipulating the gingiva to facilitate impression making. This involves a **transient displacement (retraction) of the circumferential gingivae** surrounding the prepared tooth, or implant abutment to:

- **Visualise the finish line**
- **Maintain an arid environment,** particularly for addition silicone (VPS) materials and digital impressions
- **Record an area apical to the finish line** to create a correct **emergence profile** of the artificial prosthesis
- **Accommodate a sufficient bulk of intrasulcular impression material** (at least 0.2 mm thickness) for analogue impressions

Periodontal health

The primary determinant for achieving a successful impression is achieving and maintaining periodontal health. A healthy periodontium is a prerequisite for facilitating not only impression making but also subsequent stages such as the try-in and cementation procedures. There are **two aspects influencing periodontal health: patient and operator factors**. The **patient factors** are predominately beyond the patient's and clinician's control, including:

- **Genetic predisposition** or constitution
- **Age, race, gender,** e.g. pregnancy and osteoporosis
- **Systemic illnesses**, e.g. diabetes, compromised immune system, psychological stress, bisphosphonate or radiation therapy
- **Dental biotype and bioform**
- **Oral pathogens**
- **Local trauma or previously compromised vascularity**, e.g. periapical lesions, apicectomies
- **Socio-economic status**
- **Oral hygiene, local irritants,** e.g. smoking, alcohol abuse

Conversely, the **operator factors** are within the clinician's control, and are remediable with proper techniques, including:

- **Oral hygiene, smoking cessation** counselling and meticulous prophylaxis
- **Maintaining biologic width integrity**
- **Ensuring correct emergence profiles** of all provisional and definitive restorations
- **Precision fitting of provisionals** to encourage gingival health

Gingival healing can be as rapid as a few days, or prolonged over several weeks, depending on the prevailing patient factors, or the degree of iatrogenic insult during restorative procedures. Therefore, impressions should be deferred until a stable and healthy gingival architecture is evident. This is particularly important for anterior pink aesthetics, where erratic gingival contours following gingival recession can compromise aesthetic outcomes.

Chemical retraction

Chemical retraction is the least traumatic method for achieving gingival retraction using **hygroscopic gels**, usually incorporating haemostatic agents, e.g. Expasyl (KerrHawe SA, Switzerland). This method is **ideal for equigingival or shallow subgingival preparation margins,** where minimal retraction is necessary, but may be challenging for deeper, subgingival finish lines.

Physical retraction

The most predictable and **widely practised method for gingival retraction is using retractions cords**, with or without haemostatic agents. This is the **preferred method for subgingival margins** using either the **single or double retraction cord technique**. The potential drawbacks are gingival injury and recession, especially with thin biotypes due to inadvertent trauma during cord placement and removal. If gingival bleeding is present, the cords can be presoaked in **haemostatic agents** such as **buffered aluminium chloride, aluminium potassium sulphate** or **ferric sulphate**. Adrenaline is contraindicated due to its undesirable effects of raising heart rate and blood pressure.

Surgical retraction

There **are two circumstances when surgical intervention is necessary**: first, **gingival enlargement or overgrowth**, and second, **violation of the biological width**. Gingival enlargement may be due to systemic (including medication) or local causes, e.g. occur in the presence of open, defective restoration margins or if a previous restoration has been dislodged for a considerable time. If the preparation margins are approaching the alveolar crest, **surgical crown lengthening** is required for osseous resection to re-establish the biologic width. However, all forms of surgery is unpredictable with thin biotypes, with possible ensuing gingival recession. The **surgical methods** include:

- **Scalpel** – conventional full thickness flap elevation and ostectomy is the ideal procedure for crown lengthening, either for aesthetic gingival margin contouring and re-establishing the biologic width
- **Electrosurgery** – using radio frequencies of greater than 1 MHz, electrosurgery is conducive for gingivectomy, widening of the gingival sulcus and coagulation
- **Piezo surgery** diamond coated tips to perform ostectomy and osteoplasty
- **Lasers (Chapters 43 and 44)** – e.g. argon, KTP, diode, Nd : YAG and microsecond-pulsed CO_2 lasers have similar functions to electrosurgery and are useful for soft tissue incisions and sulcular debridement
- **Rotary curettage** – using diamond burs for gingival resection or sulcus widening. However, this is a highly destructive procedure, and the lack of tactile sensation can lead to widespread gingival trauma and prolonged haemorrhage

Key points

- Soft tissue management is essential for facilitating and producing accurate analogue or digital impressions.
- The primary determinant for precise impressions is achieving and maintaining periodontal health.
- Soft tissue manipulation is achieved by a variety of gingival retraction methods including chemical, physical and surgical.
- Surgical intervention is necessary for gingival overgrowth and re-establishing the biological width.

53 Impression materials

Choice of impression materials

Removable prosthodontics

Full dentures: ZnO/eugenol paste, light body VPS or polyether

Partial dentures: Monophase VPS or polyether

Fixed prosthodontics

Teeth: Dual-phase VPS or polyether

Implants: Monophase/dual-phase VPS or polyether

Preliminary impressions

Alginate dental compound

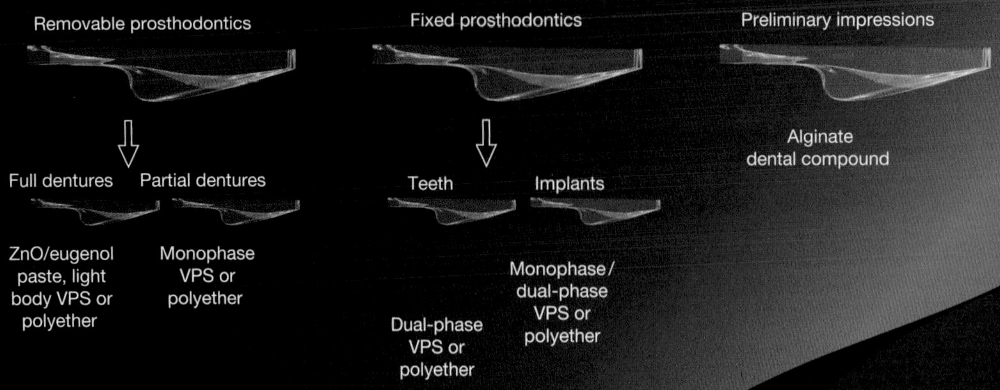

Definitions

Tear resistance	Ability of a material to resist tearing in small cross sections, e.g. deep subgingival margins
Elastic recovery	The degree of recoil of a material without permanent elastic deformation, e.g. from tooth preparation undercuts
Dimensional stability	Ability to withstand stress without permanent deformation, e.g. heavy body or putty formulations

Contact angle (wettability) of impression materials

Low – Hydrophilic

Medium – Intermediate

High – Hydrophobic

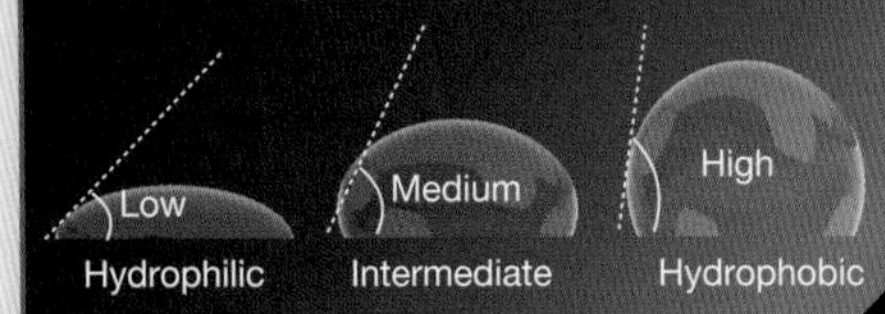

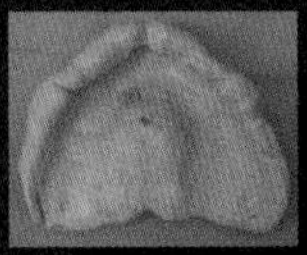

ZnO/eugenaol for RFD

Monophase VPS for RPD (below)

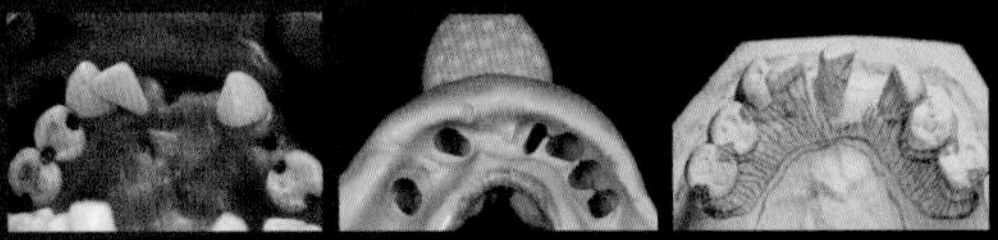

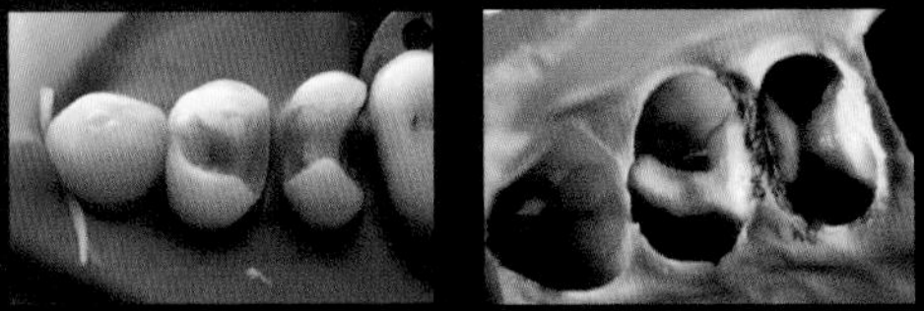

Heavy/light VPS for inlays

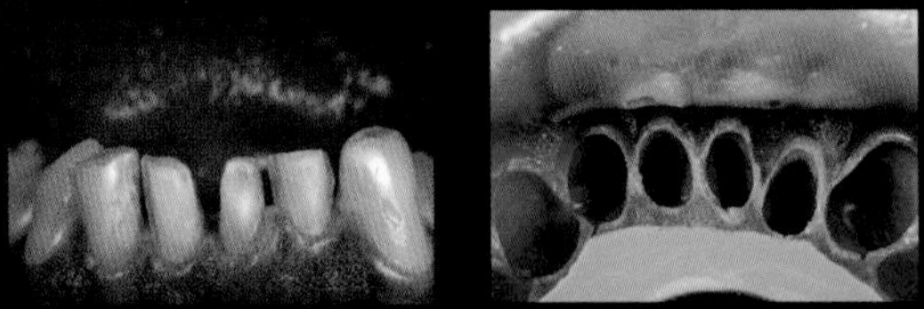

Heavy/light VPS for PLVs

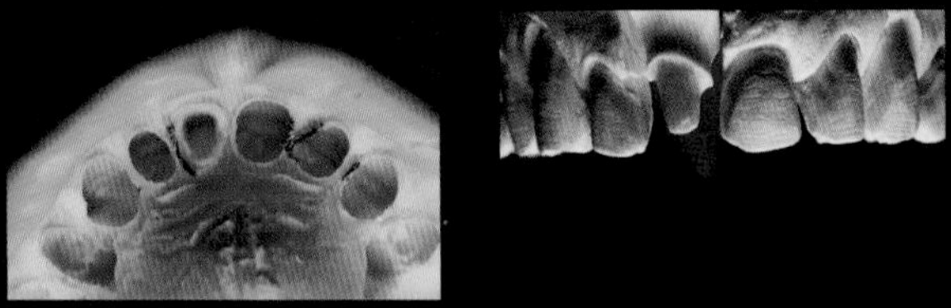

Heavy/light VPS for crowns & PLVs

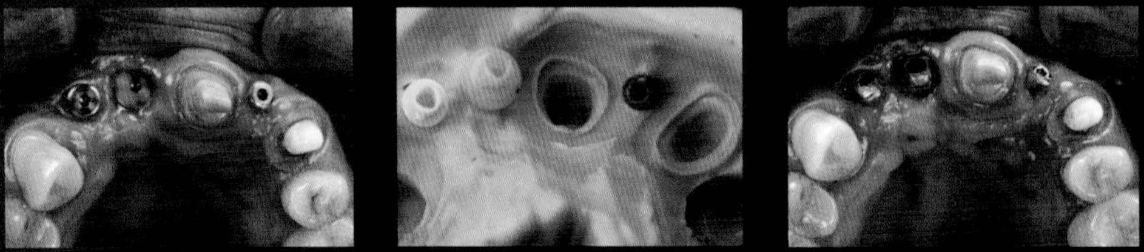

Heavy/light VPS for crowns & implants

Impressions or negative imprints of the teeth and surrounding soft tissues anatomy and required for fabricating indirect fixed or removable restorations/prostheses. The choice of **impression material** depends on the type of prosthesis. While some materials have multiple uses, predictable and precise impressions are achieved using specific materials for removable and fixed prosthodontics. Regrettably, substandard impressions are often accepted by clinicians in the expectation that the dental technician can 'fake and make' missing or inadequate details of intra-oral anatomy. Precise and accurate impressions are challenging and require knowledge of:

- **Visualising the finish line**
- **Soft tissue management** (Chapter 52)
- **Materials for analogue impressions** (this chapter)
- **Analogue impression techniques and armamentarium** (Chapters 54)
- **Digital impressions** (Chapter 55)

Many impression materials used in dentistry since the 1950s are now **archaic or redundant, including plaster, polysulphides (rubber base), reversible hydrocolloids and condensation silicones**. However, a minority of older generation or esoteric clinicians still find use for these materials. There are **various classification of dental impression materials.** They can be classified according to viscosity (low, light body, medium, monophase, high and putty), **elastic** (alginates, VPS and polyetehr), **non-elastic** (zinc-oxide eugenol, dental compound and waxes), **mucodisplacive** (high viscosity elastomers, high viscosity alginates and dental compound) or **mucostatic** (zinc-oxide eugenol or low viscosity alginate); the former records the oral mucosa under load, while the latter records a [relatively] undispalced mucosa. The impression materials discussed below are the most popular in contemporary prosthodontics.

Dental compound

Dental compound is a **thermodynamic** material that softens with heat and sets to a rigid consistency in the oral cavity. Due to its thermodynamic behaviour, **additions or corrections are relatively easy.** However, its **low strength, poor surface detail and brittleness** are drawbacks, often causing breakage, and uses include **customising stock trays, preliminary impressions** for full dentures or **supporting areas of deep sulci and edentulous ridges.**

Zinc oxide (ZnO) eugenol paste

The use of **zinc oxide/eugenol paste** is exclusively for **tissue-supported removable full dentures (RFD)**. The material's enduring property is that it **does not displace soft tissues of edentulous ridges**, or buccal sulci (**mucostatic**), thus avoiding pressure spots on fitting surfaces, and overextended buccal flanges, respectively. Furthermore, voids are readily corrected by adding wax without repeating the impression. However, the material is **unsuitable where there are profound ridge undercuts**; it is also contraindicated in patients who object to its pungent taste and odour, or who suffer from **eugenol allergy.**

Irreversible hydrocolloids

Alginates are **irreversible hydrocolloids**, frequently used for **preliminary impressions** for custom tray fabrication, opposing arch impressions, diagnostics (study models), making extra-oral provisional restorations and for orthodontic cast records. Alginates are **inexpensive** and relatively **technique-insensitive**, offer good surface detail, but are incompatible with some dental stones, and **dimensionally unstable** requiring almost immediate pouring.

Vinyl polysiloxane (VPS)

Vinyl polysiloxanes (VPS), and **polyethers (elastomers),** are the **most popular impression materials for fixed prosthodontics**, including implant-supported prostheses. VPS materials, also known as addition silicones or poly-vinyl siloxane (PVS), were introduced in the 1970s, as addition reaction silicone elastomers. Their popularity is attributed to **ease of use** (automix and cartridge delivery systems), **patient-friendliness** (odourless, insipid), **accuracy** (excellent surface detail), **dimensional stability**, **average tear resistance**, **good elastic recovery**, **long-term storage, multiple pouring**, immersible in **aqueous disinfectants** and availability in a **range of viscosities** and working/setting times for innumerable impression procedures. In addition, VPS materials are suitable for many impression techniques including quadrant, full arch and one- and two-stage protocols using either dual or monophase consistencies. Some disadvantages of VPS materials are that the **setting reaction is retarded by latex glove contamination,** which can be mitigated using an automix machine or washing the tooth preparation with 3% hydrogen peroxide. Another issue is that high viscosity VPS can **engage ridge undercuts,** making the impression tray difficult to remove from the mouth. Silicones are **hydrophobic (high contact angle)** and therefore impressions of subgingival crown margins may be problematic. However, as discussed in Chapter 52, efficient soft tissue management negates this unfavourable property.

Polyethers

Polyethers are the second most popular impression materials for fixed prosthodontics. They offer **excellent accuracy, dimensional stability, superior tear resistance and elastic recovery**. Another benefit is their **hydrophilic (low contact angle)** property, facilitating impressions of deep intracrevicular (subgingival) restorative margins. Earlier polyethers had disadvantages of high rigidity and pungent odour/taste, but newer versions offer lower viscosities and are tasteless. A major drawback is that **multiple pours are not possible,** which are essential for modern laboratory fabrication procedures, especially when using CAD/CAM methods. Finally, due to their hydrophilicity, [illegible] soluble disinfectant is necessary.

Key points

- Impressions are required for indirectly fabricated prostheses.
- Choosing the correct impression material for a specific prosthesis is essential for success.
- Contemporary materials for analogue impressions yield reliable and predictable impressions.
- The most popular impression materials for prosthodontics are alginate, VPS and polyethers.

54 Analogue impressions

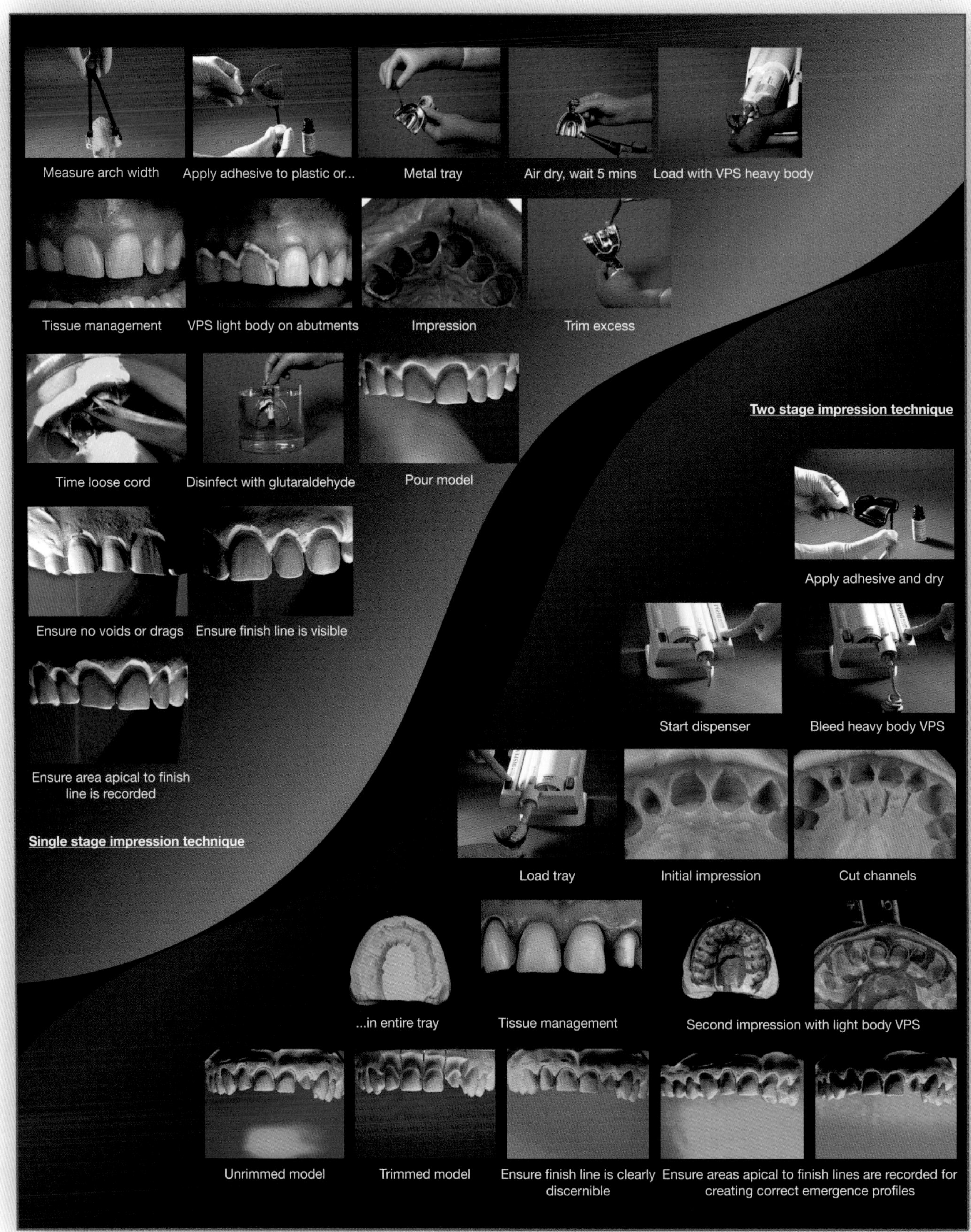

Single stage impression technique

Measure arch width

Apply adhesive to plastic or...

Metal tray

Air dry, wait 5 mins

Load with VPS heavy body

Tissue management

VPS light body on abutments

Impression

Trim excess

Time loose cord

Disinfect with glutaraldehyde

Pour model

Ensure no voids or drags

Ensure finish line is visible

Ensure area apical to finish line is recorded

Two stage impression technique

Apply adhesive and dry

Start dispenser

Bleed heavy body VPS

Load tray

Initial impression

Cut channels

...in entire tray

Tissue management

Second impression with light body VPS

Unrimmed model

Trimmed model

Ensure finish line is clearly discernible

Ensure areas apical to finish lines are recorded for creating correct emergence profiles

Prosthodontics at a Glance, Second Edition. Irfan Ahmad.

Besides choosing the correct impression material for a specific restoration, the technique and armamentarium also influence the accuracy of an analogue or tray/material impression.

Tray selection

The choice of trays are:

- **Rigid *vs.* non-rigid:** the rationale for using a rigid tray is to avoid distortion by controlling dimensional stability and minimising polymerisation shrinkage. Conversely, plastic or non-rigid trays cause distortion, even if using heavy-bodied materials. As a general rule, plastic trays are suitable for single units, but **metal trays are preferable for multiple units**
- **Stock *vs.* custom:** stock trays offer convenience and disposability (plastic variety). Most fixed prosthodontic impressions are feasible with metal stock trays with or without modifications using dental compound material. However, well-adapted, uniformly spaced (4 mm) **custom (special) trays** fabricated from autopolymerising/light-cured resins or 3D printed are an ideal choice for removable prostheses, complex cases involving a combination of teeth and implant-supported restorations, or if voids and drags are persistent in a stock tray impression. Also, care is necessary when using rigid materials, e.g. polyethers or putty-wash techniques, especially in the presence of undercuts, which may prevent removal of the custom tray after the material has set
- **Perforated *vs.* closed:** the reasoning for using a perforated tray is that the holes act as vents for excess material. However, the drawback is that material seepage may elicit a gagging reflex
- **Inter-arch *vs.* intra-arch**: Full or intra-arch trays are essential for removable, and preferred for fixed, prosthodontics. In some countries, there is a penchant for using inter-arch trays, which simultaneously act as a bite registration. While this may be useful for single units, the disadvantages include ensuring complete closure in maximum intercuspation position, distortion of the delicate 'triple tray' (plastic variety), inability to assess jaw excursions and technically challenging laboratory procedures

Tray adhesive

The function of a **tray adhesive** is to prevent material lifting off the tray and causing mass discrepancies. The tray adhesive should be compatible with the given impression material, i.e. alginate, VPS or polyether. Furthermore, to ensure efficacy of the adhesive, it should be applied and **allowed to dry** before making an impression, otherwise it will act as a lubricant rather than an adhesive.

Material manipulation

Most contemporary materials are available in **cartridges for automatic electronic mixing units** or **auto-mixing hand-held dispensers**. **Manual mixing is almost redundant** due to infection control concerns, heterogeneous mix, inadequate mixture of base and catalyst and the introduction of porosity. Heating impression materials was often used with older generations of materials to manipulate the setting time and alter viscosity. However, these practices alter the chemical composition of the material, and result in erratic setting reactions. Furthermore, newer materials are available in a range of setting times and viscosities, obviating the need to heat or chill to alter flowability or setting times. One of the drawbacks of VPS materials is that the setting reaction is affected by latex. Therefore, handing VPS should be limited to non-latex nitrile or polyethylene gloves. Also, complete setting of most elastomers is affected by residual acrylic monomer of some provisional restorative materials, but is unaffected by haemostatic agents used for gingival retraction.

Undercuts

Undercuts present a problem for impressions and may be present due to:

- **Inadequate tooth preparation**
- **Interproximal gingival embrasures** (black triangles)
- **Deep sulci**
- **Atrophic alveolar ridges**, **pontic sites**
- **Malaligned teeth**

Most softer varieties of elastomers are sufficiently flexible to overcome minor discrepancies, but blatant and profound undercuts should be blocked beforehand with wax to avoid locking of the impression tray on the teeth, or tearing the material at crucial areas such as finish lines.

Moisture control

Moisture control entails controlling salivary flow, intracrevicular fluid and gingival haemorrhage. The former is accomplished using salivary ejectors and high volume aspiration, while the latter is by soft tissue management (discussed in Chapter 52). An **arid environment is essential for recording subgingival margins using hydrophobic impressions materials,** e.g. VPS. Some VPS impression material can be pretreated with surfactants or topical agents to encourage hydrophilicity or wettability. However, hydrophilic polyethers are better suited for moisture environments.

Single vs. two stage

The most commonly practised protocol is the **putty-wash technique, either single-stage or two-stage**:

- **Single-stage:** the tray is loaded with a heavy-body material while a light-body wash is simultaneously dispensed onto the prepared abutment(s). The advantage is expediency, but the downside is distortion of the tray and excessive displacement of the soft tissues
- **Two-stage**: the first step involves taking a heavy-body or putty impression, either before or after tooth preparation, with or without an appropriate spacer, or using individual tooth copings. The second step is dispensing a light-body wash onto the abutment(s) and relocating the tray with the set putty into the mouth. The rationale is that shrinkage is minimised, since the heavy- and light-body materials set separately, but accurately relocating the tray may be challenging.

Recoil

All **elastomeric impression materials** suffer from **recoil**, which may result in a prosthesis fitting a die on a model, but not the intra-oral abutment. To minimise this effect, the impression material should be allowed to polymerise passively by not applying excessive pressure while holding the tray in the mouth, and removing rapidly once the material(s) has/have set.

Key points

- Technique and armamentarium determine the accuracy of an analogue or tray/material impression including tray selection, tray adhesive, material manipulation, undercuts, moisture control, single-stage or two-stage technique, and passive setting of the material.

Digital impressions

Advantages of digital impressions

Instant transmission via internet for improved communication/marketing

Patient comfort

Reduce treatment time

Output to CAM and 3D printing devices

Save material & transport cost

CAD

Real-time instant visualisation

Merge DICOM, facial scan and 2D image files

Minimise distortion of analogue impressions

Digital storage & retrievability

Eliminate delayed chemical reactions of impression materials

Mitigate gag reflex

Mucostatic impressions, ideal for mobile or structurally compromised teeth

Bite registration

Shade analysis

Digital impression errors

Missing contact area

Cotton wool roll

Missing crown margin

Gloved finger

Extraneous sulcus

Failure to occlude arches

Poorly scanned interproximal areas

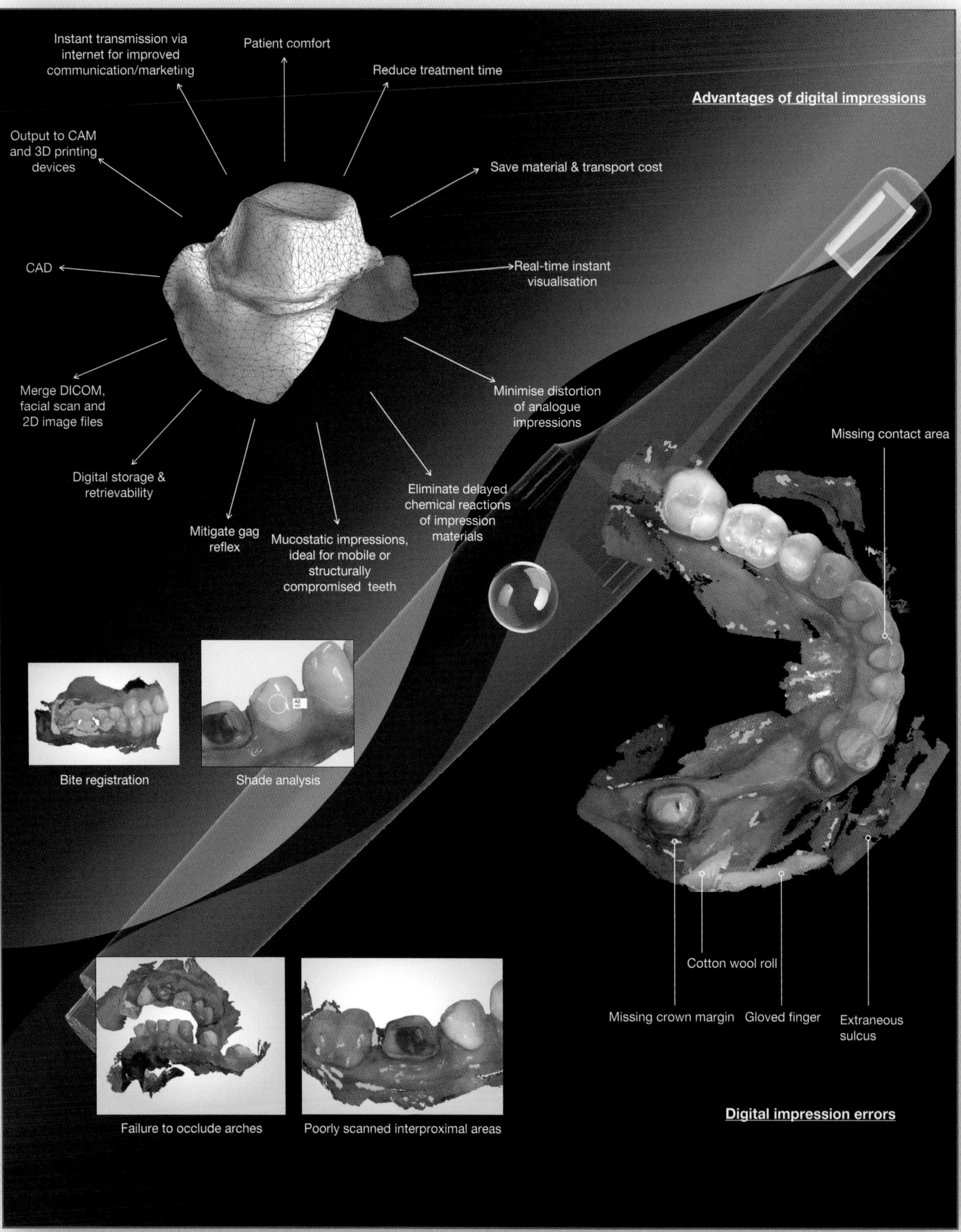

Prosthodontics at a Glance, Second Edition. Irfan Ahmad.

A **digital impression** reproduces a **positive 3D dimensional imprint the teeth and surrounding soft tissues** using an intra-oral scanner (**IOS**) **instead of a negative imprint by analogue tray/material impression.** It is advisable to read Chapters 10 and 11 to be familiar with the terminology used below.

Dental scanner specifications

As well as digitising individual arches, IOS can record the **inter-maxillary relationship** for **virtual articulation,** and tooth colour for **shade analysis**. There are several properties of **IOS** that require consideration:

- **Type of technology** – determines the application for a specific dental discipline
- **Accuracy, trueness, precision and resolution** – discussed in Chapter 11
- **Powder** – Both natural teeth and artificial restorations possess highly polished surfaces that encourage **specular reflections** or shimmering glare. This unwanted glare causes overexposed areas that affects the accuracy of the scan. In order to mitigate the visual noises from these reflections, several protocols have been proposed, e.g. orientating the scanner to encourage diffuse rather than specular reflections, placing a polarising filer in front of the sensor lens, **powdering surfaces with titanium dioxide (TiO_2)**, or asking the patient to rinse beforehand to ephemerally coat the intra-oral surfaces with a mouthwash residue. However, the particle size of opacifiers (around 20–40 μm), may be greater than the resolution of the scanner, and therefore result in decreased accuracy. Another disadvantage with using powder is that the resulting images are monochromatic, reminiscent of plaster casts. Finally, the type of technology of the scanner also determines whether or not powder is necessary, e.g. **AFI is unaffected by shiny surfaces**
- **Prompts** – visual and auditory prompts to facilitate scanning
- **Scan times** – The time to scan a complete arch varies from 4 to 15 minutes, but is influenced by the IOS technology, experience of the operator, familiarity with a particular system, and patient compliance
- **Cross-infection control** – disposable or autoclavable scanner tips
- **Ergonomics** – size, weight, interchange tip sizes to accommodate varying mouth sizes and mouth opening
- **Hardware** – wireless wand, touch screen operation, size of workstation, connection to laptop computer
- **IOS software** – Windows or AppleMac operating systems, black and white or colour imaging, speed of processing to view image, trim tools to remove extraneous items such as cotton wool rolls, sulci, etc., correcting errors such as missed parts, caries detection mode, shade selection facility
- **File format** – determines the accuracy and the type of data recorded. While the popular is an open **.stl file format** that is readily opened in the proprietary software of the scanner or in any third-party CAD software, other formats such as **.obj** and **.ply** are more accurate and also contain colour information. In addition, the scanner software should readily integrate with the chosen CAD software
- **Open or closed system** – this determines whether proprietary software is required to view the resultant 3D files, and whether a subscription is necessary to output an 'open generic' file format such as .stl
- **HIPAA** – Health Insurance Portability and Accountability Act (HIPAA) of 1996 is a US legislation that provides data privacy and security provisions for safeguarding medical information. Therefore, all scan files should be compliant with the HIPAA guidelines for electronic disseminated to a recipient, e.g. by flash drives or via the Internet
- **Cost** – The cost of an IOS is riddled with surreptitious & elusive computations. Although the initial purchase price may be alluring, but additional cost of yearly subscriptions/maintenance packages, software updates, training, CAD designing and CAM facilities can make an innocuous investment spiral out of control. A handheld IOS device ranges from US$ 20K to US$ 40K, plus annual fees of around US$ 4K

Scanning strategies

The **scanning protocol adopted influences accuracy of the final scan**. The first perquisite is proper **tissue management,** as well as maintaining a **clean, dry and clear field of view**, without contamination by oral fluids and adequate cheek and tongue retraction. The scanning path and speed should be at a tempered pace, without shaking to avoid blurring. Several scanning strategies are proposed including **linear fashion** traversing across the occlusal, lingual and buccal surfaces, or a **S/sweep zig-zag motion** over successive teeth in the arch. The former ensures spacial accuracy, while the latter ensures that hidden crevices such as proximal surfaces or contact points/areas are not missed. An **adequate depth of field** is essential to allow the scanner to maintain a reasonable distance above the teeth or oral mucosa without compromising sharply focused images. Most IOS manufacturers suggest a **scanning distance of between 5 mm to 10 mm above the surface** for ensuring that the images are not blurred, while maintaining a comfortable mouth opening for the patient.

Scanning errors

Although digital impressions offer innumerable benefits, they are not without faults. Many scanners provide visual and/or optical prompts for guiding the operator, and display on-screen **missed areas** as white, black or coloured voids. Particular attention is required at **interproximal areas, distal free-end sandals, retromolar areas** and **tooth preparation finish lines.** If missing areas are present, these need to be re-scanned or corrected by software algorithms. Another issue is if posterior teeth are missing, this often results in **failure to occlude the aches.** In addition, **extraneous or unwanted areas** or items that are unintentionally captured such as lips, tongue, cotton wool rolls, saliva ejectors, 6-in-1 syringe tip, gloves, etc., need to be erased after scanning with the 'trim' tool in the scanner or CAD software. Finally, it is worth remembering that **short span scans yield greater accuracy** since the cumulative errors are smaller compared to larger full arch digitisation.

Key points

- Digital impressions offer innumerable advantage over analogue impressions.
- Careful scanner selection and employing correct scanning strategies are essential for accurate digitisation of the oral cavity.
- Errors can be corrected by re-scanning or rectified in scanner or CAD software.
- Digital impressions will replace analogue impressions in the near future.

Dental laboratory - CAD/CAM

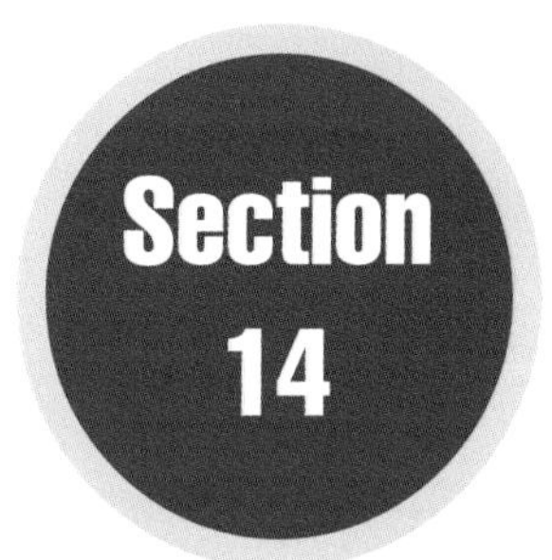

Chapters

56 CAD (computer-aided design)

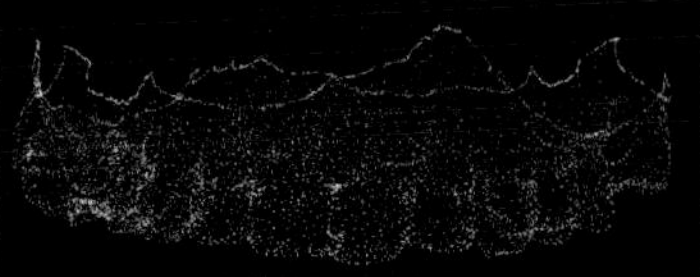

RAW 3D point cloud

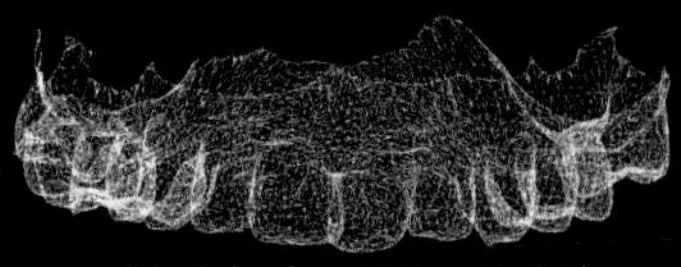

Mesh (surface reconstruction)

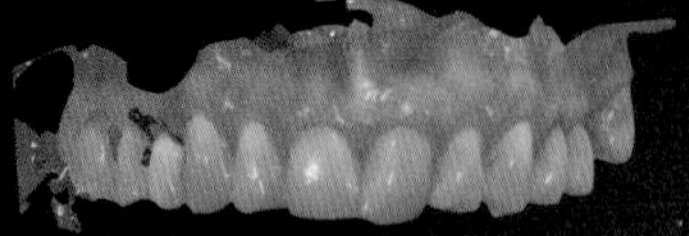

Modelling (texture mapping) by IOS software

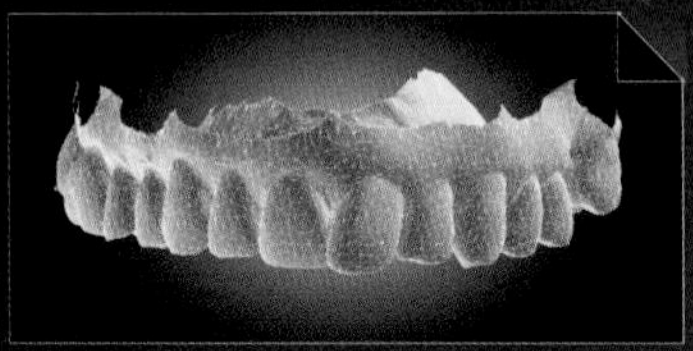

3D file, e.g., .stl

Surface reconstruction with IOS software

Format	Geometry		Physical properties				Context		Animation
	Approx	Precise	Color	Texture	Material	CGS*	Lights	Position	
.stl	ϕ								
.ply	ϕ								
.obj	ϕ	ϕ	ϕ	ϕ	ϕ				
.fbx	ϕ	ϕ	ϕ	ϕ	ϕ		ϕ	ϕ	ϕ
(COLLADA) .dae	ϕ	ϕ	ϕ	ϕ	ϕ		ϕ	ϕ	ϕ
.3DS	ϕ		ϕ	ϕ	ϕ		ϕ	ϕ	
.igs (.ijes)	ϕ	ϕ	ϕ			ϕ		ϕ	
.stp (STEP)	ϕ	ϕ	ϕ	ϕ	ϕ	ϕ		ϕ	
.dxf		ϕ	ϕ				ϕ	ϕ	ϕ
.U3D	ϕ	ϕ	ϕ	ϕ	ϕ	ϕ	ϕ	ϕ	ϕ
.wrl (.X3D)	ϕ	ϕ	ϕ	ϕ	ϕ	ϕ	ϕ	ϕ	ϕ
.3MF	ϕ	ϕ	ϕ	ϕ	ϕ	ϕ			

Attributes of 3D file formats

* CSG - constructive solid geometry

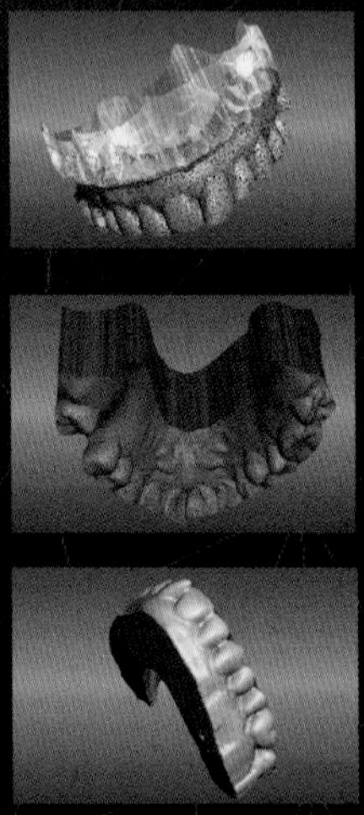

G-CAD software for adding a base to an arch scan

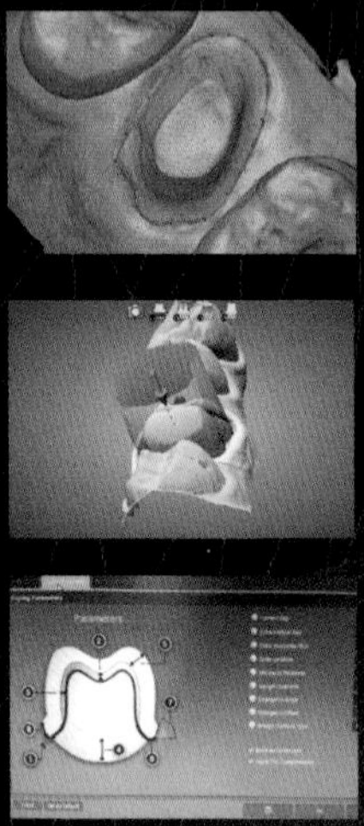

D-CAD software for plotting margins, specifying path of insertion and designing indirect restorations

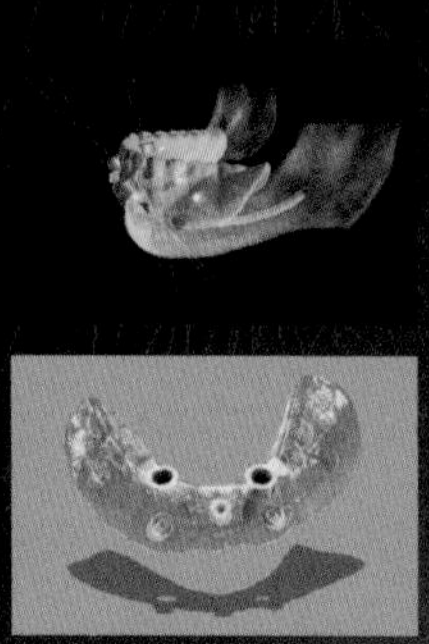

D-CAD software for designing an implant surgical guide

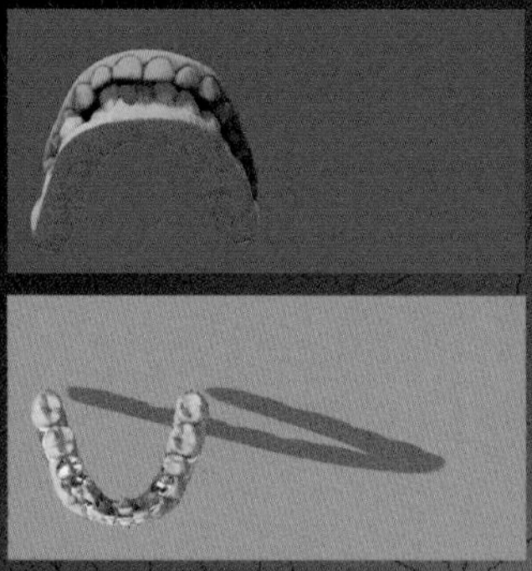

D-CAD software for planning orthodontic treatment and sequential appliances for clear aligner therapy (CAT)

Prosthodontics at a Glance, Second Edition. Irfan Ahmad.

CAD (computer-aided design) software is categorised into **two types** for performing two distinct tasks. The first type is for **reconstructing a point cloud** to a visible geometric surface (surface reconstruction), often referred to as reverse engineering, and creating 3D files that are used in CAD programmes. The second type of CAD is used for manipulating the 3D file **for surface or solid modelling**, animating, etc. However, the distinction between reconstruction and manipulation CAD software is nebulous, and many programmes are capable of performing both functions, although to varying degrees of complexity.

CAD software

Most routinely used software for word-processing, spreadsheets, drawing, databases, photo/movie-editing, etc. are based on two-dimensional (2D) interfaces. This means that only the **x (horizontal) and y (vertical) axes** are represented to form a 2D workspace. However, CAD software is capable of both 2D layouts as well as 3D modelling. For 3D modelling, a third dimension is incorporated and represented by the **z (upward and downward) axis.** This allows an object to be rotated, scaled, manipulated or altered infinitely in all three dimensions. Although the user interface of 3D CAD software is essentially 2D, but the third dimension is graphically represented to convey a 3D rendition of the model. **In dentistry, CAD is used for a variety of procedures** across several disciplines, from relatively simple tasks such as adding a base to a scan for a **study model** or a **virtual wax-up**, to complex tasks such as **virtual dynamic articulation**, **designing fixed/removable prosthesis frameworks**, **orthodontic treatment** planning and constructing precision **guides for implant or maxillofacial surgery.** Unlike many CAD designing that create an object from scratch, dental applications usually begin with an initial 'working model' to start with, i.e. a **digital acquisition of the dentition** by an IOS. Most dental scanners automatically convert a point cloud to a visible and texture mapped surface (**surface reconstruction**) plus a 3D file that is ready for CAD manipulation. There are **two CAD software options for dentistry**, either using a **generic 3D manipulation software (generic CAD or G-CAD)** or a **dedicated dental programme (dental CAD or D-CAD)** tailored specifically for dental needs.

Generic CAD (G-CAD) software

The first option of a **G-CAD software** is tempting since the price is relatively modest, but since generic programmes are designed for a wide range of applications, configuring them for dental use is onerous and requires an innate graphic designing affinity. In addition, substantial training is essential for deciphering the sophisticated and powerful features offered by these products for exploiting them to their full potential. The choice of G-CAD software ranges from **low-end, mid-range to professional levels.** Some **open-source free downloads** include Meshmixer, Blender and Meshlab offering simple but practical feature that are sufficient for many designs. However, for complex and intricate specialist designs, a paid mid-range or professional software is worth considering. The market share is dominated by protagonists Dassault Systèmes, Autodesk, PTC, Siemens (UGS), Mentor Graphics and ANSYS, all offering packages geared for every level of CAD sophistication.

Dedicated dental CAD (D-CAD) software

The second option is a **D-CAD software**, which offers the advantage of being user friendly with familiar dental terminology, but comes at a **hefty initial outlay**, and often endless support and update fees. Most D-CAD software needs to be purchased from specialist dental companies or dealers. The major companies supplying packages are **Sirona, 3 Shape, Planmeca, Exocad, Dental Wings, Kavo, Zirkon Zahn, Nobel Biocare and Straumann.** These programmes are usually available as starter kits with several add-on modules for different applications such as designing study models, indirect restorations, dentures, orthodontic aligners, smile design templates and implant surgical guides.

3D file formats

There are literally hundreds of **3D file formats**, and similar to digital image file formats, each serves a different purpose. A 3D file stores digital or **binary attributes** about an object, broadly be divided into **geometry, physical properties, context and animation**. Before choosing a particular format, the three main factors to consider are the **type of application** (3D printing/milling, computer graphics or high-precision designing), **CAD software support** for a particular file format and lastly, **interoperability** for sharing and disseminating designs. The type of application influences the type of 3D file. For example, if **only geometry** is necessary, then an **open source .stl (STereoLithography)** file is the ideal choice. However, if all four attributes are essential, then a COLLADA (.dae extension) is worth considering. The most **popular file type in dentistry is .stl** that has many **backronyms** including standard tessellation language, surface tessellation language, standard triangle language, solid-to-layer or standard template library. The .stl format is one of the oldest, simplest and leanest 3D file formats dating back to the late 1980s. The file is essentially a **black-and-white triangular representation of the surface geometry** of an object using the **approximation mesh** encoding method. It has been ubiquitously adopted as a 'generic' format for IOS, G-CAD and D-CAD software. Although the file is considered **relatively low resolution**, its **accuracy is acceptable for most dental applications** that require only morphological geometry, without colour, context or animation. However, in the near future, the .stl file may be superseded by other formats, e.g. **.ply (polygon)**, **.obj**, or **.3MF,** which offer greater resolution and support colour and texture. This will allow a crown to be 3D printed in a single run with a high-strength opaque coping (substructure or framework), and layered with various translucent shades of porcelain [illegible] natural tooth characterisations such as nuances of colour, staining, mamelons and incisal halos. In addition, many adjunct dental items such as oral hygiene products (e.g. tooth brushes) or orthodontic retainers could potentially benefit from **polychromatic 3D printing**.

Key points

- CAD software performs two function: surface reconstruction and manipulation (designing).
- CAD software options are either generic CAD (G-CAD) or dental CAD (D-CAD).
- The attributes of 3D file formats determines the type of file to use for a given application.
- CAD software is utilised for a variety of dental applications.

57 CAM (computer-aided manufacturing)

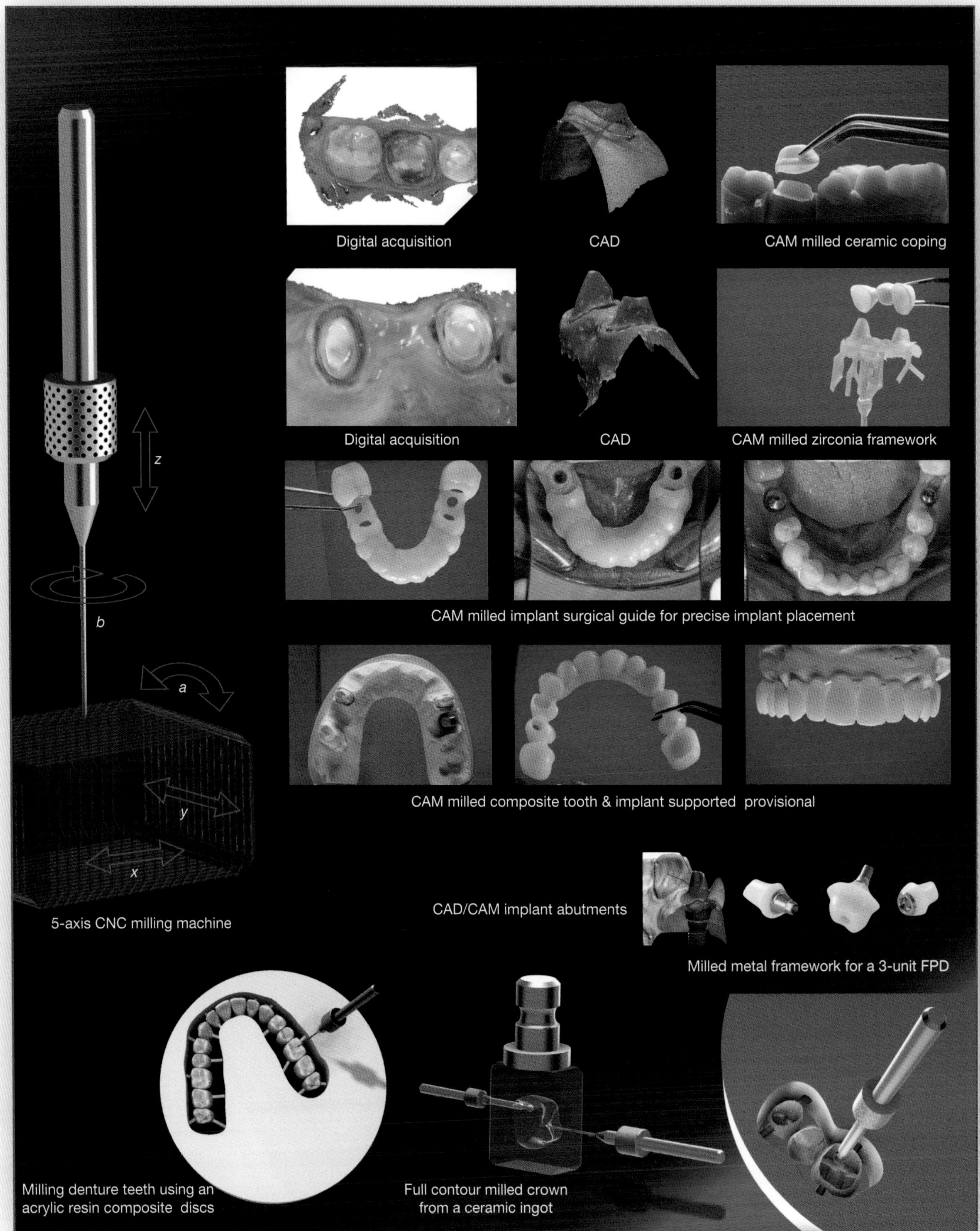

Prosthodontics at a Glance, Second Edition. Irfan Ahmad.

CAM (computer-aided manufacture) is the suffix of the acronym **CAD/CAM**, a trailblazing technology that is heralding a new age of **digital dentistry**. CAD/CAM involves three distinct processes: digital acquisition (prepared tooth/teeth or complete arch, antagonist arch and occlusal registration) – Chapters 10, 11, 12 and 55, designing in CAD software using the 3D file(s) generated from the scanner – Chapter 56 and outputting to a manufacturing device (CAM).

CAM overview

The **birth of CAD/CAM dentistry** can be traced back to the **early 1970s**, when Drs. Francois Duret and Christian Termoz patented the first dental digital workflow for indirect prostheses. This was followed by Drs. Werner Mőrmann and Marco Brandestini in the late 1980 **who introduced the first intra-oral scanner for digital impressions,** which was commercialised as CEREC 1, acronym for Chairside Economical Restoration of Esthetic Ceramics or CEramic REConstruction (Siemens, Bensheim, Germany). The CEREC system consists of a chairside IOS that is linked to a **CAM milling** machine for fabricating ceramic inlays, veneers or full-contour crowns by **subtractive manufacturing**. CAM is manufacturing a restoration by converting data from a 3D file into a set of commands that are sent to the **computer numeric-controlled (CNC)** unit, which can be **chairside** (e.g. inalys, onlay, PLVs, full-contour crowns, mock-up templates, occlusal appliances, periodontal splints and orthodontic retainers), **dental laboratory** (indirect restorations, surgical guides, complex frameworks and copings) or a **centralised production plant** (frameworks, copings, orthodontic clear aligners, implant surgical guides). The **methods for CAM** include:

- **Subtractive manufacturing** – milling ingots or discs (blocks) to the desired restoration/appliance (discussed in this chapter)
- **Additive manufacturing** – 3D printing (Chapters 58 and 59)
- Combination of subtractive and additive methods with to without analogue methods (e.g. veneering copings and frameworks)

CAM milling process

A **CNC device is a multi-axes milling unit**, which can be a **3** (*x, y, z*), **4** (*x, y, z* and *a*) or **5** *(x, y, z, a* and *b)* **axis system**. The 3-axis systems are the most widely used in dentistry, offering faster milling speeds, but are unable to recreate convergence, divergences and intricate features, and limited to [illegible] prostheses. In addition, most dental CAM machines use two burs for faster milling and 180 rotation of the blocks to allow milling of the intaglio surface. The 4- and 5-axis systems allow more complex and longer span units to be produced with a smoother surface finish. There are two types of milling: **hard and soft machining**. The hard type produces full contoured restorations from metal, sintered zirconia and acrylic resin/composite blocks, while soft machining is exclusively for presintered zirconia. Since hard machining produces elevated temperatures, water-cooling is essential. The alternative, soft machining, is carried out in dry environment and mills an **oversized presintered zirconia block**, which is subsequently sintered to the correct dimensions, usually with 25–30% shrinkage. This method is faster, prolongs cutting tool life and has a smoother surface compared to hard machining. However, the drawback is ensuring the predetermined shrinkage is precisely calculated to avoid compromising the accuracy of the restoration. The entire process is automated with a user interface displaying information about the percentage of completion, cutting efficiency and when to replace degraded burs. A typical cycle for a single restoration is around 4–7 minutes.

Pros and cons

The **advantages** of CAD/CAM fabrication are:

- **Instantly review tooth preparations** to allow refinements (e.g. removing undercuts and sharp line angles and ensuring correct path of insertion/withdrawal) before designing and fabrication
- **Removable prosthesis** that can either be designed and directly fabricated as metal frameworks and/or milled resin teeth and bases, or produce wax-patterns for conventional investing and casting
- **Precision fit** – marginal opening of <10–50 µm. Inputting parameters for ensuring accurate design of copings, cement space, adequate support for the overlying veneering porcelain, correct FPD connector and pontics dimensions, and bespoke implant abutments
- **Expedience and predictability** – access to vast biogeneric database for creating occlusal morphology for full contour restorations and implant abutments, virtual wax-up simulations, eliminating human error during onerous laboratory stages
- **Chairside units** offering 'single-appointment' treatment options, avoiding temporaries, particularly for non-retentive PLVs preparations, simultaneous implant fixture and abutment placement for immediate loading, and reduced manpower costs
- **Aesthetic and durability** – full anatomical restorations, e.g. inlays, onlays, veneers and crowns using polychromatic and polytranslucent ingots of various materials for aesthetic and functional needs, reduced porosity and more homogenous restorations, three decades of clinical performance
- **Versatility** – besides indirect provisional and definitive restorations, CAD/CAM technology can also be utilised for surgical guides, customised implant abutments, orthodontic retainers, virtual occlusal articulation, ever increasing choice of materials including metals, ceramics, resins and waxes

The **drawbacks** of CAD/CAM include:

- **Unforgiving clinical protocols** – precise tooth preparation without undercuts or shape line angles
- **Inaccuracies** may be introduced due to improper tissue management, substandard digital impression or erroneous plotting of restorative margins
- **Hard or dense materials such as titanium and zirconia are difficult to mill** and may result in under-milled intaglio surfaces resulting in poor fit
- **Frequent replacement of milling burs**, especially with hard machining
- **Time consuming post-production** such as trimming sprues, characterisation, staining, polishing and glazing
- **Milled tooth supported frameworks have greater marginal opening ([illegible] to [illegible] μm) compared to milled implant frameworks (1 to 27 μm)**
- **Limitation of 3-axis milling machines** that are unable to reproduce intricate designs
- **Poor aesthetics with monochromatic ingots** or unrealistic external staining and characterisation
- **Initial substantial capital investment**
- **Perpetual cost of subscriptions** for software updates, equipment maintenance and training

Key points

- CAD/CAM is divided into digitisation, designing (CAD) and manufacturing (CAM).
- CAM offers a wide spectrum of materials for a variety of restorations and appliances.
- CAD/CAM is beginning to supersede many analogue clinical and laboratory procedures.

58 3D printing - additive manufacturing (AM): technology

Schematic representation of the 3D printing process

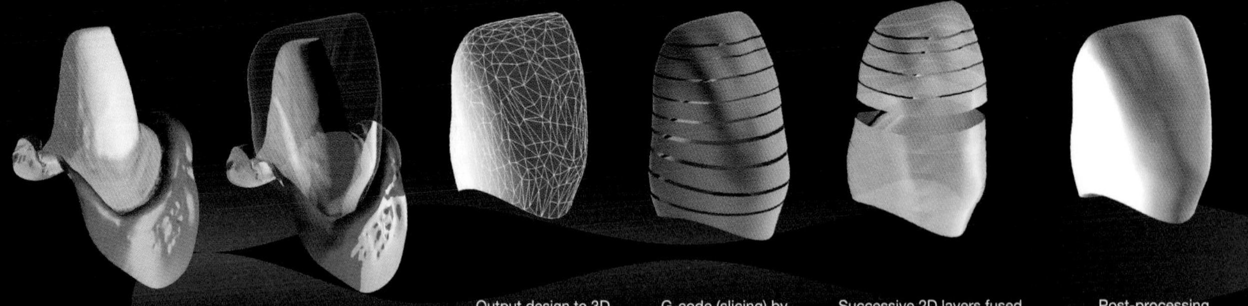

Digital acquisition
Designing in CAD software
Output design to 3D printer as a 3D file format
G-code (slicing) by printer software
Successive 2D layers fused to form a 3D object
Post-processing

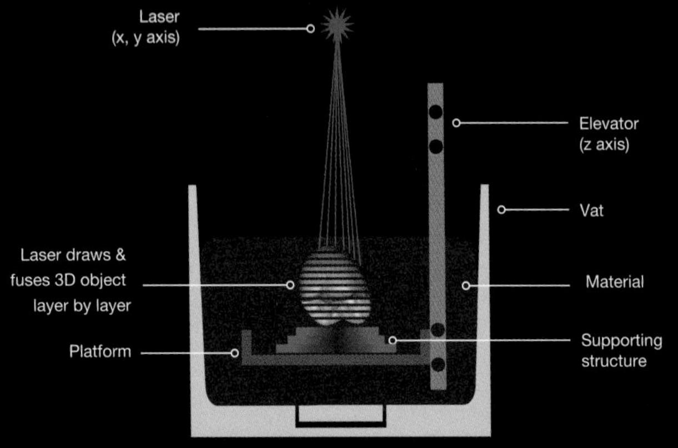

Laser (x, y axis)
Elevator (z axis)
Vat
Laser draws & fuses 3D object layer by layer
Material
Platform
Supporting structure

SLA (stereolithographic apparatus)

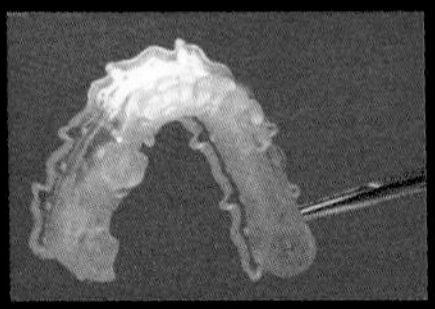

Post-processing stages involve trimming the supporting structure

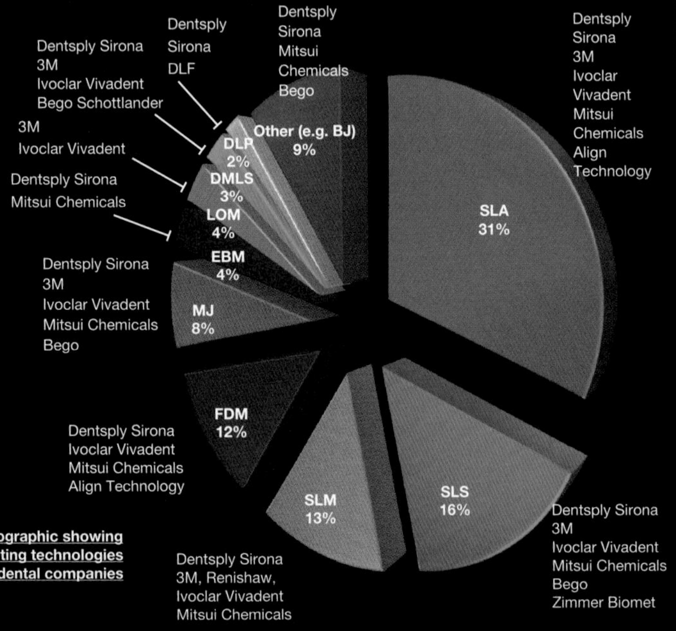

Infographic showing types of 3D printing technologies used by dental companies

SLA 31% – Dentsply Sirona, 3M, Ivoclar Vivadent, Mitsui Chemicals, Align Technology
SLS 16% – Dentsply Sirona, 3M, Ivoclar Vivadent, Mitsui Chemicals, Bego, Zimmer Biomet
SLM 13% – Dentsply Sirona, 3M, Renishaw, Ivoclar Vivadent, Mitsui Chemicals
FDM 12% – Dentsply Sirona, Ivoclar Vivadent, Mitsui Chemicals, Align Technology
MJ 8% – Dentsply Sirona, 3M, Ivoclar Vivadent, Mitsui Chemicals, Bego
EBM 4%
LOM 4% – Dentsply Sirona, Mitsui Chemicals
DMLS 3% – 3M, Ivoclar Vivadent
DLP 2% – Dentsply Sirona, 3M, Ivoclar Vivadent, Bego Schottlander
Other (e.g. BJ) 9% – Dentsply Sirona, Mitsui Chemicals, Bego
Dentsply Sirona DLF

3D Printing Process	Resolution (z axis)	Surface Roughness (Ra)
SLA	<1 μm	≈2 μm
SLS	1–150 μm	10–100 μm
DLP	10–100 μm	< 0.5 μm
MJ	16–100 μm	<1 μm
FDM	100–400 μm	3–43 μm
BJ	≈170 μm	15 μm

Resolution & Ra of 3D printing processes

3D Printing Technology	Complexity	Post-process	Duration
DLP (digital light processing)	Simple	Trimming off support, compressed air, UV curing, polishing	<15 minutes
FDM (fused deposition modeling)	Simple	Trimming & rinsing off support with detergent, polishing	< 1 hour
MJ (PolyJet or MultiJet Modelling)	Simple/Complex	Washing with H_2O, NaOH soaking	< 1 hour/ > 1 day
SLA (stereolithography)	Complex	Trimming off support, alcohol rinsing, UV curing, polishing	>1 hour
SLS (selective laser sintering)	Complex	Thermal, compressed air, polishing	> 1 day
BJ (binder jetting)	Complex	Post-sintering, infiltration, characterisation with stains, polishing, glazing	> 1 day

Post-processing for 3D printing technologies

Adapted from '3D Printing in Dentistry 2019/2020', Quintessence Publishing, UK, 2019

Prosthodontics at a Glance, Second Edition. Irfan Ahmad.

3D printing or additive manufacturing (**AM**) has several synonyms including rapid prototyping, direct digital manufacturing, solid-free form fabrication, generative manufacturing or layered manufacturing. Unlike **subtractive manufacturing (SM)** that removes or mills a material to form an object, **AM adds consecutive 2D layers to form customised three-dimensional solid object.** The first method of 3D printing, **SLA (stereolithographic apparatus)**, was developed by Charles Hull in 1984 who commercially introduced and patented the process, co-founding 3D Systems. Today, there are **many types of 3D printing technologies** that have not only been embraced by major dental companies but also permeated diverse sectors such as aerospace, medicine, automotive, telecommunications, subassemblies, food and consumer products.

3D printing technologies

3D printing can be **in-house** (chairside, or dedicated room), **outsourced** to a dental laboratory, online printing bureau and/or industrial manufacturer. Some popular printing methods in used dentistry are as follows:

- **SLA (stereolithographic apparatus)** consists of a vat or tank with photosensitive polymer that is cured by a light source termed **photo-polymerisation**, not unlike curing a resin-based composite restoration. The SLA method utilises a laser to 'draw' or trace the pattern of the object design layer-by-layer until printing is finished. Each consecutive layer is cured by UV light and the platform moves up so that the uncured resin below can be mapped by the laser for creating the subsequent layer. In this manner, several layers are chemically bonded to each other to produce a precise and functional rendition of the CAD designed object. The process is analogous to incremental layering of a direct composite filling. The advantages of this method are that the object can incorporate intricate details, is **very accurate and has a smooth surface**. SLA is ideal for small items that require fine detail reproduction (**resolution of 5 μm**) which includes fabricating complex facial anatomy replicas for cranioplasties, orbital floors, onlay grafts, customised implants, surgical guides and simple items such as dental arch models, orthodontic aligners and temporary restorations. The **drawbacks** of SLA are potentially irritant resins by contact and inhalation, plus an involved and **protracted post-printing process.** The major players in the dental field are Formlabs, DWS, 3D Systems, Zenith and Bego.
- **DLP (digital light processing)** – sometimes referred to as the masking process, is a variation of SLA but uses a digital projector to expose and cure the resin by projecting an image of each layer, rather than mapping or 'drawing' each layer with a laser. DLP **reduces the print time** as the resin is exposed to an entire layer, light cured and the process repeated for successive layers. One of the endearing qualities of DLP printing is the ability to create **optically transparent items**, ideal for making indices for directly **restoring Class IV cavities** or guides for **aesthetic crown lengthening procedures**. The main dental companies are EnvisonTec, RapidShape, B9 Creator, MoonRay and DWS.
- **FDM – fused deposition modelling** or **FFF** (fused filament fabrication) is the most popular method of 3D printing. The process involves heating a high-grade thermoplastic filament (e.g. **PEEK** – polyether ether ketone), which is extruded via a nozzle to create individual layers. Each layer rapidly cools (less than 1/10 second) before the next later is deposited and cold welds to the previous layer. FDM is used for **bioprinting** biodegradable scaffolds for **tissue engineering** and reconstructing osseous defects. FDM items have **excellent thermal, physical and chemical properties**, but **lower resolution compared to SLA**, and limited geometric complexity items, making it unsuitable for prosthetic units. Several dental printers are available from Stratasys, UniMaker and MakerBot.
- **SLS (Selective laser sintering) and SLM and DMLS** – uses a vat of powder instead of a liquid resin. The powder is selectively sintered by a laser and layers built to complete the object. Unlike other methods, no supporting structure or platform is required since the object is constantly encased in powder. After completion, the residual unsintered powder is removed with brushes and pressurised air to expose the 3D object. Since several materials of different properties can be used, e.g. **ceramics, polyamides, flexible PrimePart® (flexible nylon) and alloys, PEEK, SLS offers greater versatility for customisation.** This technology is used for constructing **all-ceramic dental restorations, metal partial denture frameworks, framework copings and acrylic provisional prostheses**. The disadvantages of SLS are the protracted post-processing time, and the nanoparticle powder, which is a potential health risk if inhaled. Selective laser melting (SLM) and direct metal laser sintering (DMLS) are similar processes to SLS, but exclusively use metals.
- **MJF – Multi-jet fusion** is the innovation of Hewlett-Packard (hp) using a high-end industrial printer for prototyping as well as manufacturing. The concept is based on molecular-level **voxels** (short for "volumetric elements"), the building blocks of there-dimensional objects. The process involves thermal energy, rather than a laser, to selectively fuse powder particles with a detailing agent to form individual layers that are cooled before ensuing layers are added. One of the **dental applications** is printing heat-resistant sequential computer generated models, which are used for fabricating **clear orthodontic aligners** by thermoforming, e.g. Invisalign.®
- **MJ (material jetting)** – also referred to as PolyJet or MultiJet Modelling (MJM), is similar to 2D inkjet printing and delivers materials through a nozzle, drop by drop, to form layers that are cured by UV light. The uniqueness of MJ is that **multicolour** and **multi-property materials** can be selected for a single object. This allows products such as a tooth brush with a rigid handle and flexible bristles of different colours to be fabricated in a single print run. The choices of material include transparent, flexible or rigid polymers that can be mixed together in a single object to create composite materials with varying properties and colour. In addition, several **biocompatible materials are available** for medical and dental purposes from companies such as Stratasys. The drawback is poor accuracy, high cost and potentially **weak products**.
- **BJ – binder jetting** uses a bonding agent to stick particles together to form the successive layers, and is an inexpensive process ideal for prototypes, **mould making, casting patterns** or **green structures** that can be **infiltrated afterwards to enhance mechanical properties**. The choice of materials is impressive, e.g. lucite-reinforced glass ceramics, polyamides, PMMA (polymethyl methacrylate), gypsum, plaster of Paris, silica, stainless steel and tungsten-carbide, but the prints lack structural integrity and are unsuitable for end use unless post-processed, e.g. by infiltration with cyanoacrylate or epoxy resin to enhance physical and mechanical properties

Key points

- 3D printing is a broad term to describe several technologies using a variety of materials.
- In dentistry, 3D printing at present is in its nascent stage, but with ever-increasing novel applications.

3D printing: materials and applications

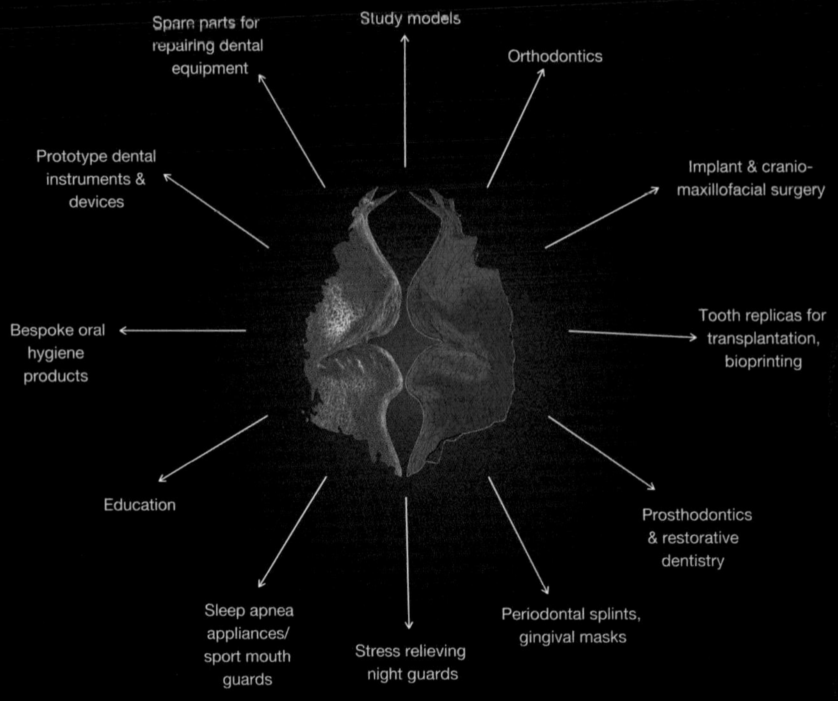

Spare parts for repairing dental equipment

Study models

Orthodontics

Prototype dental instruments & devices

Implant & cranio-maxillofacial surgery

Bespoke oral hygiene products

Tooth replicas for transplantation, bioprinting

Education

Prosthodontics & restorative dentistry

Sleep apnea appliances/ sport mouth guards

Stress relieving night guards

Periodontal splints, gingival masks

Dental applications of 3D printing

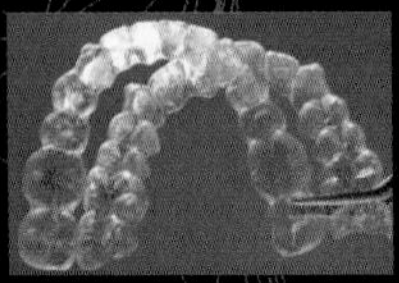

Sequential aligners for orthodontic clear aligner therapy (CAT)

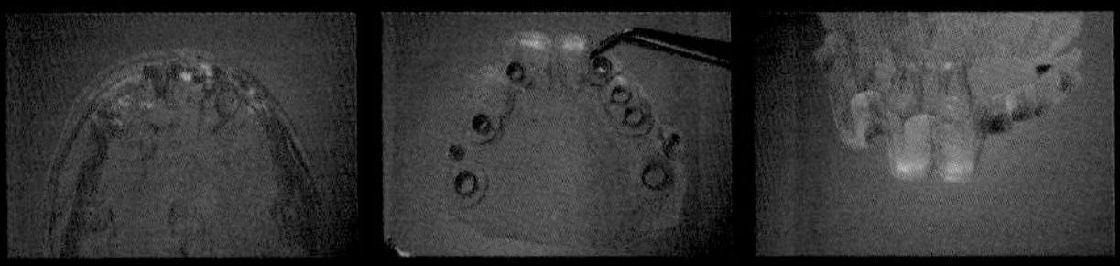

SLA printed study models, and surgical guide for implant placement

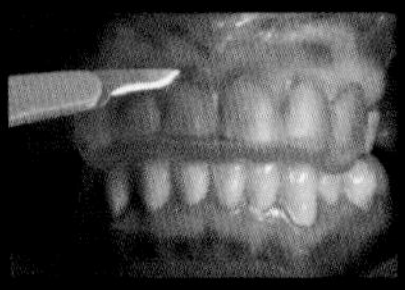

SLA printed guide for crown lengthening

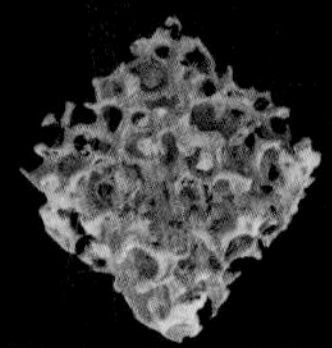

Bioprinted ceramic bone lattice for osseous defect reconstruction

Materials for 3D printing

3D Printing Process	Materials
SLA (stereolithography)	ABS, PMMA, hybrid composite resin
SLS (selective laser sintering)	Titanium, stainless steel, dental gold alloys, Co-Cr, nylon, PEEK
SLM & DMLS	SLM (melting base metals) DMLS (sintering alloys)
DLP (digital light processing)	ABS, PEG
MJ (PolyJet or MultiJet Modelling)	Waxes, flexible silicones
FDM (fused deposition modeling)	ABS, PLA
BJ (binder jetting)	Cyanoacrylate, epoxy resin, dental ceramic powders

ABS–acrylonitrile butadiene styrene, PMMA–polymethyl methacrylate, PEEK–polyether ether ketone, PEG–polyethyl glycol, PLA–poly-lactic acid

Adapted from '3D Printing in Dentistry 2019/2020', Quintessence Publishing, UK, 2019

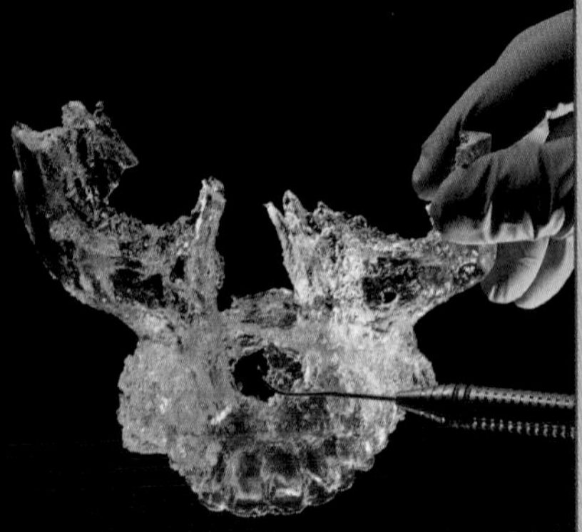

DLP printed maxilla showing a through-and-through osseous defect

Prosthodontics at a Glance, Second Edition. Irfan Ahmad.

The **applications of 3D printing** are increasing exponentially, not only for the provision of dental care, but also for making spare parts for repairing broken equipment, or even prototypes for inventions such as designing new dental instruments and devices.

Orthodontics

Digital orthodontics has taken the most advantage of 3D printing. The major use is printing **study models** to replace plaster casts. The difference between analogue plaster casts and 3D printed models is assessed by the thickness of the layers using different 3D printing processes. For example, **SLA printers** have a layer thickness of around **0.15 mm (vertical resolution)**, while **DLP or MJ methods produce models with thinner layers with superior accuracy.** The **clinical tolerance** that is satisfactory between plaster casts and 3D printed models is **0.25 mm**, which is readily achievable by most additive manufacturing processes. Other applications are appliances for clear aligner therapy (CAT), retainers, indirect bracket guides and replicating artificial teeth (using CBCT scans) for autotransplantation.

Oral surgery and implantology

Cranio-maxillofacial and implant surgery has benefited enormously from 3D printing, which started **as early as 1985.** The concepts of **computer-aided implant planning (CAIP)** and **computer-guided implant surgery (CGIS)** have transformed implantology. The utilisation of 3D printed surgical guides for implant osteotomies is now widely accepted as the standard of care. Also, printed anatomical models are used for analysing pathology, vital structures and planning implant placement with extreme precision that minimises risk and ensuring the fixtures are ideally placed for the prosthetic components. Furthermore, guided bone regeneration (GBR) and CGIS can be practised beforehand on printed models by **tactile rehearsal treatment planning (TRTP)**, making the actual procedure a déjà vu.

Bioprinting

Bioprinting is used for printing **biomimetic scaffolds for GBR** using SLA, SLS, FDM, BJ and LOM printing that are utilised for **tissue engineering** (Chapter 74). The scaffolds are fabricated from biocompatible and osteoconductive materials such as **alginate peptide hybrid, β tricalcium phosphate (β-TCP) or porous metal/thermoplastic meshes** that are **customised** [illegible] prevailing bone defect. **EBM** is particularly useful for manufacturing **porous metal meshes** for encouraging bone growth for repairing bone defects and regenerating new bone. The **thermoplastic biodegradable** materials include **polyglycolic acid (PGA), polylactic acid (PLA) or polycaprolactone (PCL).** Similarly, **ceramic matrices**, composed of lattices with intricate microstructure or micro-channels mimicking **bone architecture,** have also been printed with a variety of materials such as hydroxyapatite, using different technologies such as SLA, SLS, LOM and BJ. For extensive defects, **customised 3D printed titanium scaffolds** (e.g. Yxoss CBR®, ReOss® GmbH and Filderstadt) are tailored using CBCT scans to precisely conform to the local anatomy. In addition, AM is utilised for **facial prostheses** for replacing congenitally missing or deformed facial features such as ears or orbital rim defects. Taking a leap into the future, bioprinting could synthesise **artificial tissues or entire organs with stem cell coatings for transplantation**.

Prosthodontics and restorative dentistry

As well as study models, the prosthodontic applications include both **temporary and definitive units** made of **resins, ceramics** (e.g. lithium disilicate, zirconia) and **metals** with **accuracies of 30 µm.** Also, digitally manufactured lithium disilicate crowns display an accuracy comparable to those using a conventional lost-wax-process. Also, **DMLS can fabricate metal copings** and **frameworks for FPD**, and construct cobalt-chrome **superstructures** for implant-supported prostheses with superior precision than conventional casting methods. 3D printed resins can fabricating **acrylic bases** for interim, **immediate or implant retained dentures.** As technology evolves, using processes such as MJ (PolyJet), it will become possible to simultaneously print both the denture base and teeth in a single print cycle. **RPD frameworks are printed with castable wax-like resins**, and subsequently invested and cast in metal or **directly printed** using SLA, SLM and DMLS. For restorative dentistry, the ability to instantly construct **resin indices** are enormously beneficial for direct composite restorations, e.g. Class IV cavies.

Periodontics

A simple and effective method for stabilising mobile teeth is printing **periodontal splints**, which are adhesively bonded to the lingual or palatal surfaces. Another use is fabricating **gingival masks** for prosthetic rehabilitation of Miller's Class III and IV gingival recession, which are not amenable to perioplastic surgery, and reproducing the **sculpted tissues around implants so** that the definitive restorations have the same contour and **emergence profile** as the precursor temporary restorations. Also, many **perioplastic corrective procedures** such as **aesthetic crown lengthening** can be guided by templates fabricated from virtual wax-ups for performing precise gingivectomy, ostectomy and osteoplasty. Finally, the ability to **individualise toothbrushes** or oral hygiene adjuncts is invaluable for the elderly, infirm and disabled patients, who have deteriorating manual dexterity, trismus or a pronounced gag reflex.

Education

Rather than dissecting cadavers, **printed anatomical models** can be used for **interactive teaching** with greater comprehension of osseous anatomy, vital structures, nerve and blood vessel trajectories, tooth morphology, occlusion, etc. This can also **facilitate understanding** of complex procedures for educating patients before gaining **informed consent.** Furthermore, having a 'hard copy' of the jaws rather than virtual models, supplements teaching using a **'touch to comprehend' approach**. For example, tooth preparation, endodontic canal configuration and surgical procedures can be rehearsed in vitro by **tactile rehearsal treatment planning (TRTP)** to anticipate complications and risks before performing the procedures in vivo. The use of printed anatomical models for education is shifting the **emphasis from a virtual teaching to a tactile teaching environment.** This approach is invaluable for CGIS or cranio-maxillofacial surgery where tangible printed models provide a facsimile of the jaws for appreciating the limitations or complications of a particular procedure, devise contingency plans, as well as performing a tactile rehearsal beforehand.

Key points

- 3D printing is used in many dental disciplines, including teaching and patient education.
- The current applications of 3D printing in dentistry represent 'the tip of the iceberg'.

60 Digital workflows

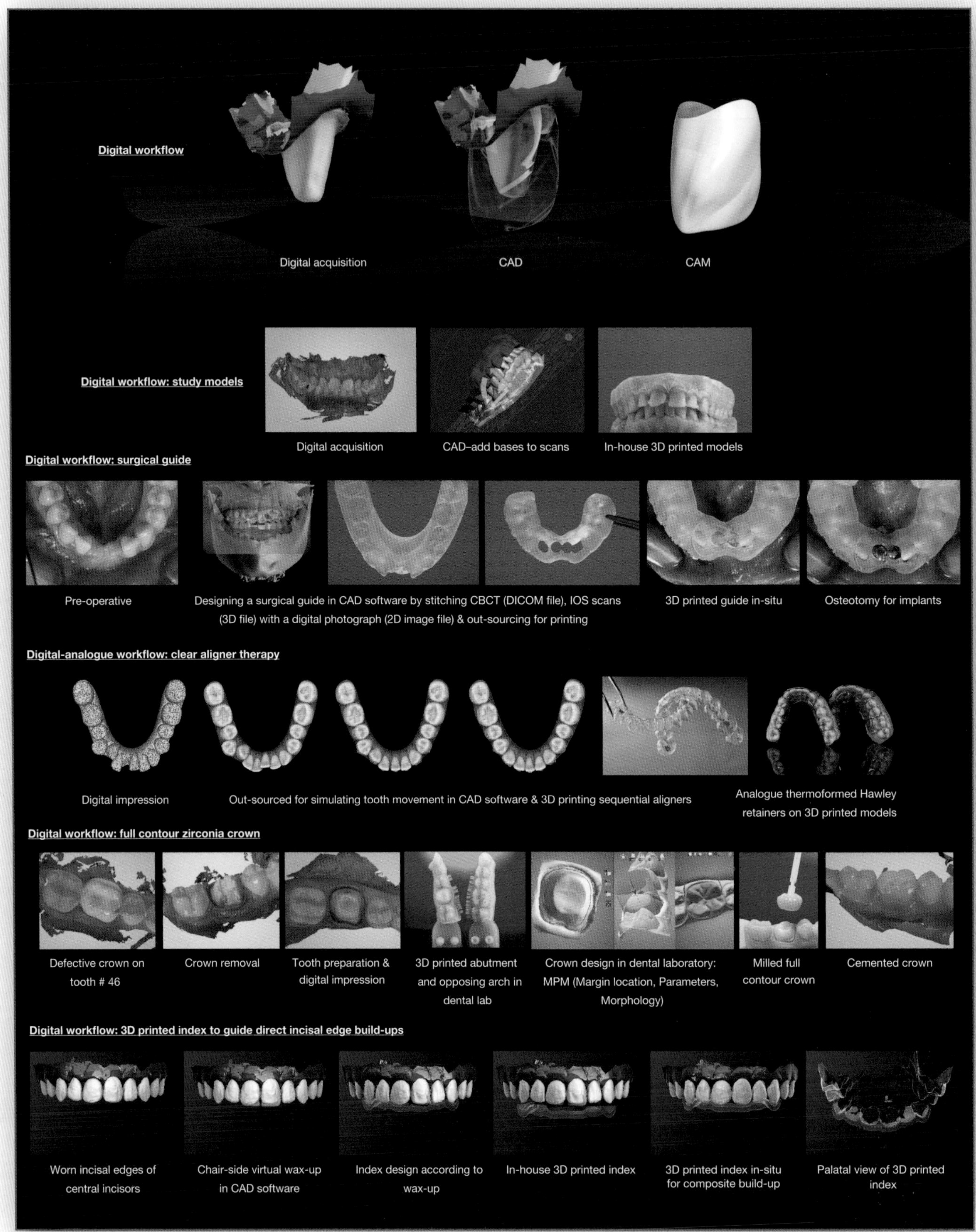

Digital workflow

Digital acquisition | CAD | CAM

Digital workflow: study models

Digital acquisition | CAD–add bases to scans | In-house 3D printed models

Digital workflow: surgical guide

Pre-operative | Designing a surgical guide in CAD software by stitching CBCT (DICOM file), IOS scans (3D file) with a digital photograph (2D image file) & out-sourcing for printing | 3D printed guide in-situ | Osteotomy for implants

Digital-analogue workflow: clear aligner therapy

Digital impression | Out-sourced for simulating tooth movement in CAD software & 3D printing sequential aligners | Analogue thermoformed Hawley retainers on 3D printed models

Digital workflow: full contour zirconia crown

Defective crown on tooth # 46 | Crown removal | Tooth preparation & digital impression | 3D printed abutment and opposing arch in dental lab | Crown design in dental laboratory: MPM (Margin location, Parameters, Morphology) | Milled full contour crown | Cemented crown

Digital workflow: 3D printed index to guide direct incisal edge build-ups

Worn incisal edges of central incisors | Chair-side virtual wax-up in CAD software | Index design according to wax-up | In-house 3D printed index | 3D printed index in-situ for composite build-up | Palatal view of 3D printed index

Prosthodontics at a Glance, Second Edition. Irfan Ahmad.

Today, nearly every dental discipline uses some form of **digital workflow** for providing patient care. In its **svelte chain sequence**, a digital workflow consists of **digital acquisition** (optical or radiographic), **CAD** and **CAM**. However, this schematic is somewhat simplistic, and often the digital continuum is interspersed with analogue processes.

Digital workflow

The fabrication of **3D printed models** of the dental arches is becoming commonplace using an entirely digital workflow consisting of a digital impressions, CAD and CAM. Also, it is now possible to digitise the patient, plan treatment in CAD software and produce sequential aligners for **clear aligner orthodontic therapy** without any analogue procedure. Similarly, an implant **surgical guide** can be generated entirely by digital means using CBCT and intra-oral scans, and outputting the design to a 3D printer. In addition, **monolithic full contour restorations** such as inlays, onlays, PLVs, crowns, implant abutments and even 3-unit FPD are entirely produced using CAD/CAM technology. Some of these procedures can be performed **in-house (chairside)** or **outsourced** to a dental laboratory or company specialising in a particular discipline such as orthodontics, prosthodontics or implants. If an office or institution does not have access to CAM devices such as a milling unit or 3D printer, a **digital impression** can be forwarded to the dental laboratory via the internet to continue the digital workflow.

Digital–analogue workflow

The **permutations of a combined digital–analogue workflow are limitless.** An office or institution can delegate the **'digital responsibility'** to a dental laboratory or company by forwarding a conventional (analogue) impression that can be digitised by an extra-oral scanners (EOS) to begin the CAD/CAM process. Furthermore, a digital–analogue offers advantages such as designing and milling a precision fit ceramic coping or framework that is subsequently veneered by an artisan ceramist to create nuances of colour, translucency and characterisations which are presently impossible with an entirely digital workflow. Another example is a removable partial denture framework, which can be designed in CAD software and a resin pattern 3D printed for conventional investing and casting with chrome-cobalt.

The digital dental revolution

Adopting new technologies [illegible] tools requiring patience and perseverance, as well as stepping **out of one's comfort zone.** Although CAD/CAM methods for fabricating restorations have been available for nearly four decades, **only a third of the dental profession has embraced this technology on a routine basis.** At present, many treatments combine both the tried and tested analogue methods infused with novel digital technologies as adjuncts.

The precision of **CGIS (computer-guided implant surgery)** is unquestionable, ensuring accurate positioning of implants in relation to the definitive prosthetic units. One study has reported that **error of implant placement with surgical guides is 6%, compared to freehand surgery error of 88%.** Also, the benefits of pre-planning flapless surgical procedures reduces post-operative discomfort, swelling and expedites healing by ensuring integrity of vascularisation, a profusion of growth factors, and preserving keratinised gingiva and inter-dental papilla. As well as implant placement, the provision of the final restoration via a digital approach has been shown to be three times more efficient than conventional methods of fabrication. Furthermore, a digital workflow is twice as fast compared to a combined analogue–digital method. Finally, another emerging technology is **navigational or robotic surgery** that allows precise implant placement with computer guided real-time surgery.

Confronting challenges

Although an entirely digital workflow offers innumerable advantages, however, can it effectively replace an analogue or even a mixed digital–analogue approach? It is obvious that the **rate of technological innovation in digital dentistry is outpacing the RCTs (randomised controlled trials)** in the dental literature. The pace at which new applications and new materials are being introduced far outstrips research in this field. However, in spite of the paucity of scientific backup, the digital workflow is being aggressively marketed by manufacturers, dental dealers [and leaders] as the next industrial revolution. However, **it is important to view these technological breakthroughs with some trepidation**, and to bear in mind that digital dentistry is not a panacea for every dental modality. A regime of regular followups, combined with scientific validation, is essential before a complete digital workflow can be unequivocally recommended for widespread and routine use.

While there is a plethora of literature documenting the benefits of a digital workflow for implantology and orthodontics, there is spare scientific data to support this protocol for prosthodontic procedures. A recent literature review revealed few significant RCTs that reported a complete digital workflow for single units on tooth and implant abutments, and no RCTs were available for multiunit prostheses. An important issue to consider with a digital workflow is the numerous factors susceptible to error. This starts with image **defects during digital acquisition** by optical scanners (both intra-oral and extra-oral). The next stage in the chain **prone to error is the painstaking designing**, geometric complexity of the object and the subsequent **slicing when using a 3D printer.** Finally, the r**esolution of the chosen CAM process (additive or subtractive method)** also has inherent inaccuracies that must be counteracted or compensated with careful designing in CAD software. Therefore, further investigation regarding efficacy, economics, ethics and long-term survival rate of restorations using a complete digital workflow is essential for complementing and substantiating the burgeoning manufacturers' claims about **the magic of digital dentistry.**

Key points

- A complete digital workflow has many advantages but at present cannot replace all analogue procedures.
- The rate of technological developments are outpacing research and many new digital protocols have little clinical track record.

Cementation

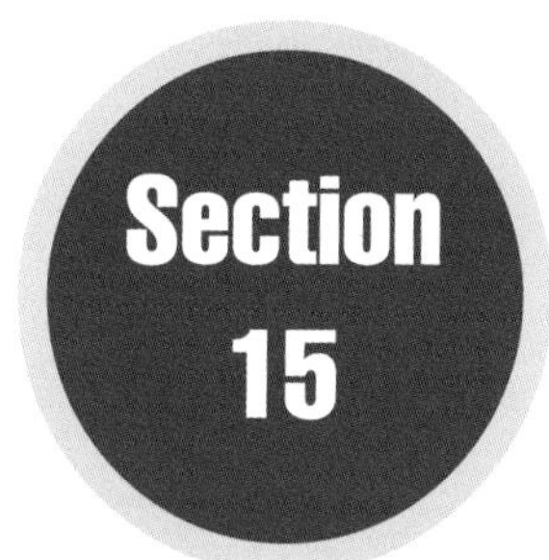

Chapters

61 Cements: overview

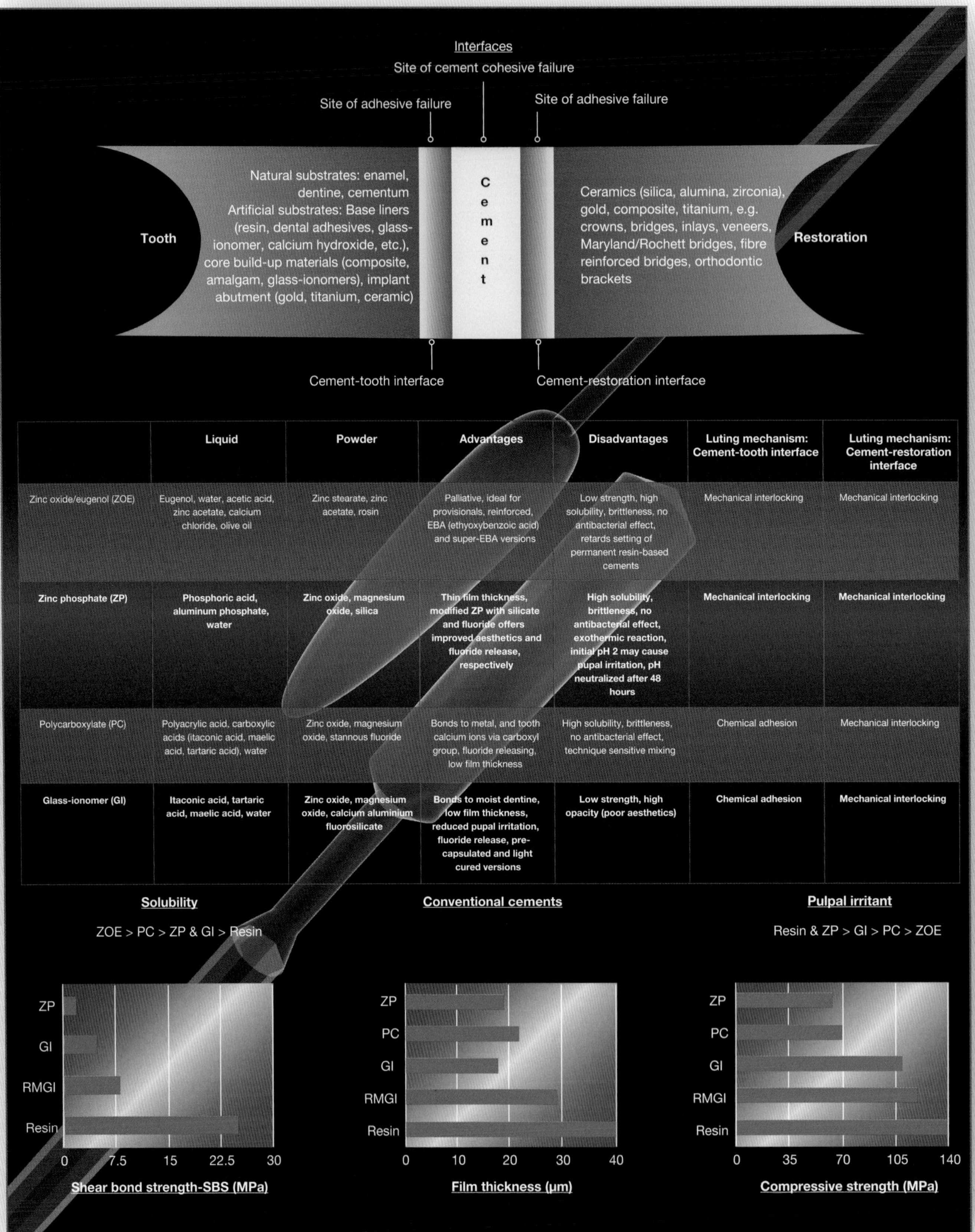

	Liquid	Powder	Advantages	Disadvantages	Luting mechanism: Cement-tooth interface	Luting mechanism: Cement-restoration interface
Zinc oxide/eugenol (ZOE)	Eugenol, water, acetic acid, zinc acetate, calcium chloride, olive oil	Zinc stearate, zinc acetate, rosin	Palliative, ideal for provisionals, reinforced, EBA (ethyoxybenzoic acid) and super-EBA versions	Low strength, high solubility, brittleness, no antibacterial effect, retards setting of permanent resin-based cements	Mechanical interlocking	Mechanical interlocking
Zinc phosphate (ZP)	Phosphoric acid, aluminum phosphate, water	Zinc oxide, magnesium oxide, silica	Thin film thickness, modified ZP with silicate and fluoride offers improved aesthetics and fluoride release, respectively	High solubility, brittleness, no antibacterial effect, exothermic reaction, initial pH 2 may cause pupal irritation, pH neutralized after 48 hours	Mechanical interlocking	Mechanical interlocking
Polycarboxylate (PC)	Polyacrylic acid, carboxylic acids (itaconic acid, maelic acid, tartaric acid), water	Zinc oxide, magnesium oxide, stannous fluoride	Bonds to metal, and tooth calcium ions via carboxyl group, fluoride releasing, low film thickness	High solubility, brittleness, no antibacterial effect, technique sensitive mixing	Chemical adhesion	Mechanical interlocking
Glass-ionomer (GI)	Itaconic acid, tartaric acid, maelic acid, water	Zinc oxide, magnesium oxide, calcium aluminium fluorosilicate	Bonds to moist dentine, low film thickness, reduced pupal irritation, fluoride release, pre-capsulated and light cured versions	Low strength, high opacity (poor aesthetics)	Chemical adhesion	Mechanical interlocking

Prosthodontics at a Glance, Second Edition. Irfan Ahmad.

Cements or luting agents are used for **retaining indirect restorations** on teeth or implant abutments. The functions of a luting agent are:

- **Retention** for preventing dislodgement of the restoration. However, retention alone is insufficient for success. A restoration may be in situ but, if microleakage is present, this may lead to pulpal and gingival irritation, requiring removal of the offending restoration
- **'Hermetic seal'** between the tooth and restoration to minimise microleakage, prevent secondary caries and pulpal and gingival inflammation. In addition, an efficacious seal retards dentinal fluid movement, mitigating hypersensitivity
- **Resist oral functional and parafunctional forces**, which are particularly significant for tooth preparations with inadequate resistance form

Mechanism

The cementation mechanism of cements is classified as:

- **Non-adhesive or mechanical interlocking retention** by engaging tooth surface and restoration intaglio surface irregularities, measuring 20–100 µm. This mechanism is applicable for all dental cements
- **Micromechanical interlocking (or 'adhesion')** is engaging finer surface irregularities of < 2 µm created by etching, air abrasion and usually in combination with a dental adhesive to form a hybrid layer (0.5–10 µm) – Chapter 62
- **Chemical (molecular) adhesion** by hydrogen bonding, Van der Waals forces and primary and secondary chemical interaction, which is the ideal adhesion, and contemporary cements strive to achieve this ideal

Interfaces

The **mechanism** of retention by cements can broadly be termed **luting** or **bonding**. **Luting provides non-adhesive retention**, while **bonding** implies a closer approximation of the cement with the tooth and restoration, which includes **micromechanical and chemical adhesion.**

There are two interfaces between cements and the tooth/restoration complex. On the tooth side, the substrate is either dentine, enamel or cementum, and is called the **cement–tooth interface**. On the opposing side is the artificial restoration, termed the **cement–restoration interface.** Certain resin cements in conjunction with dental adhesives offer chemical adhesion at both interfaces. A large number of interfaces are possible depending on the substrate on the tooth and restoration sides. These interfaces are the weakest link, accounting for **adhesive failure** of the restoration. Conversely, **cohesive failure** occurs either due to cement breakdown, or fracture within the tooth or the restoration.

A seal is essential to prevent microleakage between the *concealed interfaces* beneath the bulk of the restoration, as well as at the **open margins** exposed to the oral cavity. Furthermore, the exposed margins are also vulnerable to occlusal stresses transmitted from the coronal part of the restoration to the cervical aspect, and the cement should be resilient enough to resist these forces and maintain a long-lasting seal.

Properties

Most properties of cements are assessed by laboratory tests that are useful for comparison, but not for clinical performance, e.g. zinc phosphate dissolves in experimental tests, but provides long-term retention in clinical practice, impeding toxins and preventing dentinal fluid flow. Also, the methodologies of various studies are rarely identical, making a judicious comparison very difficult. The **favourable properties of a dental cement** include:

- **Physical** – similar elastic modulus, shade and optical properties to natural teeth, and provide thermal insulation
- **Mechanical** – high compressive, fatigue, tensile and shear bond strengths (SBS), and promoting increased fracture resistance of restoration and the supporting abutment
- **Chemical** – insoluble in oral fluids and resisting water sorption
- **Biological** – biocompatible and bioactivity with dental and surrounding soft tissues, bacteriostatic and/or bactericidal, bioregenerative (fluoride releasing)
- **Minimum film thickness** – 25 µm is often quoted as an ideal, but realistic in vivo values range from 50 µm to 350 µm
- **Radiopaque**
- **Aesthetic**
- **Handling properties** – ease of mixing or dispensing, sufficient working time, rapid setting time, adequate fluidity (low viscosity) for thin film thickness

Classification

Dental cements can broadly be classified into **conventional** (zinc oxide/eugenol, zinc phosphate, polycarboxylate and glass ionomer), and **contemporary** (resins and resin-modified glass ionomers – Chapter 63). All dental cements consist of a matrix infiltrated by filler particles to confer favourable properties. The salient properties of some popular **conventional cements** are as follows:

- **Zinc oxide/eugenol (ZOE)** – palliative temporary cement used for provisionals, but caution is necessary when using a subsequent definitive resin cement since eugenol is a radical scavenger, possibly retarding polymerisation of resin-based luting agents
- **Zinc phosphate (ZP)** – the first permanent cement, introduced in the 1920s, and was considered the gold standard for nearly half a century. ZP offers good mechanical properties, but poor marginal seal due to dissolution in oral fluids
- **Polycarboxylate (PC)** – invented in the 1960s, based on ZP, but with the added benefit of being more biocompatible and the ability to bond to tooth substrate and metal. However, the technique-sensitive mixing procedure has made this cement almost redundant
- **Glass ionomer (GI)** – introduced in the 1970s by Wilson, this polyacrylic acid composition offers chemical adhesion to dentine, fluoride release and a thin film thickness. The drawbacks are poor mechanical properties and unaesthetic opaque appearance, limiting its use to base liners. However, resin-modified glass ionomers (RMGI) have overcome many physical and mechanical limitations of GI

Key points

- Luting agents are used to adhere indirect dental restoration to teeth or implants.
- An ideal cement should seal and retain a restoration, as well as resisting occlusal forces.
- Dental cements can be classified into either conventional (ZOE, ZP, PC and GI), or contemporary (resins and RMGI).

62 Dental adhesives

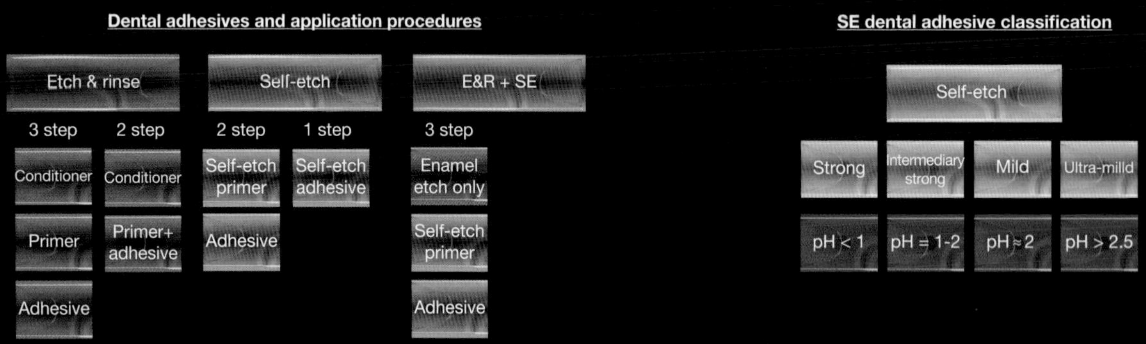

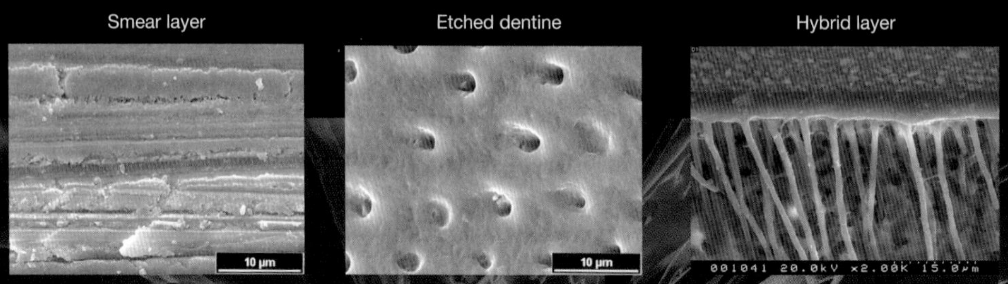

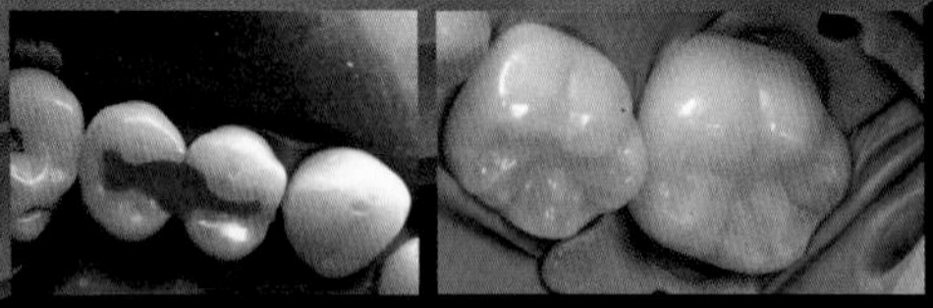

Dental adhesives and application procedures

SE dental adhesive classification

Smear layer

Etched dentine

Hybrid layer

Total etching

Frosty white enamel appearance

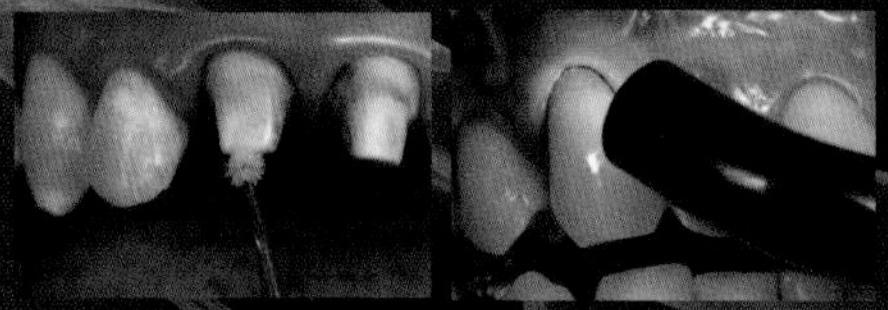

Immediate dentine sealing

Desensitising

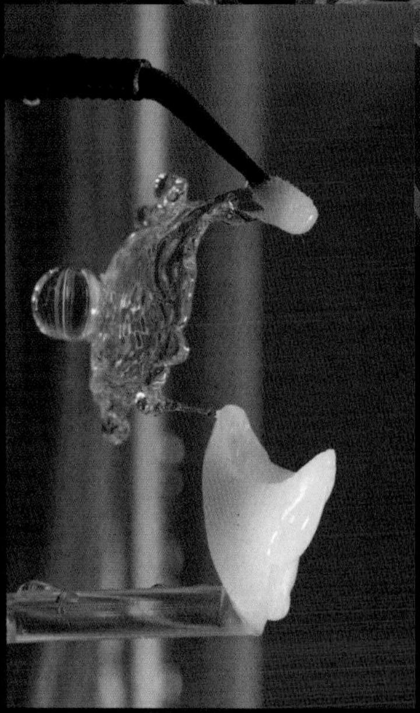

	Water	Ethanol	Acetone
Boilling point	100 °C	78.5 °C	56.5 °C
Rehydrates collagen fibres	Yes	Partially	No
Facilitates resin penetration	No	Partially	Yes
Requires moist dentine	No	Partially	Yes
Technique sensitive	Low	Intermediate	High

Dental adhesive solvents

Bonding indirect restorations

	E&R	SE
Smear layer removal	Yes interlocking +2°	Partially
Type of adhesion	Micromechanical interlocking + 2° chemical	Micromechanical interlocking +1° chemical
Penetration into dentine	3–6 µm	≈1 µm
Hybrid layer	Thick	Thin
Selective etching?	No	Recommended
Best adhesion for...	Enamel	Dentine

E&R vs. SE

Prosthodontics at a Glance, Second Edition. Irfan Ahmad.

Resin-based restoratives and cements require an intermediary **dental adhesive** to adhere to enamel and dentine. The nomenclature and categorisation of dental adhesives (or dentine bonding agents) are perpetually changing to reflect advances in material science and refinement of clinical techniques. The current classification of dental adhesives is **etch and rinse (E&R)**, formerly known as total-etch, and **self-etching (SE)**.

Historical

In 1955, Buonocore introduced the **acid-etch technique** for adhering acrylic restoratives to tooth substrate. While adhering to enamel has changed little since its inception, adhering to dentine has proved far more elusive. The **breakthrough came in the 1990s with the fourth and fifth generation of dental adhesives** with the **acceptance of etching dentine**, and now the state-of-the-art **eighth-generation universal adhesives (UAs)** introduced in the last decade, which **allow both E&R and SE**, as well as **selective enamel etching modes**.

Adhesion mechanism

Adhering to enamel and dentine are fundamentally different processes, involving **surface wetting, micromechanical interlocking** (micro-retention) and **chemical interaction**. To achieve an efficacious adhesion to tooth substrate, an adhesive should **initially be hydrophobic for enhanced wettability to dentine**, and **hydrophobic after polymerisation to prevent hydrolytic bond degradation.** To achieve micromechanical interlocking, the surface needs to be **mechanically (tooth preparation) or chemically (etching) roughened.** Enamel etching by the E&R provides a substrate that is amenable to micromechanical interlocking but **demineralises 3–6 µm of the dentine layer** that is **poorly infiltrated by the resin adhesive**, and results in a weak dentine bond. Alternately, **mild-SE agents only penetrate the dentine layer by 1 µm** that is fully engulfed by resin combined with **ionic (chemical) interaction** with the remaining **dentine hydroxyapatite (HA)**, and therefore, produces a more durable bond. Hence, **E&R offers a superior bond to enamel but not to dentine,** and **vice versa for mild SE agents.** The **adhesion-decalicification (AD concept)** proposes the formation of Ca-monomer bonds with HA by an **adhesive or decalicification route with monomers such as phosphorylated pullulan (PPL) or 10-methacryloyloxydecyl dihydrogen phosphate (10-MDP).**

The **E&R approach is described as diffusion-based micromechanical interlocking without primary chemical interaction.** Both enamel and dentine are etched with phosphoric acid to completely remove the smear layer, giving the proverbial frosted white appearance. On enamel, the resin penetrates the etched pits to create macro-resin tags and micro-tags by capillary action. Ideally, the dentine should neither be over etched, nor over dried as the resin cannot infiltrate into deeper etched dentine. An ethanol/water (solvent)-based primer is massaged and air dried to rehydrate the dentine and promotes resin infiltration to form the **hybrid layer** (also known as an interdiffusion zone or resin-infiltrated dentine layer). The **thickness of the hybrid layer can vary from 0.5 µm to 10 µm.** However, the thickness and morphology of the hybrid layer seems less important than its consistency and integrity (lack of gaps, porosity and voids), which are paramount for achieving efficacious and durable dentine sealing and bonding.

The **advantages of E&R** (3-step, e.g. Optibond FL) are **superior and durable enamel bonding, shock absorbing potential,** and 20+ years clinical performance. The **disadvantages** are that all the **smear layer [with HA] is removed from dentine**, and therefore, only **secondary chemical interaction is possible**, producing thick hybrid layers that are prone to degradation. The **mild SE approach** combines a conditioner and primer for partial demineralisation but not completely removing the smear layer. Therefore, adhesion to enamel is less efficacious to enamel than with E&R, but superior to dentine since some HA remains to produce both micromechanical interlocking and **chemical bonding using functional monomers such as 10-MDP** for form ionic binding and stable **nanolayering**. The partial demineralisation (≈1 µm) and retention of HA around the collagen fibres are advantageous for complete resin penetration and primary chemical interaction with functional monomers (two-step SE, e.g. Clearfil SE Bond). The limitations are **poor enamel adhesion** due to poor etching pattern, and therefore, **selective enamel etching is recommended**, and 10-MDP shows poor hydrolytic stability.

Efficacy

The **efficacy** of an adhesive is assessed by the **shear bond strength (SBS)** and **marginal gap** formation at the restoration–tooth interface, resulting in secondary caries, pulpal pathologies and discolouration. The SBS should be sufficient to counteract the polymerisation stresses generated by the resin-based restorative material and, therefore, prevent breakdown of the bond. The gold standard for **SBS** comparison is the bond **to enamel, ranging from 23 MPa to 25 MPa. Dentine SBS are erratic, ranging from as little as 3 MPa to 25 MPa.** The reported **marginal gap ranges from 0 to 10 µm.** Failure of the dental adhesives is multifactorial, depending on both the material properties and clinical techniques (adequate isolation, preparation design, mode of light curing, etc.).

Clinical procedures and applications

The **current gold standard for E&R is a three-step procedure** as follows:

- **Etch both enamel and dentine** with 30–40% phosphoric acid for 15s, rinse for 10s and dry (frosty white dull appearance)
- **Rub primer** (e.g. HEMA, PENTA or 4-META, preferably with a water-based solvent [to overcome wet-bonding] and photo-initiator), dry for 15s
- **Apply resin adhesive** (e.g. bis- GMA, UDMA), air dry and immediately polymerise (light cure) to prevent water sorption by osmosis from dentine layer. An optional step is to cover with a flowable composite as a stress-absorbing layer

The **current gold standard for mild-SE is a three-step procedure** as follows:

- **Selectively etch enamel** with 30–40% phosphoric acid for 15s, rinse for 10s and dry (frosty white dull appearance)
- **Rub 10-MDP self-etch primer** (for chemical adhesion to dentine) for 15s, dry to evaporate solvent
- **Apply resin and immediately polymerise**, optional flowable

The recently introduced **UAs contain a primer and adhesive resin, and are aimed to simplify clinical procedures** with the option to use either E&R, SE or selective etching modes of application. The clinical applications of dental adhesives include direct restorations, luting indirect prostheses, desensitising and immediate dentine sealing (IDS).

Key points

- Dental adhesives are categorised as E&R, SE, and selective enamel etching
- The gold standard for E&R and SE is a three-step approach
- Chemical interaction with dentine is possible using 10-MDP

63 Contemporary cements

Contemporary cements

	Formulation	Varieties	Advantages	Disadvantages	Cementation mechanism: Cement-tooth interface	Cementation mechanism: Cement-restoration interface
Resin-modified glass ionomer (RMGI)	Polyalkenoic acid with addition of a methacrylate component (e.g. HEMA) and fillers	Pre-capsulated, chemical and light cured	Adhesion to dentine, thin film thickness, antimicrobial, fluoride releasing, low solubility, adheres to moist tooth substrate, reduced chemical trauma to pulp	Mechanically weaker than resins, significant post cementation dimensional changes may fracture weak ceramics	Chemical adhesion	Mechanical interlocking
Conventional resins (CR)	Polymer infiltrated with filler particles	Chemical, light and dual cured, low and high viscosities, shade tints to modify colour	High compressive strength, superior optical properties	Technique sensitive, hydrolytic degradation, shade shift over time, possible post-operative sensitivity with poor technique	Micromechanical adhesion and/or chemical adhesion	Chemical adhesion
Adhesive resins (AR)	Polymer infiltrated with filler particles with the addition of an adhesive functional phosphate monomer e.g. MPD (10-Methacryloyloxydecyl dihydrogen phosphate)	Dual cured, self-etching, self-adhesive, antibacterial, fluoride releasing	High compressive strength, superior optical properties, chemical bonding to cast metal , alumina and zirconia substructures	Technique sensitive, hydrolytic degradation, shade shift over time, lower bond strength compared to CR, reduced post-operative sensitivity compared to CR	Micromechanical adhesion and/or chemical adhesion	Chemical adhesion

Type of restoration	Restorative material	Ideal cement	Possible cement
Cast metal crowns & inlays, intra-radicular posts, porcelain fused to metal crowns & fixed partial dentures (bridges)	High gold & semi-precious alloys	AR, RMGI	ZP, PC, CR
Maryland/Rochette bridges & splints	Semi-precious alloys	AR	CRD
Fibre-reinforced composite bridges and splints	Composite, fibre	AR	CRD
Light transmitting intra-radicular posts	Fibre, zirconia	AR	CRD
Orthodontic fixed brackets	Metal alloy	AR	CRD
Inlays and onlays	Composite or silica-based ceramic	AR	CRD
Porcelain laminate veneers (feldspathic)	Silica-based ceramics	CRL	AR
All-ceramic crowns, e.g. feldspathic, leucite-reinforced pressed glass, lithium disilicate	Silica-based ceramics	AR, RMGI	–
All-ceramic crowns and fixed partial dentures of glass infiltrated alumina, densely sintered alumina, zirconia substructures	Alumina & zirconia-based ceramics	AR, RMGI	–
Implant supported crowns or fixed partial dentures	Porcelain fused to metal, or alumina & zirconia-based ceramics	AR, RMGI	ZOE

ZOE - zinc/oxide eugenol, ZP - zinc phosphate, PC - polycarboxylate, RMGI - resin-modified glass ionomer, CRL - conventional resin light-cured, CRD - conventional resin dual-cured, AR - adhesive resins

Choice of cements

Prosthodontics at a Glance, Second Edition. Irfan Ahmad.

Contemporary cements for indirect definitive restorations can broadly be categorised as **resin-modified glass ionomers (RMGI)** and **resins**. The latter can be further subdivided into **conventional resins (CR)** and **adhesive resins (AR)**.

Resin-modified glass-ionomers (RMGI)

RMGIs exploit the benefits of both glass ionomers (GIs) and resins. **RMGIs bond to dentine**, have a **thin film thickness, release fluoride and are less prone to ageing degradatio**n, while the **resin part confers improved physical, mechanical and aesthetic properties**. These materials are the **most popular luting agents used in clinical practice** due to **ease of use**, and are **less technique-sensitive compared to resins**. The indications include cast metal and high strength ceramic core restorations such as alumina and zirconia for tooth abutments and implant-supported titanium and zirconia abutments.

Conventional resins (CR)

Resin-based cements have a similar chemistry to resin-based restorative composites. An o**rganic resin matrix** (e.g. Bis-GMA) is i**nfiltrated with inorganic filler** (e.g. silica) particles, which are coated with silane to bind with the surrounding polymer (matrix). The **type and amount of filler particles determine the physical, mechanical and optical properties** of the cement. The major **advantage** of resins is **superior mechanical and optical properties,** and they are particularly indicated for **bonding aesthetic ceramic restorations** such as inlays, PLVs, all-ceramic crowns and fixed partial dentures (FPD).

The **adhesion mechanism at the cement–tooth interface** is **micromechanical interlocking** in conjunction with a **dental adhesive** by forming a **hybrid layer**. Some dental adhesives offer **chemical adhesion** by bonding with calcium ions from the hydroxyapatite of the tooth substrate. To resist the polymerisation stresses of the overlying resin cement, the **bond strength of the adhesive should exceed 25 MPa**. The dental adhesive can either be separately applied beforehand or incorporated within the cement (adhesive resins [AR]). Caution is necessary with self-etching adhesives since the acidic inhibition layer may be incompatible with the setting reaction of some resin cements. Cement can contain a self-etching primers to eliminate the etching and priming stages, while the self-adhesive varieties also incorporate a bonding agent to simplify clinical protocols. However, the self-etching/self-adhesive cements are more efficacious bonding to dentine than enamel, while enamel bonding benefits from a separate etch and rinse adhesive applied beforehand.

Conventional resins (CR) are recommended for silica-based ceramics where aesthetics are a paramount concern. Silica is a low-strength ceramic (flexural strength 100–300 MPa) with a high glass content, offering increased translucency and superior aesthetics (assuming the underlying tooth substrate is an acceptable colour). In addition, **silica is amenable to etching with hydrofluoric acid (HF)** to increase mechanical retention, and when treated with silane, creates **silica–silane chemical bonds at the cement–restoration interface**. **A separate dental adhesive**, either an **etch and rinse** or **self-etch system,** is necessary to prepare the tooth substrate before cementation. CR cements are available in a **large selection of tooth-coloured shades**, enabling accurate colour matching. Furthermore, **try-in pastes** corresponding to the definitive cement shades allow colour assessment and alteration before final cementation.

Adhesive resins (AR)

Adhesive resins (AR) have similar chemistry to CR, but with the addition of an **adhesive phosphate monomer, e.g. MDP** (10-methacryloyloxydecyl dihydrogen phosphate) or **4-META** (methacry-loxyethyl trimellitic anhydride), e.g. RelyX™ Unicem, G-Cem, Maxcem, SmartCem2, PermaCem 2, BiFix SE and Panavia SA. This allows the cement to have broader applications for cementing **cast metal as well as alumina and zirconia core restorations**. The latter are classified as high-strength ceramics (flexural strength ranging from 400 MPa to >1000 MPa), **not etchable with HF,** and the lower glass content results in increased opacity with poorer optical properties, but greater masking capability for underlying tooth discolouration. The self-etching, self-adhesive AR are contraindicated for bonding PLVs since their higher pH of 2 is insufficient to adequately etch enamel compared to etching with 37% phosphoric acid that has a lower pH of 1.

Choice of cements

The **choice of cement depends upon the type of restoration**, the **restorative material** and prevailing **clinical scenario**. Non-retentive prostheses, such as Maryland/Rochette or RBFPD, PLVs and inlays/onlays, rely solely on the cement for retention. Furthermore, proper shade matching is critical for aesthetics restorations such as PLVs, ceramic inlays/onlay or crowns. In these circumstances, resin cements are ideal candidates, offering superior adhesion and enhanced aesthetics.

The basic rule when using **porcelain** in the oral cavity is that it **must be supported.** This is because porcelain is inherently brittle (high modulus of elasticity), making it **vulnerable to fractures**. **Fractures** in the hostile oral cavity are caused by the **aqueous environment** and **physiological and pathological occlusal stresses**. The weaker-strength materials such as silica-based ceramics must therefore be supported by the natural **underlying tooth substrate**. Alternately, instead of gaining support from tooth substrate, a weak silica ceramic can be supported by a **dense core or substructure, which can either be metal (PFM) or ceramic,** e.g. alumina or zirconia ceramics. Therefore, these **bilayers restorations** can either be **bonded** with resin cements, or **luted** with RMGI. Lastly, the clinical scenario dictates the choice of cement. **If the resistance and retention form of the tooth abutment is less than the ideal of 4° axial tapers (8° convergence angle), a resin cement is the prudent choice.** Similarly, poor marginal integrity of the restoration may be sealed by resins, if a remake is unpractical. Finally, **for deep subgingival margins where an arid environment is challenging, RMGIs that are less sensitive to moisture are a better option.**

Key points

- Contemporary definitive cements can be categorised as resin-modified glass ionomers (RMGI), conventional resins (CR) and adhesive resins (AR).
- The choice of cement depends on the type of restoration, restorative material and prevailing clinical scenario.
- The self-etching, self-adhesive resin cements simplify the exacting clinical protocols associated with an adhesive technique.

Cementing techniques

Pre-treatment of intra-oral abutment

Cement/ abutment surface	RMGI	CR + etch & rinse (E&R)	CR + self-etching (SE)	AR
Enamel	None	30–40% phosphoric acid	30–40% phosphoric acid	30–40% phosphoric acid
Dentine	None	30–40% phosphoric acid	None	None
Composite/amalgam	Air abrasion + 30–40% phosphoric acid (for cleansing)	Air abrasion + 30–40% phosphoric acid + silane (depends on dental adhesive)		Air abrasion + 30–40% phosphoric acid (for cleansing)

Pre-treatment of restoration intaglio surface

Restorative material	High gold content alloy	Base or semi-precious alloy	Silica ceramics	Alumina ceramics	Zirconia ceramics
Pre-treatment of intaglio surface	Air abrasion + alloy primer (or tin plate or silica/ silane coat) + 30–40% phosphoric acid	Air abrasion + 30–40% phosphoric acid	4–10% hydrofluoric acid (for etching) + silane	4–10% hydrofluoric or 30–40% phosphoric acid (for cleansing)	4–10 % hydrofluoric or 30–40% phosphoric acid (for cleansing)

Clinical cementation procedure for CR cement

Isolate abutments with retraction cord & wedges

Etch

Rinse and dry

Apply dental adhesive of choice

Seat restoration & mop cement

Floss contact areas

Try-in paste to stop O_2 inhibition layer

Remove cord & light cure

Trim with #12 blade

Polish, e.g. with EVA tips

Check occlusion

Irrigate with saline to flush out set cement

Prosthodontics at a Glance, Second Edition. Irfan Ahmad.

The **performance of a cement** depends on **clinical factors and pretreatment of the indirect restoration intaglio surface and the intra-oral abutment.** The cementation technique is both time-consuming and exacting, and any omissions will compromise the durability and long-term survival of the restoration.

Clinical factors

Clinical performance of cements is influenced by:

- **Operator variables** – mixing, dispensing and loading cement accounts for more than 50% of all risk factors
- **Tooth preparation design** – ideal 8° convergence angle and adequate resistance form
- **Material properties** – accounts for approximately 5% of risk factors
- **Location of tooth** – anterior (aesthetic considerations) or posterior (mechanical considerations)
- **Patient factors** – oral hygiene, habits, e.g. sport activities, playing wind instruments, etc.

Pretreatment of intra-oral abutment

Preconditioning of the intra-oral abutment starts by **removing the temporary cement,** which is accomplished mechanically using hand instruments, rotary plastic burs (OptiClean, KerrHawe SA, Switzerland), air abrasion, pumice paste or ultrasonic devices. Total removal is essential to avoid compromising the bond strength between the natural tooth substrate (or artificial abutment, e.g. intra-radicular post/cores or implant abutments) and the definitive cement.

The next stage is **isolation**, either with rubber dam or intra-sulcular gingival retraction cords and interproximal wooden wedges. An **arid environment** is essential for resin-based cements, but less critical for RMGI. Rubber dam is the ideal choice for cementing inlays in posterior teeth, but for anterior teeth the retaining **rubber dam** metal clamps can potentially traumatise the gingival margin, leading to recession, especially for teeth in the aesthetic zone with thin periodontal biotypes. **Gingival retraction cords**, dry or impregnated with an astringent, not only allows visualisation of the abutment margins, but also acts as a physical barrier to avoid excess cement entering the delicate gingival sulcus. However, retraction cords may be inappropriate around implant abutments, since the latter can damage the friable epithelial attachment.

Tooth abutment pretreatment depends on the type of cement being used. If RMGI is employed, no further conditioning is necessary irrespective of whether the abutment is dentine, enamel or artificial restorative material, e.g. composite, amalgam, cast metal, ceramic cores or implant abutments made of titanium, alumina and zirconia. If a **conventional resin (CR)** is chosen and the abutment is natural tooth substrate, the **gold standard is a three-step etch and rinse, self-etching (SE) or universal adhesive procedures** (Chapter 62). If a **SE or adhesive resin (AR) cement** is chosen, it is prudent to **selectively etch enamel** (to create an adequate etching pattern, especially with uncut, aprismatic enamel). Etching dentine with phosphoric acid when using a SE dental adhesive is superfluous, since this may over etch the dentine and if the adhesive resin fails to penetrate the dentine tubules, the result in postoperative sensitivity.

For **artificial intra-oral abutments, the pretreatment depends on the restorative material,** e.g. for composite and amalgam core build-ups, the pretreatment is air abrasion followed by etching with 30–40% phosphoric acid.

Pretreatment of intaglio surface

The conditioning of the fitting, or **intaglio surface**, depends on the **restorative material** and the **choice of cement** (RMGI, CR or AR). The methods available are:

- **Mechanical**: rotary diamond burs, only indicated for cast metal surfaces
- **Air abrasion**: aluminium oxide powder (30–50 µm Al_2O_3 powder at 60–100 psi pressure for 2–3 seconds per cm^2). It has been suggested to use this method on high-strength ceramics such as alumina and zirconia, but not on weaker ceramics (feldspathic, leucite) since air abrasion can reduce strength by 30% by forming microscopic cracks that propagate at the fitting surface and during function
- **Chemical**: hydrofluoric acid (HF; 4–10% for 3 minutes) for silica-based ceramics, followed by application of **warm silane**. HF and phosphoric acid cannot etch metal, alumina or zirconia, but are used for cleansing to ensure a contamination-free intaglio surface, especially following air abrasion. Other chemical agents include alloy primers or tin plating for some cast alloys
- **Dental adhesive** – or unfilled resin, can be applied (but not light cured) onto the intaglio surface, irrespective of the type of restorative material if a resin-based cement is used

Cementation procedure

After pretreatment of the abutment and intaglio surfaces, the next stage is dispensing the chosen cement. One of the major factors that reduces cement strength is introduction of air into the cement. For example, **10% porosity can reduce strength by 55%. Porosity** is primarily due to the **method of mixing, polymerisation shrinkage** during the setting reaction and **disintegration due to fatigue and thermocycling.** For this reason, auto-mixing dispensers and precapsulated cartridges are ideal for a smooth, reduced porosity mix.

For **inlays/onlays, Maryland/Rochette or RBFPD and orthodontic brackets, the cement is placed on the recipient tooth or teeth.** For **intraradicular posts, crowns, FPDs and PLVs, the cement is dispensed onto the intaglio surface of the restoration.** The restoration is correctly located and seated with gentle pressure. Excess cement is immediately mopped, and floss is used to clean the interproximal areas. If a retraction cord or wooden wedges were placed beforehand, they are now removed together with excess cement, and the restoration firmly held in place, and light cured from all aspects with an appropriate light intensity and duration (20 seconds for halogen lights and 10 seconds for LED lights of 800 mW/cm^2). After setting, a #12 blade is used to trim set excess cement and the margins polished with silicone tips, interproximal diamond or alumina strips, and the sulcus irrigated with saline to flush out remnants of set cement. Finally, the occlusion is checked and adjusted as required.

Key points

- Successful cementation depends on clinical factors, and appropriate pretreatment of the intra-oral abutment and intaglio surface of the restoration.
- Pretreatment of both the abutment and intaglio surface depends on the restorative material and choice of cement.
- The cementation procedure should be executed meticulously for long-term survival of the restoration or prosthesis.

Removable prostheses

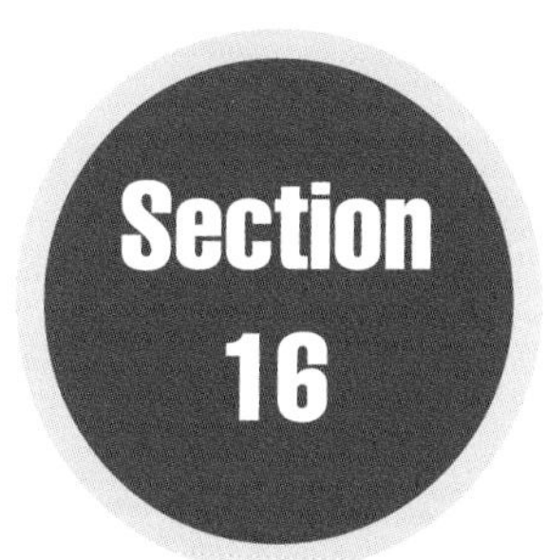

Chapter

65 Removable prostheses

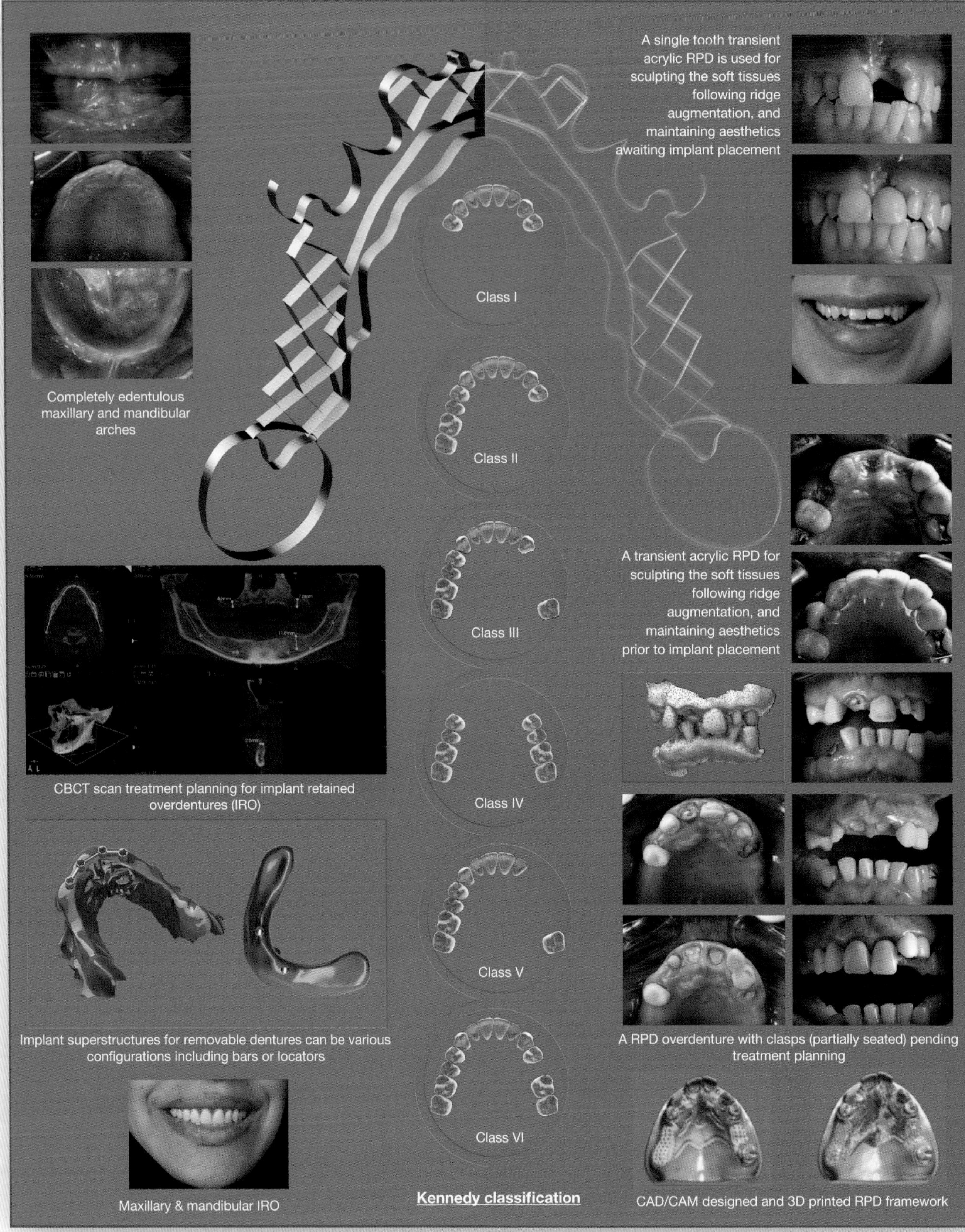

Completely edentulous maxillary and mandibular arches

A single tooth transient acrylic RPD is used for sculpting the soft tissues following ridge augmentation, and maintaining aesthetics awaiting implant placement

A transient acrylic RPD for sculpting the soft tissues following ridge augmentation, and maintaining aesthetics prior to implant placement

CBCT scan treatment planning for implant retained overdentures (IRO)

Implant superstructures for removable dentures can be various configurations including bars or locators

A RPD overdenture with clasps (partially seated) pending treatment planning

Maxillary & mandibular IRO

CAD/CAM designed and 3D printed RPD framework

Prosthodontics at a Glance, Second Edition. Irfan Ahmad.

Removable dentures are categorised as **full (complete) – RFD or partial (RPD)**, and can either be **immediate, delayed or replacement dentures**. Due to the increase in implant-stabilised removable dentures in the last few decades, there has been a significant decline in the provision of exclusively tissue-borne removable dentures. This has resulted in diminishing clinical knowledge plus reduced expertise of technicians (and less experience), and a reluctance to provide these prostheses when alternative solutions with implants are available for oral rehabilitation. Furthermore, the **success of removable dentures relies on psychological acceptance and tolerance by the patient**, more than prosthodontic factors. Also, there is little evidence to support that removable dentures allow patients to pursue a more healthy diet. However, this type of modality is valuable and indispensable for both **transitional phases of treatment**, and as a **definitive prosthesis** when extensive grafting procedures for implants are contraindicated due to medical history, intra-oral factors or financial considerations.

Indications

The **indications for removable prostheses** include:

- **Transitional** full or partial dentures awaiting osseointegration for definitive fixed or removable **implant retained overdentures (IRO)**
- **Periodontal splints**
- **Training bases** for assessing altered VDO and anterior guidance
- **Templates** (with radiographic markers) for preoperative CBCT scans for implant treatment planning
- **Definitive oral rehabilitation**

Edentulism

The **sequelae following tooth extraction** are **alveolar bone loss and remodelling**, resulting in:

- **Pseudo class III** and cross-bites of dental ridges
- **Differential or site-specific bone loss**, e.g. flabby anterior maxillary ridge, atrophic mandibular ridge
- **Prominence of muscle attachments** hindering a denture prescription
- **Reduced lower third facial height**
- **Inadequate lip support**
- **Premature ageing** by formation of facial grooves and fissures
- **Social embarrassment**
- **Psychological trauma**

These factors can contribute to poor denture support, poor stability, lack of retention, compromised aesthetics and inadequate lip support. **Further complications after fitting the denture(s)** include denture stomatitis, inappropriate occlusal schemes (balanced occlusion or balanced articulation), altered taste sensation, painful TMJ (incorrect VDO, inadequate freeway space (2–3 mm advisable), correct position of maxillary central incisors relative to incisal papilla (9 mm anterior and 12 mm below), instability due to incorrect position of posterior teeth and continual ridge resorption requiring relines or rebases.

Removable full dentures (RFD)

Edentulous ridges have varied presentation depending on the degree of resorption. For a **well-preserved ridge, a denture is merely replacing teeth**, while for an **atrophic ridge, a denture replaces both the lost bone and teeth**. However, full-denture success is not only dependent on ridge morphology, but as mentioned above, also on patient compliance and psychology. **Retention of a maxillary full denture** relies on suction from the palatal mucosa, peripheral flanges, tuberosities and a suitable post-dam. In contrast, **retention of a mandibular denture** is more challenging, depending on the patient's neuromuscular adaptability, extension onto the retromolar and buccal shelves, flanges, denture fixatives or retention from strategically placed **implants (for IRO) or retained roots**. RFD bases and teeth can be **milled or 3D printed**, or alternately the bases can be 3D printed or milled and stock teeth cemented into the 'sockets'. Both upper and lower dentures can be reinforced with **chrome-cobalt frameworks**, or preferably **lighter weight titanium** for additional strength. This is especially useful for full-dentures opposing a natural dentate arch, and for patients with a history of bruxism and fracturing acrylic dentures. In these circumstances, the ridges, flanges and peripheral extensions, including post-dam, are kept in acrylic for future relines. Another precarious situation is a removable full denture opposing a full arch of fixed prosthesis, which can potentially cause **pressure necrosis** of the opposing edentulous ridge.

Removable partial dentures (RPD)

Partially edentulous arches are described according to the **Kennedy classification**. Before replacing any missing teeth, it is important to consider the **shortened dental arch concept** (Chapter 19), and if functional and aesthetic needs are met, replacing molar teeth is superfluous. If a fixed solution for replacing missing teeth is precluded, a removable prosthodontic alternative should be considered for oral rehabilitation. **RPDs can be both tissue and teeth/implant supported**. All supporting teeth require endodontic, periodontal and occlusal assessment for suitability. Also, **it is not a fait accompli that a RPD denture will cause periodontal problems if meticulous oral hygiene is addressed beforehand.** Furthermore, RPDs offer the benefits of adding further teeth, or overdentures with retained roots (or implants using locator or bars). They are relatively inexpensive, and have shorter treatment time compared to fixed options. Many types are possible depending on number and location of the missing teeth, for example:

- **Entirely acrylic bases** are ideal as transitional, training or templates for scans and fabricating surgical guides. In addition, clasps and rests can be incorporated to improve stability and retention
- **Metal framework with acrylic bases**. This variety is suited for long-term usage, and semi-permanent periodontal splinting. **CAD/CAM** technology can design frameworks, which can be 3D printed as a **burnout resin** and invested and cast by conventional means, or directly **milled/3D printed in a choice of metals** such as chrome-cobalt or titanium. In addition, the design can incorporate clasps, reciprocating bracing rests, milled guiding planes, anti-rotational features, precision attachments and correct paths of insertion/removal to cater for a wide range of clinical situations.

Key points

- Removable prostheses are not an antiquated treatment modality, but have many uses in contemporary prosthodontics.
- The negative aspects of edentulism should be considered before extractions are planned.
- Partial dentures are classified as RFD and RPD, and supported by soft tissues, teeth or implants.
- Both RFD and RPD can be definitive prostheses if implants are contraindicated.

Dental implants

Section 17

Chapters

66 Osseointegration

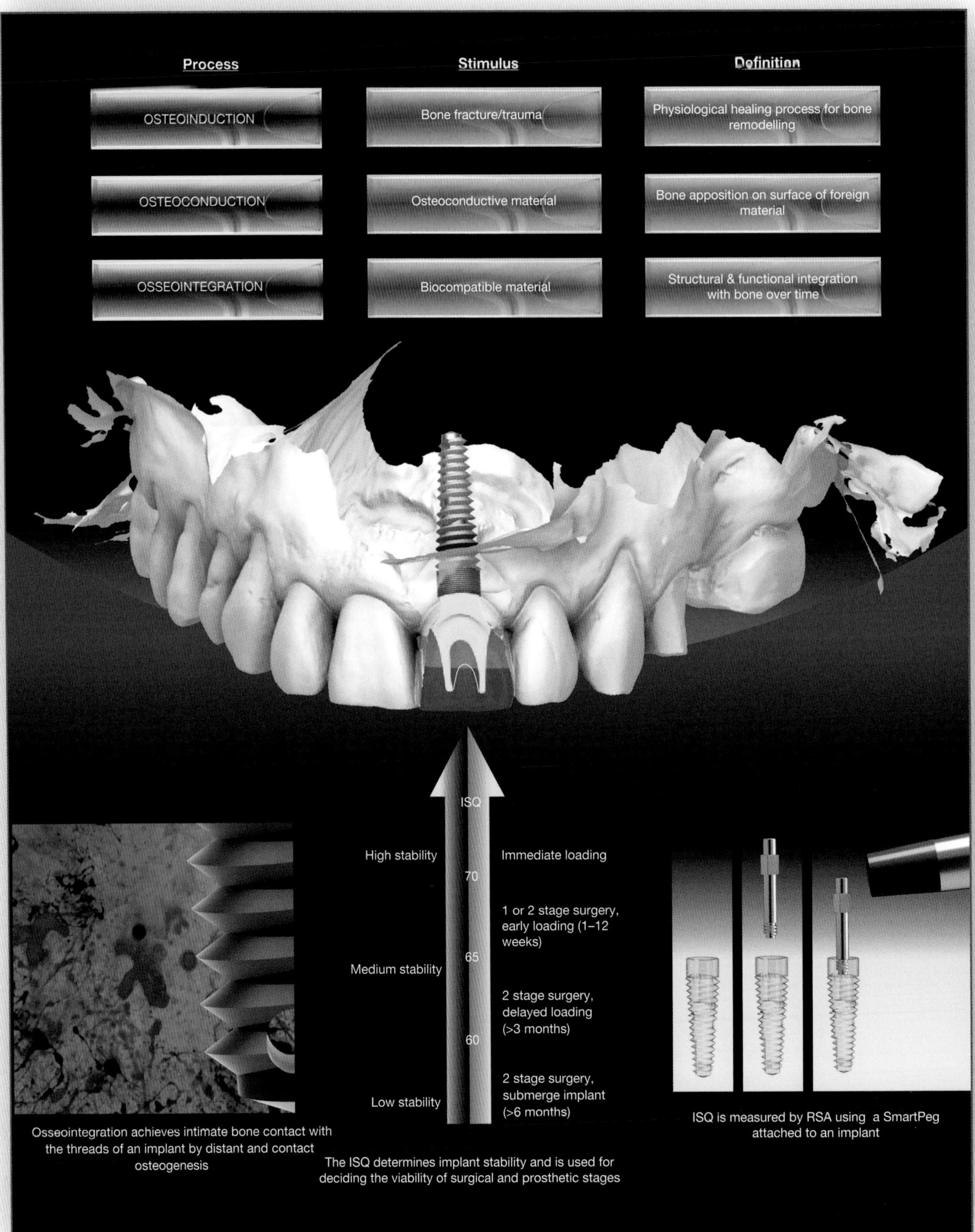

Osseointegration achieves intimate bone contact with the threads of an implant by distant and contact osteogenesis

The ISQ determines implant stability and is used for deciding the viability of surgical and prosthetic stages

ISQ is measured by RSA using a SmartPeg attached to an implant

Apart from G.V. Black, **P.-I. Brånemark** has made the most significant contribution to dentistry in the last century. Although 'dental implants' can be traced back as far as 4000 BCE in China, it was Brånemark who laid the foundation for modern dental implantology. His invention of dental implants has revolutionised the replacement of single teeth, partial edentulous segments and totally edentulous dental arches with both fixed and removable prostheses. In addition, implants are also used for providing anchorage for orthodontic, orthopaedic and orthognathic movements.

Definitions

Three distinct processes describe bone healing and remodelling: osteoinduction, osteoconduction and osseointegration. These three mechanisms are interrelated but not interchangeable. The definitions for the above are as follows:

- **Osteoinduction** – physiological process of bone healing and repair by osteogenesis following traumatic fractures
- **Osteoconduction** – bone growth on the surface of osteoconductive foreign bodies, e.g. implants or synthetic bone grafting materials
- **Osseointegration** – direct contact of living bone with an implant surface (without formation of fibrous tissue), which is maintained during functional loading over a long period, and is accomplished by **distance and contact osteogenesis**

Processes

The **osteoinduction** healing process is initiated **following trauma** to bone. Undifferentiated, mesenchymal cells are converted to pre-osteoblasts, which are eventually transformed to bone-forming osteoblasts and osteocytes by stimulation from inductive transformation growth factors such as bone **BMP (bone morphogenic proteins)**. This is the normal mechanism that occurs during repair of a bone fracture and implant integration.

Osteoconduction is bone **apposition on the surface of implants from pre-existing osteoblasts or immature mesenchymal cells** that have been transformed by the osteoinduction process. The surface of the implant is said to be osteoconductive and promotes, in combination with the trauma of osteotomy, the stimulation of bone growth. Bone remodelling requires **sufficient vascularisation** and is signalled by **bone growth factors, such as insulin-like growth factor (IGF I, IGF II), fibroblast growth factor (FGF) and platelet-derived growth factor (PDGF).** Bone conduction requires highly biocompatible materials such as commercially pure titanium or demineralised bone, and is not possible with incompatible materials such as copper or silver.

Osseointegration is a term coined by Brånemark to describe the **structural and functional integration of implants with surrounding bone.** The process of **osseointegration is preceded by osteoinduction and osteoconduction,** and implies that anchored implants are functionally maintained over time. **Osteoconduction is short-lived,** while **osseointegration maintains bone anchorage of the implant over a long period.** This was a monumental breakthrough in oral and craniofacial implantology, paving the way for replacing missing or lost teeth with dental implants. **Osseointegration is a histological concept**, involving formation of an amorphous layer measuring **20–40 µm at the bone–implant interface,** which has similar density to surrounding bone. The speed of **osseointegration can be accelerated by pretreatment of the titanium implant surface by roughening, coating with bio-affinity layers such as titanium oxides or hydroxyapatite.** Furthermore, osseoperception is evident in patients that have implant-supported dental prostheses, i.e. there is **sensory feedback from the loaded implant(s),** similar to natural teeth.

Clinical assessment

Osseointegration per se is a histological principle that cannot be visualised clinically. However, it is essential to **confirm osseointegration and stability of an implant before it can be prosthetically restored**. Some methodologies proposed for assessing clinical osseointegration, and its subsequent monitoring, are as follows:

- **Visual** – healthy soft tissues around the fixture without inflammation, suppuration or pain
- **Radiographic** – periapical or panoramic assessment of bone levels around implants, but because the images are 2D, buccal dehiscences may be concealed. However, 3D CBCT or radio-stereo-photogrammetric analysis (RSA) techniques offer better evaluation
- **Percussion** is probably the crudest method, involving tapping the implant with a hand instrument (similar to tapping a tooth suspected of endodontic lesions), and listening to the pitch of the tone. A high pitch indicates implant stability, while a low, dull pitch infers poorly integrated implant fixtures
- **Periotest** (e.g. wireless Periotest M) – quantifies implant mobility in response to an electronically controlled translational hammer. However, readings are erratic and highly dependent on position and angulation of the testing instrument
- **Dynamic modal testing**, e.g. Dental mobility checker (DMC)® – using a rotational hammer that produces an electric voltage to plot a force vs. time graph for assessing mobility. However, similar to the Periotest, the readings do not measure the implant in its free state and are highly apparatus-dependent
- **Reverse torque** – a surgical handpiece attached to the implant head applies a reverse torque of 20 N cm to 'remove' the fixture. This test is traumatic and may disrupt healing or lead to failure of an implant that has been slow to integrate
- **Pulsed oscillation waveform (POWF)** – measures the vibrations produced at the implant–bone interface by a steady-state wave, but readings depends on the direction and position of the applied load from a steady-state wave at the implant-bone interface
- **Resonance frequency analysis (RFA)**, e.g. Osstell ISQ, Implomates or Penguin RFA – measures the resonance frequency of implants to assess the healing process. A drawback with this method is that it fails to account for the initial bone quality and density, which greatly influences integration. RFA categorises implant stability by the implant stability quotient (ISQ)
- **Impulse testing**, e.g. Implatest – tests an implant in its free state without being encumbered with the testing apparatus. The implant is percussed with a floating calibrated hammer housed in a probe that records the **acceleration time history (ATH)**. The latter is translated by a computer using the fast Fourier transform (FFT) algorithm. A comparison is made between an ideal graph and the testing graph to ascertain the 'stiffness' of the implant. This test is useful for both unloaded and loaded implants. However, assessing implants with multiple unit FPDs still requires further refinement

Key points

- Dental implants have revolutionised the replacement of missing teeth.
- Osseointegration is defined as structural and functional integration over time of an implant with the surrounding bone.
- Various clinical tests are available for assessing osseointegration before restoring implant(s) with prosthetic unit(s).

67 Implants: general considerations

Benefits	Precautions
Restore mastication, speech, aesthetics and support of facial soft tissues	Specialist training and liaison with various dental specialists is mandatory
Prevent alveolar bone loss	Medical history may complicate surgical procedures
Prevent destruction of adjacent teeth for FPDs	Thorough preoperative dental assessment and treatment planning are key to success
Avoid inflammation of soft tissues and decay of natural teeth, associated with removable prostheses	Protracted surgical phases may deter many patients
Predicable treatment modality with good long-term success rates	Unsuitable for very young and elderly patients
Versatile treatment options, including single tooth replacement, rehabilitation of partially edentulous and fully edentulous ridges with either fixed or removable prostheses	Failure may cause local morbidity, and involve further surgical trauma to rectify problems
Extensive choice of restorative materials for prosthetic units including cast alloys, titanium, ceramics and resin-based composites	Costly

Pre-op missing #11

Failing #12, graft & implant

Implant fixture

Fit crown

Healing abutment

9 years later

Fit crown

Implant supported FPD

8 years later

Implant replacing missing # 25

Implant at #24 placed too apical to curve of Spee

Poor implant positioning and angulation resulting in proximity to adjacent tooth

Two failing implants in the anterior maxilla due to gross bone loss

Peri-implantitis and suppuration causing mobility of implant fixtures

Prosthodontics at a Glance, Second Edition. Irfan Ahmad.

Dental implants are increasingly becoming the first choice of treatment for replacing missing teeth, and represent a step along the road to **regenerative medicine**, and future research in **genomics** and **proteomics** will perhaps offer even greater benefits than titanium cylinders for the replacement of missing teeth.

Rationale and indications

Dental implants are no longer an esoteric treatment modality limited to a few specialised practices. The last few decades have witnessed a burgeoning demand for dental implants which is now pervading general dental practices. Furthermore, innumerable studies and **controlled clinical trials report encouraging mean survival rates of endosseous implants greater than 90% over 10 years.** Due to this high level of predictability, implant fixtures offer treatment options that were once implausible. The benefits of implants are as follows:

- **Maintenance of alveolar bone** – bone requires stimulation to maintain its form and density. Tooth extraction leads to both soft and hard tissue defects. For example, **bone loss in the fully edentulous maxilla occurs in a medial and superior direction, while in the mandible, the resorption is lateral and inferior.** This results in a **narrow maxilla, often tending to a class III skeletal relationship**
- **Soft tissue support** – edentulism results in reduced support for facial soft tissues, causing premature ageing
- **Improved mastication** – the bite force of implant-supported prostheses is similar to the natural dentition, unlike the reduced masticatory function experienced with removable dentures
- **Improved phonetics** – because implant supported prostheses offer better stability compared to soft tissue-borne dentures
- **Preservation of natural teeth** – in partially edentulous patients, adjacent healthy teeth are spared preparation
- **Prevention of dental and soft tissue lesions** – both fixed and removable prostheses are potentially harmful to teeth (decay, endodontic and periodontal problems) and the soft tissues (inflammation and continual ridge atrophy). Preventing these unwanted pathologies improves oral comfort
- **Improved aesthetics** – for both teeth and facial contours due to soft tissue support
- **Replacing existing fixed or removable dentures** – a failing FPD with decayed, endodontic or periodontally compromised abutments is potentially ideal for implant therapy. Similarly, loose, uncomfortable dentures (especially mandibular) benefit by implant-retained overdentures (IRO) that offer improved mechanical stability, mastication, speech and mitigate further bone loss
- **Replacement can be a single teeth, partially edentulous ridges or fully edentulous arches.** Also, the **definitive prosthesis may be a fixed partial denture (FPD), fixed full denture (FFD) or removable full denture (RFD)**
- **Temporary anchorage devices (TADs)** to facilitate orthodontic movement. TADs are also an ideal method for intruding overerupted teeth to create occlusal clearance for replacing teeth in the opposing arch

Contraindications

As mentioned above, there is no doubt that many patients can, and do, benefit from implants rather than traditional treatment modalities. However, implantology depends on many factors for a successful outcome (see MAP – Chapter 2). Some **contraindications** that may reduce the chances for optimal prognosis, or preclude patients from implant therapy, are:

- **Medical history** – the following conditions may complicate or delay healing following surgical procedures:

Endocrine disorders, e.g. diabetes mellitus, hypothyroidism and adrenal insufficiency
Uncontrolled granulomatous diseases, e.g. tuberculosis and sarcoidosis
Cardiovascular diseases, e.g. angina, aortitis, arteriosclerosis, aortic insufficiency or aneurysms
Bone diseases, e.g. Paget's disease, fibrous dysplasia, histiocytosis X or osteoporosis
Carcinoma, e.g. oral (mouth), head or neck
Radiotherapy of the jaws, head or neck
Haematological disorders, e.g. anaemia, haemophilia (factor VIII deficiency), or factor IX, X, XII deficiencies, or reduced platelet count disorders, all predispose to poor haemorrhage control
Autoimmune diseases, e.g. HIV
Medication, e.g. bisphosphonates causing bisphosphonate-related osteonecrosis of the jaw (BRONJ) or other drugs, e.g. anti-RANKL drugs causing medication-related osteonecrosis of the jaw (MRONJ), immunosuppressant drugs following organ transplants
Other factors, e.g. xerostomia, smoking, pregnancy, psychological stress, poor oral hygiene
Very young and old patients – patients with primary or mixed dentitions are unsuitable candidates for implants, as well as the elderly or infirm, who may prefer non-surgical options
Osseous remodelling of the jaws throughout life may impact the long-term success of dental implants

- **Surgical technique and experience of the operator**
- **Skilled multidisciplinary dental specialists** – liaison and successful co-operation with the prosthodontist, cranio-maxillofacial surgeons, orthodontists and dental ceramists
- **Dental variables**, e.g. ridge anatomy, adjacent and opposing teeth, occlusal factors, soft tissue morphology
- **Previous dental history and present dental status**, oral hygiene compliance, smoking cessation
- **Duration of treatment** is usually protracted, especially if soft and hard tissue grafting is envisaged. Therefore, patients require a degree of patience and endurance to last the course
- **Cost** is a major factor to consider before embarking on implant treatment. While an mandibular IRO may be within the financial reach of many, a complex and comprehensive fixed rehabilitation may be limited to the few
- **Prognosis** depends on all the above variables, and if unfavourable factors are likely to compromise implant treatment, it may be prudent to seek alternative modalities

Although, implants offer many benefits, there is an emerging trend for overprescribing this modality. In addition, implant failures could potentially leave the patient in a worse situation that is costly and protracted to rectify.

Key points

- Dental implants are the state-of-the-art treatment modality for replacing missing teeth.
- Implants offer numerous advantages over conventional treatment options for restoring health, function and aesthetics.
- Although successful and predictable, numerous factors affect implant therapy, and contraindications should be thoroughly assessed beforehand.

68 Implants: treatment planning

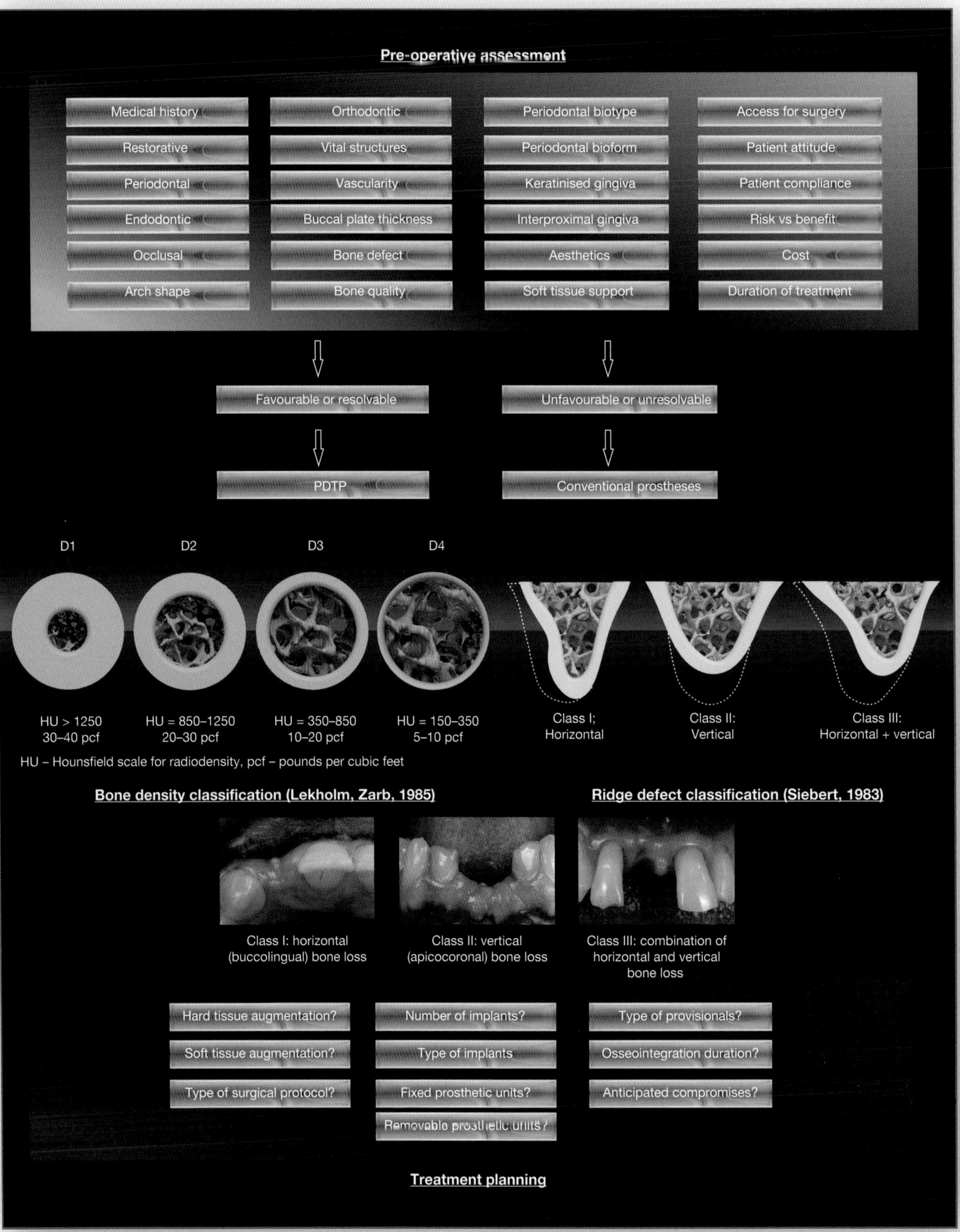

Prosthodontics at a Glance, Second Edition. Irfan Ahmad.

A patient considering dental implants should initially be assessed using **MAP (medical, anatomy, prognosis)**, discussed in Chapter 2. After this cursory evaluation, comprehensive diagnostic tests are essential (discussed in the Diagnostics section) before formulating a treatment plan. The objective of implant therapy is restoring both function and aesthetics of missing teeth, and the key to achieving this goal is **meticulous diagnosis and treatment planning**.

Pre-operative assessment

A detailed **medical and dental history** is followed by **diagnostic tests, including radiographs, CBCT scans, photographs, virtual or analogue diagnostic wax-ups and fabrication of surgical guides.** If necessary, **specialist advice** is sought from the periodontist, endodontist, orthodontist, cranio-maxillofacial surgeon, radiologist and the dental technician. The assessment should consider:

- **Medical history**
- **Existing dental status** – periodontal, endodontic and restorative status of existing teeth
- **Occlusion** – parafunctional activity, occlusal stability (avoiding lateral forces on implant-supported prostheses), and sufficient occlusal clearance for prosthetic units
- **Arch shape** – narrow, square, oval, crowding, spacing or posterior cross-bite may require orthodontic intervention
- **Proximity of vital structures** – sinuses, neurovascular bundles (e.g. inferior dental nerve, mandibular midline lingual vascular bundle, mental and incisal foramina), adjacent tooth roots
- **Reduced vascularity** – due to previous periapical infections
- **Buccal plate thickness or its absence** due to fistulas, fenestrations (intact marginal bone), or dehiscences (no marginal bone)
- **Extent of bone defect** – following tooth extraction, prevailing or previous periodontal disease, previous surgical trauma
- **Bone quality** – classified as D1 to D4 (or types I to IV); DI is highly dense cortical bone (e.g. in the mandible), and D4 is least dense cancellous bone (e.g. in the posterior maxilla)
- **Ridge defect** can either be vertical or horizontal, or a combination. For totally edentulous patients, ridge absorption often results in a transformation of class I to class III jaw relationship
- **Periodontal biotype and bioform** – thin, highly scalloped biotypes predispose to gingival recession, while thick-flat biotypes result in pocket formation following surgical trauma or inflammation. Furthermore, thin-scalloped may also result in defects due to delayed bone remodelling, while thick-flat types result in gingival notches and scarring. **Peri-implant biotypes** around dental implants are also classified as thick and thin, similar to periodontal biotypes
- **Biologic width** – a histological concept that is the sum of the linear measurements of the junctional epithelial and connective tissues attachments around natural teeth, averaging 2.04 mm. However, clinically, the biologic width **varies from as little as 0.59 mm to > 3 mm** depending on the type of tooth, and no value has been identified as an absolute minimum for gingival health. The biologic width around implants is similar to that for natural teeth but the implant–epithelium junction is shorter and thinner, influenced by implant design, the presence of adjacent teeth, and **platform switching** that shifts the position of the microgap (either in a horizontal or vertical plane) to minimise circumferential bone loss. Furthermore, the connective tissue fibres around natural teeth are perpendicular, but parallel around implants
- **Degree of keratinised gingiva** – a minimum of 3 mm is usually quoted as essential
- **Interproximal papilla** – for complete papilla fill between natural teeth, the distance of the contact point to the interproximal bone should be < 5 mm. However, between two adjacent implants, this distance needs to be reduced to a minimum of 3.4 mm for complete papilla fill. In addition, sufficient interproximal spaces are required for adequate oral hygiene procedures
- **Aesthetics** – degree of anterior maxillary tooth exposure at rest, relaxed and exaggerated smile. On average, a relaxed smile shows 75–100% of the maxillary central incisors plus the interproximal papilla. A low lip line shows < 75% tooth exposure, while a high lip line shows > 75% tooth exposure plus attached gingiva apical to the teeth (gummy smile). Also, sufficient lip support is necessary to mitigate labial grooves
- **Patient's dental literacy and attitude** – counselling about dental preventive measures, tobacco and alcohol abuse and oral hygiene. Elderly or infirm patients may not be able to tolerate protracted surgical procedures
- **Other** – oral cavity access of a least 35 mm mouth opening at the site of implant placement for adequate surgical and prosthetic instrumentation
- **Risks vs benefits** assessment and alternative treatment options, cost, anticipated treatment duration
- **Written and verbal informed consent**

Prosthetically driven treatment planning (PDTP)

Previously, implant placement was dictated by a surgical approach, i.e. implants were placed according to the existing ridge anatomy. The contemporary approach is **prosthetically driven treatment planning (PDTP)**, i.e. implant placement is dictated by the position of the final restoration(s), and a deficient ridge is augmented accordingly, ensuring that the implant(s) and subsequent restoration(s) are both functional and aesthetic.

The first stage of PDTP is a **diagnostic wax-up (analogue or digital)** for ascertaining ridge morphology, need for augmentation, number, position, angulation and type of implants (shape, size, surface treatment) and the type of prosthetic rehabilitation (fixed, removable, screw- or cement-retained prosthesis). The wax-up also provides a template for any provisional restoration(s) and a surgical guide (in conjunction with a CBCT scans for 3D assessment of ridge anatomy):

- **Mesial-distal** – minimum 1.5–2 mm distance between implant and tooth and 3–4 mm between implant and implant
- **Bucco lingual** – minimum of 1–2 mm on both aspects
- **Incisal-cervical** – head of implant should be 3 mm apical to the anticipated gingival margin or 3–5 mm apical to the cement-enamel junction of adjacent teeth, and its apex clear of vital structures. In addition, the platform should be aligned for correct emergence profile (< 25°) without compromising the occlusion

Key points

- Implant treatment planning involves meticulous assessment and diagnostic tests.
- Implant placement is prosthetically driven.
- Risk assessment is essential for realistic treatment outcomes and expectations.

69 Implants: augmentation and site preparation

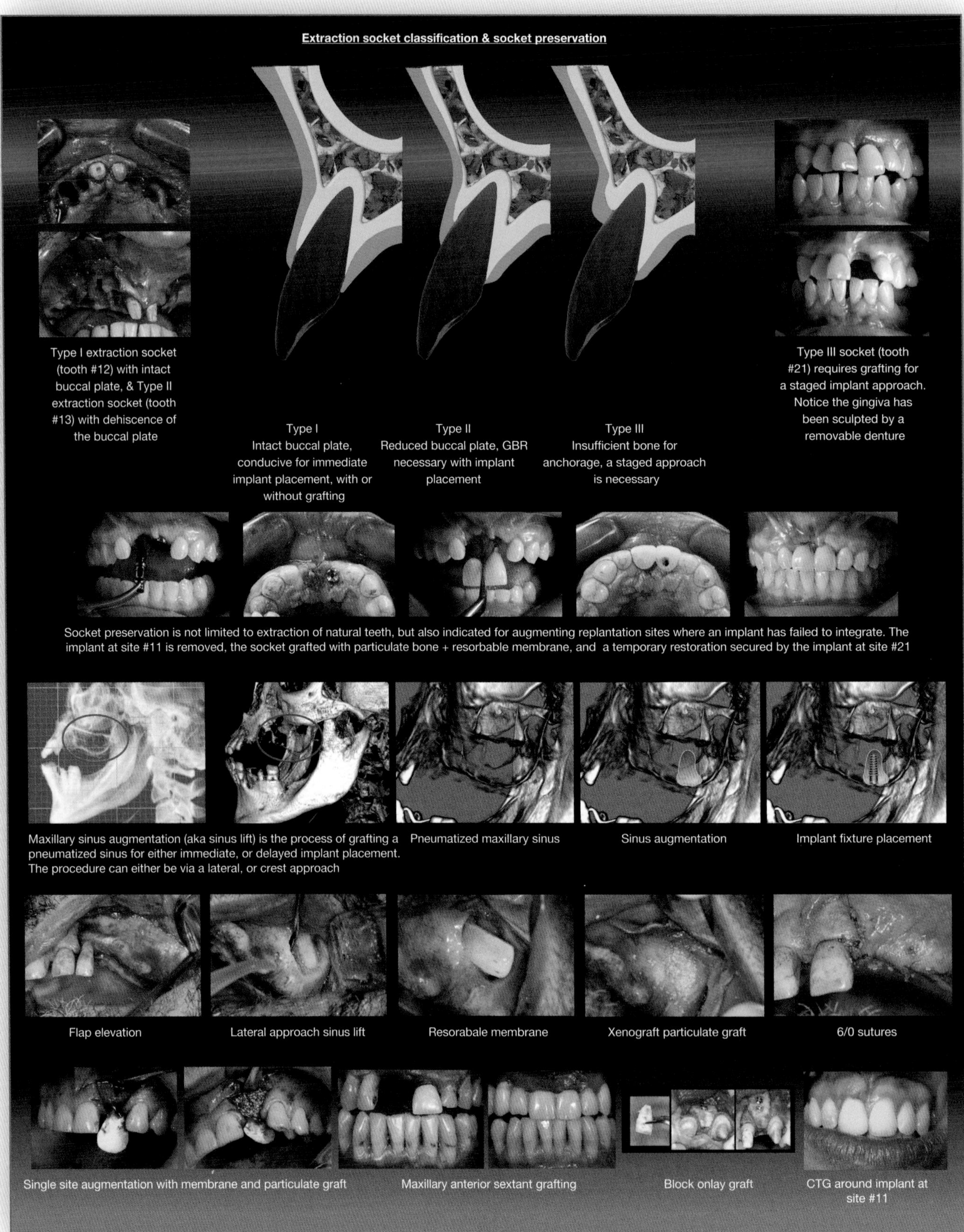

Prosthodontics at a Glance, Second Edition. Irfan Ahmad.

A CBCT scan or surgical guide of a **prosthetically driven treatment plan (PDTP)** will elucidate whether augmentation is required for ideal implant positioning for existing bone and/or soft tissue deficiencies. The **bone volume** required for standard implants is a minimum **10 mm height** with a **1.5 to 2 mm circumferential collar**.

Ridge and socket defects

Many criteria have been proposed for classifying ridge defects, for example, the **Siebert ridge deficiencies**, and systems based on **tooth extraction sockets**. Ridge defects range from a pristine ridge with no resorption, requiring no augmentation, to extensive bone loss such as atrophic ridges presenting with labial concavities and knife-edge morphologies.

Principles of GTR and GBR

Guided tissue regeneration (GTR) is **exclusion of connective and epithelial tissues** to create space for cells of the periodontal ligament to colonise the root surface. Therefore, in **GTR five components are involved:** epithelium, connective tissue, periodontal ligament cells, cementum and bone. With **guided bone regeneration (GBR),** only **two components are involved**: the connective tissue and bone. In GBR, the competing, non-osteogenic connective tissue is excluded, and a space created to encourage bone formation.

Bone-grafting materials

Bone-grafting materials offer structural stability and space to promote of osteogenesis. The mode of action can either be **osteoconductive**, acting as a scaffold for new bone regeneration, or **osteoinductive**, i.e. actively stimulating osteoblasts to form new bone. Graft materials can be used in combination to gain advantages of different materials. Examples of bone grafts include:

- **Autogenous grafts** – **osteoinductive** and nonimmunogenic, **harvested from the patient's body**, either intra-oral sites, e.g. ramus of the mandible, mandibular symphysis, nasal spine, maxillary tuberosity, zygoma or extra-oral sites, e.g. iliac crest, hip marrow, ribs, cranium and tibial metaphyses. The graft can be blocks or bone scrapings, including those from the osteotomy for implant placement
- **Allografts** – **bone grafts from another individual,** which are freeze-dried, demineralised and irradiated to prevent disease transmission. This avoids morbidity of a donor site, but the graft is less efficacious compared to an autogenous graft
- **Alloplasts** – **osteoconductive**, derived from **inorganic sources** such as synthetic calcium hydroxyapatite, calcium carbonate, tricalcium phosphate, alkaline phosphate and bioactive glass, and are absorbable or non-absorbable, acting as biocompatible fillers without the potential for disease transmission
- **Xenografts** – cancellous bone **from another species** such as bovine or porcine that are deproteinised to eliminate the chances of disease transmission, and are available as particulate granules, blocks and collagen plugs. Xenografts are **osteoconductive**, and abundant quantities obviate surgical preparation of donor site(s)
- **Barrier membranes** – usually used in conjunction with particulate grafting materials for providing space and covering graft materials. Membranes can be **resorbable** (e.g. collagen matrix, polyglycolactic membrane or Vicryl) or **non-resorbable** (e.g. expanded poly tetrafluorethylene or e-PTFE and titanium reinforced), which require a second surgical stage for removal
- **Platelet-rich plasma (PRP)** – accelerates the body's natural postsurgical wound healing by two to three times. PRP is a platelet concentrate from the patient's own blood, containing growth factors such as **platelet-derived growth factor and transforming growth factor beta**
- **Tissue engineering** (Chapter 74) – the latest and promising method for tissue regeneration by using **self-polymerising scaffold structures** placed in extraction or surgically prepared sites

Bone-grafting techniques

The techniques available include:

- **Onlay block and veneer bone grafts** – utilise autogenous bone blocks that are stabilised with screw fixation onto the residual bone. Veneer grafts are indicated for knife-edge ridges and are more predictable than block grafts
- **Particulate bone grafting** – the most popular method using a variety of grafting materials, which can be mixed together, and covered with membranes, or for extensive augmentation with customised titanium meshes. Indications include horizontal, small vertical defects, socket preservation, sinus lifts and simultaneous grafting with implant placement
- **Socket preservation** – immediately following tooth extraction for maintaining space and preventing ridge collapse with the Bio-Col technique, using particulate bone and collagen plugs
- **Sinus floor augmentation (sinus lift)** – indicated for the posterior maxilla for gaining bone volume by **lifting the Schneiderian membrane** and grafting the floor of the maxillary sinuses. **Two techniques** are advocated, depending on the amount of residual bone thickness. For **<5 mm vertical bone thickness, the lateral wall approach** is preferred, with or without simultaneous implant placement. If the **bone thickness is 7–8 mm, the osteotome or closed technique** is less aggressive, via a crestal approach
- **Bone expansion** – by decorticalisation (split-ridge technique) with simultaneous implant placement in combination with various types of bone grafts

Other method for increasing bone volume are **orthodontic extrusion** of teeth destined for extraction and 'gaining' bone by moving the entire dentogingival complex in a coronal direction, or placing fixture devices that are periodically adjusted by the principle of **distraction osteogenesis**. Also, **lateral repositioning of neurovascular bundles**, e.g. mental and inferior dental nerves, to avoid impinging on implant fixtures. However, these procedures can potentially cause paraesthesia and partial or complete anaesthesia.

Soft tissue grafting

Reconstructive **periodontal plastic surgery** is used to compensate or pre-empt gingival recession (especially with thin periodontal biotypes). The methods include **palatal roll, free gingival graft (FGG), connective tissue grafts (CTG) and vascularised interposition periosteal connective tissue (VIP-CT)**. The most popular approach is the CTG from the palate, anterior to first molars or the tuberosities, in combination with coronally advanced flaps. **Membranes and silk-gel scaffolds** are a substitute for CTG, avoiding donor site surgery. Soft tissue grafting is more predictable when underlying bone support is present to support the gingival architecture.

Key points

- Augmentation is required for achieving functional and aesthetic implant positioning.
- Most grafting materials are osteoconductive, acting as scaffolds for new bone formation.
- Both hard and soft tissue grafting may be necessary for augmenting deficient sites.

Implants: surgical techniques

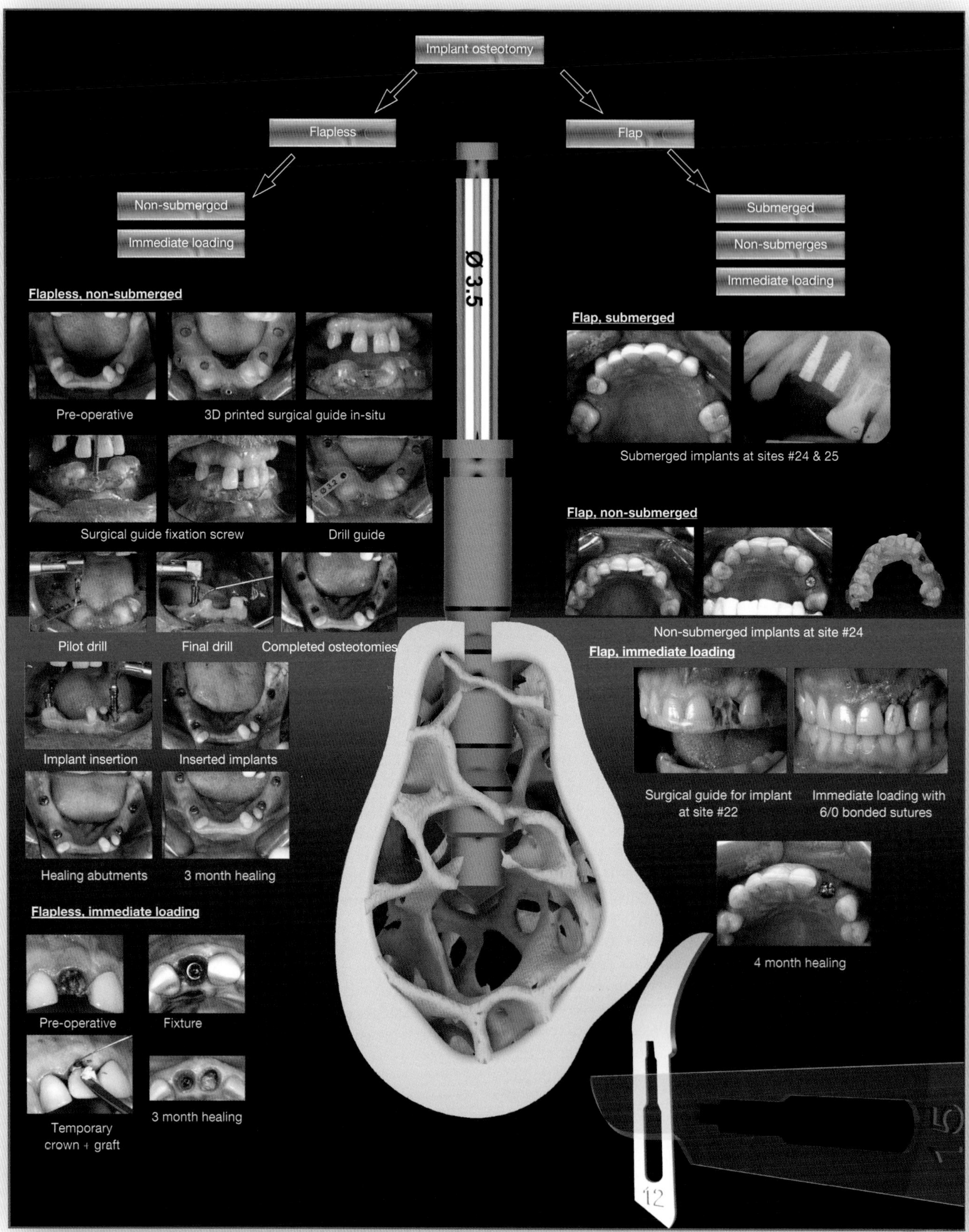

Implant osteotomy

Flapless

Flap

Non-submerged

Immediate loading

Submerged

Non-submerges

Immediate loading

Ø 3.5

Flapless, non-submerged

Pre-operative

3D printed surgical guide in-situ

Surgical guide fixation screw

Drill guide

Pilot drill

Final drill

Completed osteotomies

Implant insertion

Inserted implants

Healing abutments

3 month healing

Flapless, immediate loading

Pre-operative

Fixture

Temporary crown + graft

3 month healing

Flap, submerged

Submerged implants at sites #24 & 25

Flap, non-submerged

Non-submerged implants at site #24

Flap, immediate loading

Surgical guide for implant at site #22

Immediate loading with 6/0 bonded sutures

4 month healing

12

Surgical techniques have evolved considerably since the Brånemark protocol of distinct surgical and prosthetic phases for the delayed approach for implant rehabilitation. Most surgical approaches use a prefabricated **surgical guide, with prior CBCT assessment**. The surgical stage involves a **flap** or **flapless** preparation of an **osteotomy**. Implants are then inserted by **pre-taping** or **self-tapping** into the prepared site. The **location of the implant platform** can be **supra-crestal**, **equi-crestal** or **sub-crestal**, and either **submerged** by covering with soft tissue, **non-submerged** with a **transmucosal healing abutment**, or **immediately restored** with a provisional restoration.

Flap design

A flap should be conservative, but allow adequate access to determine morphology, size and trajectory of the alveolar bone ridge. Several designs are advocated depending on clinical manifestations and include:

- **Full thickness mucoperiosteal** buccal, lingual or crestal incision flaps, with or without vertical releasing incisions, avoiding interproximal papillae if adjacent teeth are present. These flaps are ideal for gaining access, simultaneous bone grafting and osseous contouring
- **Mini-flaps** are restricted to the area of implantation, e.g. a small buccal flap for single tooth replacement or a palatal peninsular flap to avoid buccal incisions and the ensuing scarring in aesthetically sensitive maxillary anterior regions
- **Tissue punch** – for exposing underlying bone for 'flapless' surgery. This method is ideal for broad flat ridges, with adequate attached gingiva, not requiring osseous contouring or hard or soft tissue augmentation

Flapless design

The **flapless method is the least invasive surgical protocol**, but is essentially a **blind surgical procedure**. The prerequisites are adequate bone volume and attached gingiva. A **surgical guide** accurately guides the implant to the predesignated position without needing to raise a flap. The **fixture head is non-submerged** and a transmucosal **healing cap** is placed to **sculpt the soft tissue** and allow maturation. The negative aspect of this protocol is lack of visualisation of the bone architecture, particularly if a prior CBCT scan has not been performed. Therefore, the procedure is potentially fraught with the risk of inadvertent perforations, especially of thin buccal maxillary plates leading to fenestrations and implant thread exposure. Particular care is necessary to avoid lingual perforation of the cortical plate in the anterior mandible that may cause haemorrhage at the floor of the mouth and compromise respiration.

Two-stage – submerged

The **two-stage or submerged delayed approach** was originally proposed for **stress-free integration of oral implants**. It consists of submerging the implant to allow healing for 3–6 months (average three months for mandible, six months for maxilla). Afterwards, the implant is surgically exposed, the cover screw removed and the implant prosthetically restored. This method is preferable if primary stability is unattainable, or if extensive pre-surgical or concurrent bone grafting is required.

One-stage – non-submerged

For the **one-stage, non-submerged approach** the cover screw or transmucosal healing cap (abutment) on the implant is exposed to the oral cavity during osseointegration. After a suitable healing period, the cover or abutment is removed and the implant restored without needing a second surgical procedure. Furthermore, the clinical success rate for the one-stage procedure is equally effective and predictable as the two-stage approach. Also, a single-stage procedure permits early loading, is patient friendly, reduces post-operative discomfort and is more economical. However, certain criteria must be met, e.g. minimum or no preliminary augmentations required, **greater than 30 N cm primary stability**, an adequate **circumferential zone of keratinised gingival tissue** and **adequate oral hygiene** to prevent and manage peri-implantitis and peri-implant mucositis. Peri-implantitis is defined as inflammation around an implant causing marginal bone loss, while peri-implant mucositis (precursor to peri-implantitis) is a reversible inflammatory condition without accompanying bone loss.

Post-extraction placement

Another method for **implant insertion is immediately following tooth extraction,** which can be **immediate** at time of extraction, **delayed immediate** (2–3 weeks later) or **delayed conventional** (3+ months later). Initial research findings regarding immediate placement and concurrent particulate bone grafting are promising, but long-term trials are required to establish the efficacy of this protocol.

Immediate loading

Immediate loading is placing a temporary restoration at time of fixture placement, or **early loading (1–12 weeks)** to expedite the prosthetic rehabilitation phase. After placing the implant(s), a fixed provisional restoration(s) is/are immediately fitted. Immediate loading has also been proposed for **immediate post-extraction implant placement in order to reduce treatment times,** and avoid temporary prostheses (fixed or removable) during the integration stage. The technique is extremely sensitive, and preoperative assessment is essential for success. Current research confirms good short- and medium-term survival rates compared to delayed loading (> 3 months), but long-term data are unavailable. Most of the literature reports case studies, (rather than randomised clinical trials [RCT]), carried out by experienced surgeons under stringent clinical situations on a limited number of patients. The few completed RCTs are inconclusive concerning peri-implant or marginal bone height loss. The **prerequisites for immediate loading** are:

- **Absence of acute infection or active suppuration**
- **Adequate vascularisation** of the site, which precludes sites with previous surgical traumas (e.g. apicectomies) or longstanding chronic infection
- **Good bone quality** (density), preferably D1 or D2, e.g. in the mandible
- **Primary stability >30 N cm, without micro-motion (< 50–150 μm)** at time of placement
- **Occlusal loading** is a contentious issue and some authorities distinguish between immediate provisionalisation and immediate loading. However, it is prudent to avoid undue occlusal stresses during healing, especially in lateral excursions, and in patients with a history of bruxism

Key points

- Implant placement involves a surgical osteotomy with or without flap elevation.
- Surgical protocols include two-stage submerged, one-stage non-submerged and immediate post-extraction placement.
- Immediate loading expedites the implant prosthetic phase.

71 Implants: types, configuration and design

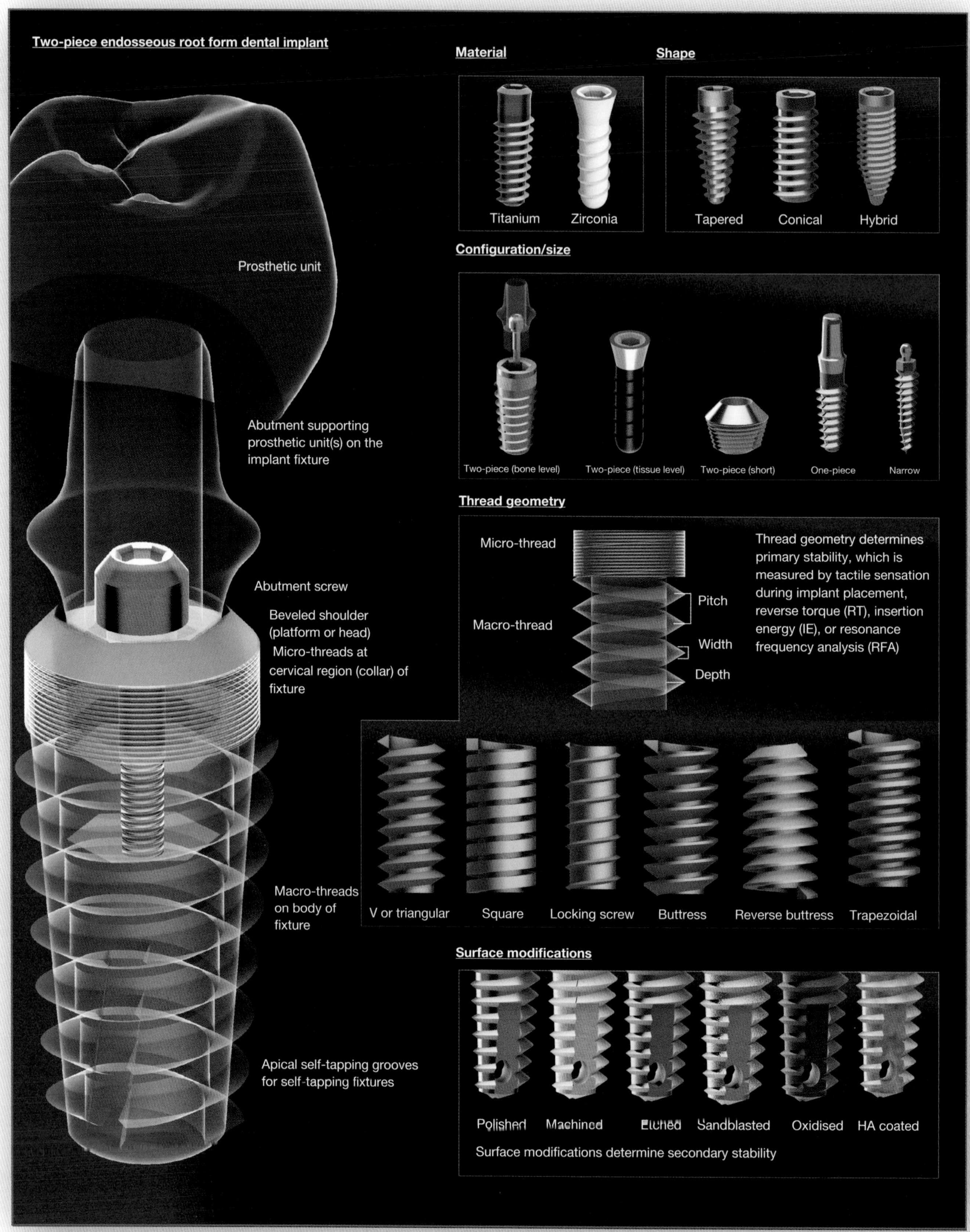

Two-piece endosseous root form dental implant

Prosthetic unit

Abutment supporting prosthetic unit(s) on the implant fixture

Abutment screw

Beveled shoulder (platform or head)

Micro-threads at cervical region (collar) of fixture

Macro-threads on body of fixture

Apical self-tapping grooves for self-tapping fixtures

Material

Titanium Zirconia

Shape

Tapered Conical Hybrid

Configuration/size

Two-piece (bone level) Two-piece (tissue level) Two-piece (short) One-piece Narrow

Thread geometry

Micro-thread

Macro-thread

Pitch

Width

Depth

Thread geometry determines primary stability, which is measured by tactile sensation during implant placement, reverse torque (RT), insertion energy (IE), or resonance frequency analysis (RFA)

V or triangular Square Locking screw Buttress Reverse buttress Trapezoidal

Surface modifications

Polished Machined Etched Sandblasted Oxidised HA coated

Surface modifications determine secondary stability

Prosthodontics at a Glance, Second Edition. Irfan Ahmad.

The aim of any implant design is to **maximise bone apposition** at the **implant–bone interface for osseointegration**.

Types of dental implants

A dental implant provides support or anchorage for an intra-oral prosthesis. The basic types of dental implants are:

- **Subperiosteal** – **placed onto the bone**, custom-made CAD/CAM titanium framework for extensively resorbed alveolar ridges
- **Transosseous** – **placed through bone**, usually in the mandible, but due to the extensive surgical protocol, their use today is almost redundant
- **Endosseous (endosteal)** – **placed into bone**:
  - Plate or blade form – thin cross-section metal pieces, 65% narrower than root form implants, indicated for narrow ridges not amenable to bone grafting
  - Ramus frame – long metal plates inserted into a resorbed mandible from the chin to ramus
  - Zygomatic – for severely resorbed maxillae
  - Basal (lateral) implants placed via a palatal approach in the maxilla
- **Root form** – mimicking the morphology of natural tooth roots, which can be **pre-taping** (screws prepared into osteotomy by a tap drill) or **self-taping.** Virtually all contemporary dental implants are endosseous root form, and the discussion below is therefore limited to these varieties

Configuration

Root form implants are mechanical modular devices with the following **configurations**:

- **Two-piece implants** – consisting of a separate fixture and abutment
- **One-piece implants** – the fixture and abutment components are incorporated into one piece
- **Mini-implants or small diameter implants** (SDIs) – diameters <3 mm for implant retaining overdentures (IRO), transitional implants for supporting provisional prostheses awaiting integration of larger diameter implants and temporary anchorage devices (TADs) for orthodontic therapy
- **Short length implants** (< 10 mm) for less than optimal bone height, such as the posterior maxilla and obviate the need for sinus augmentation

Materials

The material from which a dental implant is manufactured must be **biocompatible, promote osseointegration** and be **biofunctional** to resist oral forces (ranging from 200 N to >2000 N). The materials that meet these objectives are **commercially pure titanium (cpTi)** categorised into **grades 1–4** or **Ti-6Al-4V.** Ti spontaneously forms the **biocompatible TiO_2** surface when exposed to the atmosphere. Other materials are **yttrium-stabilized tetragonal zirconia polycrystalline ceramics** (Ceralog) and **titanium-zirconia alloy (TiZr1317).**

Geometry

Geometry refers to **macromorphology** or shape, i.e. 3D profile of the implant and is responsible for **primary stability**, which is prerequisite for osseointegration to discourage fibrous tissue formation and avoid failure due to the **stability dip phenomenon.** Primary stability depends on **bone quality, surgical technique** and **implant design** (length and platform diameter), **surface area, shape** and **thread geometry.**

Tapered implants are better adapted for immediate post-extraction placement by compressing soft bone for primary stability. The function of threads is to increase surface area and **translate tensile forces to compressive components** to favour bone preservation. The ideal **thread parameters** depend on the **type of thread**, e.g. the optimal pitch for a triangular and trapezoidal-thread shapes are 1.2 mm and 1.6 mm, respectively. Many implants incorporate **micro-threads** at the neck and **macro-threads** on the body. Finite element analysis (FEA) reveals that **the neck (cervical part) of an implant has the highest bone stresses,** causing **marginal bone remodelling (MBR)**, predominantly in the first year of loading. Similar to a natural tooth, an area above the crestal bone of an implant is necessary to form a biological width. Therefore, some designs have a polished collar at the neck to allow epithelial and connective tissue attachments, while others opt for a rough neck to reduce disuse atrophy and retain greater marginal bone.

Surface modifications

Micromorphology and **nanomorphhology** modifications determine **secondary stability** and enhance and expedite **'secondary' osseointegration by contact and distant osteogenesis.** Surface modification include:

- **Polished or machined** surface (Sa: < 0.5 µm), originally proposed by Brånemark, attract epithelial cells and fibroblasts that results in reduced bone-implant contact compared to roughened surfaces that promote osteoblastic proliferation
- **Subtractive**:
  - **Macro-modifications** (Sa: > 100 µm), e.g. pores or diffusion-bonded microspheres, and sintered porous surface for bone ingrowth
  - **Micro-modifications** (Sa: < 10 µm) to enhance interlocking of bone at a microscopic level, e.g. roughening by large-grit sandblasting (250–500 µm particles) followed by acid etching with hydrochloric, sulphuric or nitric acids (SLActive), anodic oxidisation (TiUnite), superhydrophilic conversion of Ti surface (UV photofunctionalisation), laser ablation to create to nanochannels at the cervical (collar) region of the fixture (Laser-Lok) or a combination of these processes
  - **Nano-modifications** (Sa: 1–100nm) – anodic oxidation to create TiO_2 nanotube arrays that are osteogenic, antibacterial and allow sustained drug release. However, delamination of the **nanotubular surface** has hindered this process for dental implants pending further research
- **Additive**:
  - **Surface enhancement/coatings** – bioactive coatings such as **plasma spray** to deposit hydroxyapatite [HA] (MicroVent), core functional peptides that allow adhesion of osteogenic cells, bioglass, fluoride-modified surfaces by electrochemical etching to encourage calcium and phosphate deposition (Osseospeed). Osteoattraction factors for promoting healing, e.g. human recombinant bone morphogenic protein-2 (rhBMP-2)
  - **Antibacterial coatings on the internals fixture surfaces**
  - (for internal connection implants)

Key points

- Most dental implants are endosseous root form to support prosthetic units.
- The geometry of an implant determines primary stability, while surface modifications determine secondary stability.

72 Implants: abutments

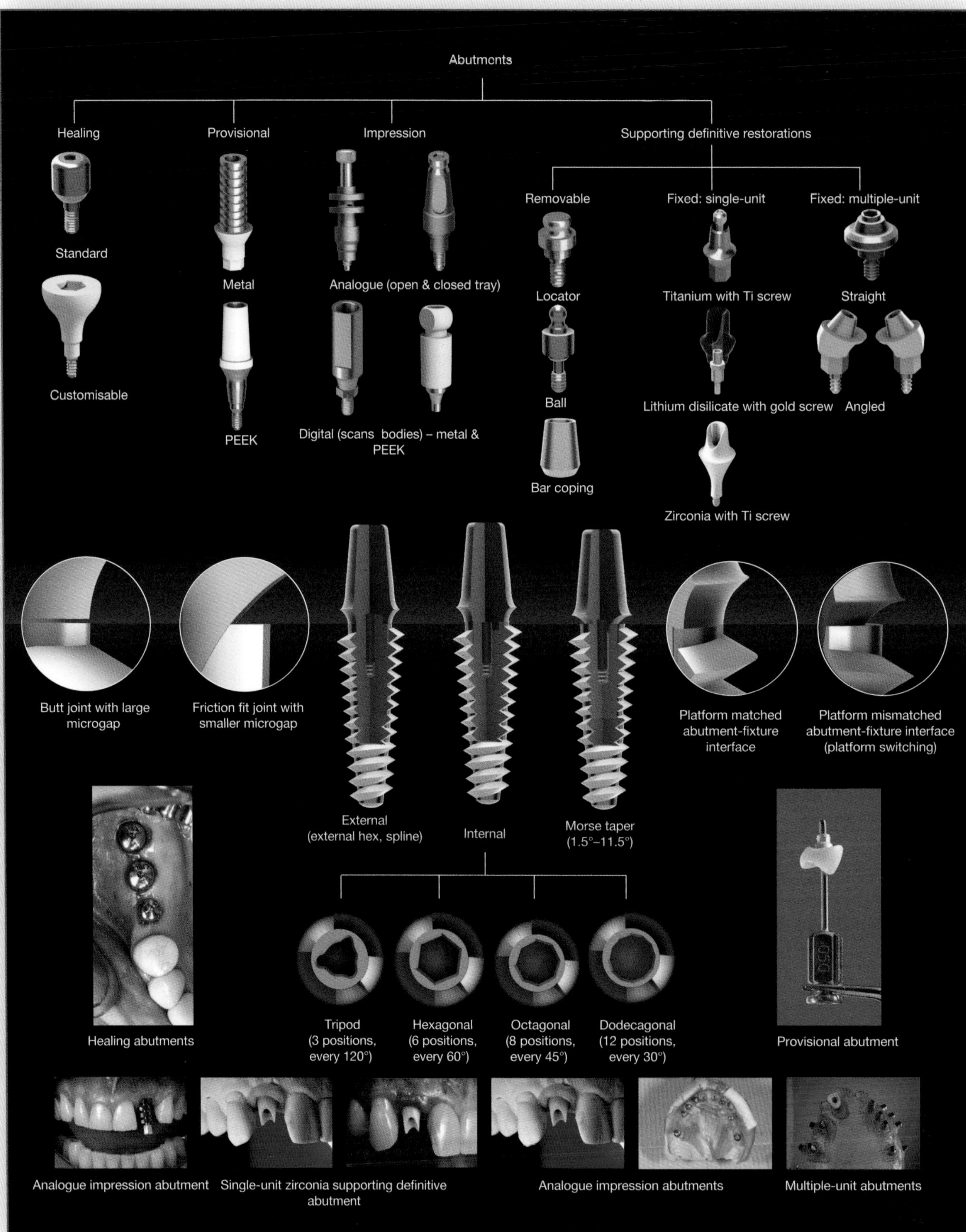

An **abutment simply links the implant fixture for a variety of purposes** including **healing**, **temporisation**, **impressions** and **supporting the definitive prosthesis** or restoration (directly or via a superstructure). There is no accepted taxonomy for dental implant abutments, which can be classified according to purpose, type of connection, anti-rotational features, engaging or non-engaging, material of manufacture, method of manufacture to name a few.

Connections

An **abutment-fixture connection or interface** should offer optimal mechanical stability, strength, fatigue resistance, anti-rotation, prevent microleakage, avoid screw loosening and provide a 'hermetic' seal with a minimum **microgap**. The connection can be a **butt-joint/slip joint (passive joint), friction fit (active joint)** or **no interface (one-piece implant)**. The butt-joint/slip joint can either be an **external or internal connection** with a relatively large microgap. Alternately, a friction fit-tapered internal connection has a smaller microgap. Abutments connect to the fixture by a **screw**, or are **screwless** relying purely on friction. Furthermore, many designs incorporate more than one type of interface along the abutment-implant connection. The broad clarification of connections are:

- **External connection**, e.g. external hexagon (hex), which was used by Brånemark for screwing a metal superstructure for supporting a prosthesis. However, due to its small external height of 0.7 mm, this connection is incapable of withstanding intra-oral forces of individual crowns, and is better suited for connecting multiple implants
- **Internal connection** – available in a variety of seating depths into fixtures (1.2–4 mm), configurations and angles for anti-rotational properties
- **Conical interface**, e.g. the **Morse taper** that relies on friction fit to achieve **cold welding**. The screw used in a Morse taper abutment is for locating the abutment to the fixture rather than retention. The original Morse taper had an angle of 2°, but the angle of the Morse taper-like connections of dental implants ranges from 1.5° to 11.5°; **the smaller the angle the higher the stability**. In addition, the length of contact into the fixture influences the degree of micromovements and contamination

Currently, **no interface prevents bacterial or endotoxin penetration into the microgap,** but a butt-joint is a potential risk for peri-implantitis. Even a precision fit **microgap of 10µm** does not prevent invasion of gram negative endotoxins measuring 1–2 µm. **Platform switching** has been proposed to minimise the routinely observed **1.5–2 mm bone resorption at the neck of diameter matched abutment-fixture** configurations. The concept is to use smaller diameter abutments than the implant fixture head to **shift the microgap either in the coronal (vertical shift) or mesial (horizontal shift)** directions to encourage a soft tissue biologic width and discourage bacterial colonisation.

Materials

Implant abutments are fabricated from various materials including **plastic (e.g. PEEK), cast gold, titanium and ceramics (e.g. alumina, lithium dilsilicate, zirconia).** PEEK can be 3D printed or milled, and is ideal for provisional restoration abutments and **scan bodies for digital implant impressions.** Bespoke cast gold abutments were popular, but in recent years have been superseded by CAD/CAM customised varieties. Titanium is unsuitable for aesthetic-sensitive regions, and especially if definitive all-ceramic restorations are planned. Furthermore, titanium is a thermal conductor and, if exposed at the periphery, may cause **marginal bone necrosis** in patients who have a habit of ingesting hot drinks. Alumina has the propensity to fracture during preparation and shaping due to relatively poor strength compared to zirconia. **Ingots of zirconia and lithium disilicate** are available in different shades and translucencies to facilitate colour matching with the surrounding dentition and used **for CAD/CAM manufacturing.** In addition, various materials are used as **mono-block abutment/restoration screw-retained** single and multiple unit for temporary as well as definitive prostheses. There is a belief that transmucosal epithelial attachment on abutments is only possible with titanium, alumina or zirconia but not with silica ceramics or cast gold. However, **epithelium will adhere to any clean and smooth surface, irrespective of the restorative material.**

Supporting abutments

A **supporting (definitive) abutment provides retention for the permanent restoration**, and the choice is dictated by the type of prosthesis (temporary or permanent, fixed or removable), tissue collar height, implant angulation, interproximal space, location in the mouth, strength for resisting both external (functional and parafunctional) and internal (preload) forces and aesthetics. The configuration of abutments are as follows:

- **Three component** – individual implant, abutment and prosthetic unit(s). A separate abutment is connected onto the implant fixture with either a retaining screw (usually at a torque of 20 N cm), locking taper or cement, and the definite restoration cemented onto the abutment, e.g. **cement retained** crown or FPD. To **prevent abutment screw loosening,** some screws are gold-plated for improved retention by creating a bond equivalent to a 'cold weld'. This is the most popular and universal system, offering versatility for **abutment angulations** and numerous materials to suit different purposes
- **Two-component** – either **implant, abutments + prosthetic unit as one entity**, e.g. a screw-retained crown, or **implant + abutment as one entity** (one-piece implant) and a separate prosthetic unit

Supporting abutments are available as:

- **Prefabricated** or stock abutments in different shapes, heights and predefined angles (10–35°) to accommodate varying interocclusal clearance and implant angulation. They can be further modified chairside or in the laboratory, to compensate for implant misalignment and/or achieve ideally emergence profiles
- **Customised castable**, e.g. **UCLA** (University of California Los Angeles) abutments that offer flexibility to compensate for misaligned implant fixtures by altering abutment angle, taper, finish line and width according to the position and emergence profile of the definitive restoration
- **Customised CAD/CAM** – The latest method is using CAD/CAM technology (e.g. NobelProcera, BellaTek Encode, Straumann CARES, Atlantis) for designing, milling or 3D printing, to produce abutments with individual parameters according to clinical needs

Key points

- Implant abutments provide a connection with the implant fixture, which can be external or internal (including conical interface).
- Abutments have several purposes during implant therapy.
- Abutments are fabricated from plastic, cast metal or ceramics.
- Customised, CAD/CAM abutments offer state-of-the art technology for bespoke designing and fabrication.

73 Implants: restorative options

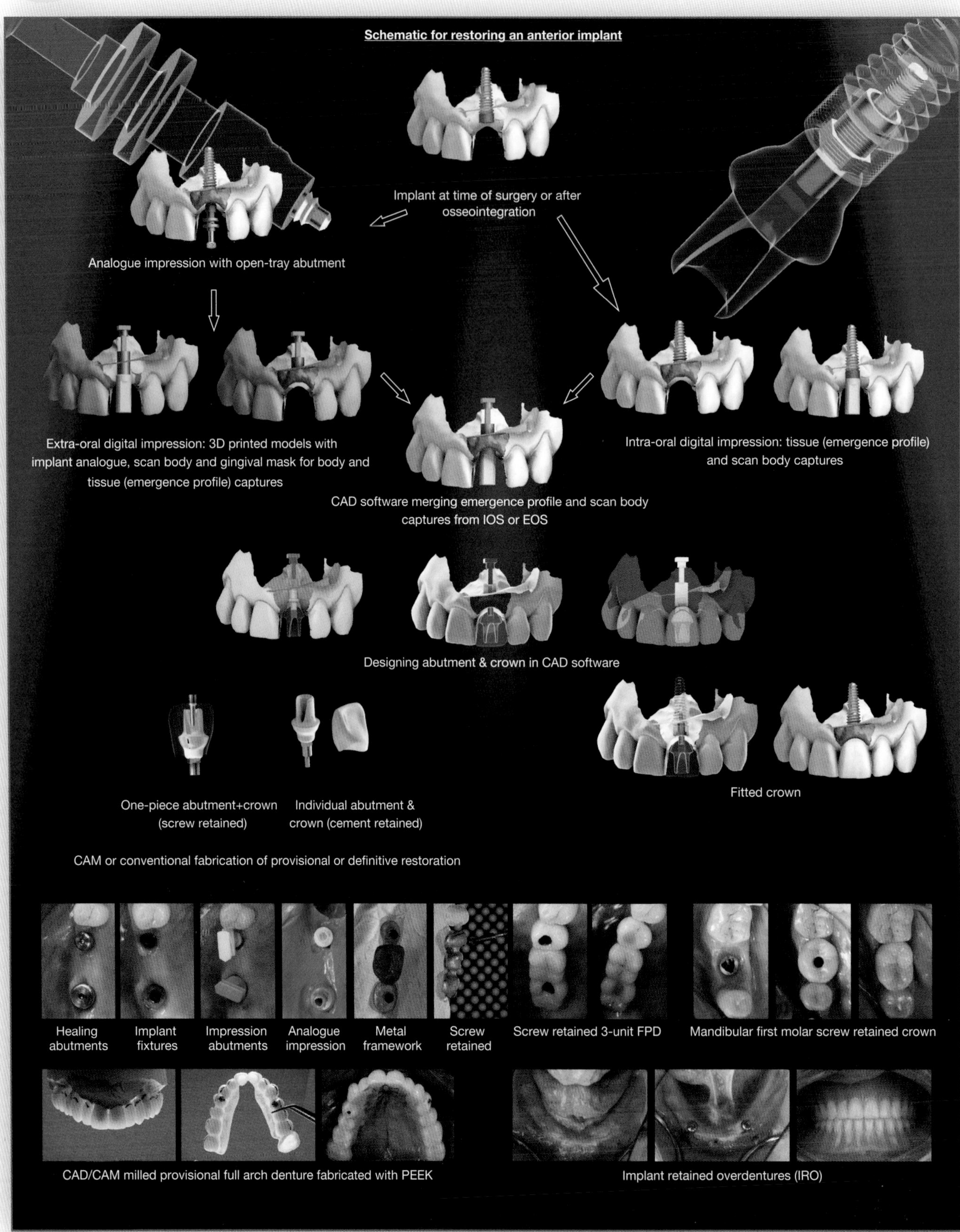

The final stage of implant rehabilitation is **transferring the intra-oral data to the dental laboratory** for the fabrication of the definitive restoration/prosthesis. The restorative permutations for implants are immense and ever expanding, ranging from a single-unit crown to complex full-arch rehabilitation with either fixed or removable prostheses, including linking implants with natural tooth abutments. The decision of the definitive restoration(s) is decided at the treatment planning stage and determines the type, number and positioning of the fixtures and abutments for supporting the final restoration(s), with or without an intervening superstructure (bar or framework).

Transferring data

The **intra-oral data include the number, location, size and angulation of implants together with surrounding soft tissues and the adjacent and opposing dentition**. This can be accomplished with an **analogue, digital or combined approach**. The **analogue method** involves taking an impression using **open or closed tray impression abutments** (copings) seated onto the fixture, pouring or 3D printing a model using the corresponding **implant analogues** in preparation for designing and fabricating the abutment(s) and restoration(s) by conventional waxing, investing and casting.

The **digital approach** involves using a **scan body** (implant-positioning-transfer abutment), either **intra-orally** torqued to the implant at 10–15 N cm, or **extra-orally** located onto implant analogues in a model. **Two scans are necessary, one with the scan body,** and the **second without the scan body (emergence profile scan) to capture the tissues profile** around the fixture (intra-oral scan) or a gingival mask (extra-oral scan). The **scanner software** uses algorithms to **merge the two scans** and **calculates the orientation axis and angle of the implant fixture,** as well as the **emergence profile**. An example of a combined analogue–digital approach is taking an analogue impression, creating a stone or 3D printed model and using an extra-oral scanner (EOS) to digitise the model with scan bodies and gingival mask. For all methods, either a provisional or permanent restoration can be fabricated as individual abutment(s) with a separate prosthetic unit **cemented onto the supporting abutment(s)**. Alternately, the abutment and prosthetic unit(s) can be produced as a single entity and seated onto the implant fixture (**screw retained**).

Fixed screw-retained

Screw-retained restorations are indicated for both single crowns and FPDs. The **abutment and crown (or FPD) is combined into a single prosthetic component**, avoiding different material interfaces with increased strength and stability, and eliminating cement remnants. The **major benefit is retrievability and accessibility**, especially for multi-unit reconstructions, without damaging the prosthetic units. Also, if occlusal clearance allows, a screw-retained restoration provides superior long-term retention compared to a cemented restoration. The **drawbacks of screw-retained** units are:

- **Implant head requires vertical orientation**, for anterior restorations the screw location should be in line with the incisal edge, and for posterior units towards the central fossa. However, **angled screw access abutments** are available to compensate for less than ideal implant angulations
- **Poor aesthetics** if screw hole is incorrectly positioned, or requires masking with an opaquer
- **Microgap** between the crown and fixture is apical to the gingival crest, predisposing to chronic gingival inflammation

Fixed cement-retained

Cement-retained restorations are also possible for single crowns or multiple-unit FPDs. First, the abutment is screwed or tapped onto the implant fixture, and second, the final restoration is subsequently cemented onto the supporting abutment. **Cement-retained restorations are recommended for:**

- **Single anterior crowns for optimal aesthetics**, especially all-ceramic units that can be adhesively bonded to an underlying ceramic abutment (e.g. zirconia) with self-adhesive resin cements
- **Severely misaligned implants** to compensate for poor emergence profile
- **Facially located screw access** holes compromising aesthetics
- **Screw access and sealing fillings interfering with occlusal stability**
- **Thin biotypes** predisposed to gingival recession
- **Limited interocclusal clearance for accessing screw hole(s)**
- **Narrow-diameter crowns with inadequate width for placing screws**

A **major problem with cement-retained restorations is gaining access to the abutment-retaining screw** if **screw loosening** is suspected, which may require **damaging the definitive restoration,** particularly for cemented multiple-unit FPDs. Another concern is **deep subgingival margins (>3 mm), making cement removal difficult.** To conclude, the **choice between a screw-retained or cemented restoration is empirical,** depending on the clinician's experience and preference, and prevailing clinical scenario. Research shows little difference between the two types of restorations with regard to peri-implant inflammation, marginal bone loss or implant survival or success rates.

Implant-retained overdentures (IRO)

Fixed implant-supported prostheses necessitating multiple implants may be contraindicated for several reasons including extensive bone grafting, anatomical obstacles, occlusal problems, elderly or infirm patients not able to tolerate protracted treatment sessions or fiscal constraints. In these circumstances, removable **IRO** provide improved retention, stability, aesthetics, phonetics and mastication. **IROs can either be entirely implant-supported, or a combination of mucosa-supported and implant-supported.** A few strategically placed implants support an overdenture with a ball abutment with O-rings, magnetic or locator abutments or a bar-superstructure retainer with corresponding female matrices on the fitting surface of the prosthesis. Bar retainers are particularly useful for non-parallel implants. For the **edentulous mandible**, usually two or four implants are placed in the interforaminal region, while for the **edentulous maxilla**, two or four implants in the canine and second premolar regions support a retentive bar attachment. Furthermore, if **conventional-diameter implants (> 3 mm)** are not feasible due to inadequate bone volume, **small-diameter implants** (SDIs) or **'mini-implants' (1.8–2.9 mm)** provide a conservative, minimally invasive alternative.

Key points

- Transferring intra-oral data requires taking an analogue or digital impressions for fabricating the abutment and restoration/prosthesis.
- Fixed single- or multiple-unit prostheses can either be cement-retained or screw-retained.
- Implant-retained overdentures provide an alternative to fixed units, especially using mini-implants.

Regenerative medicine

Section 18

Chapters

74 Tissue engineering

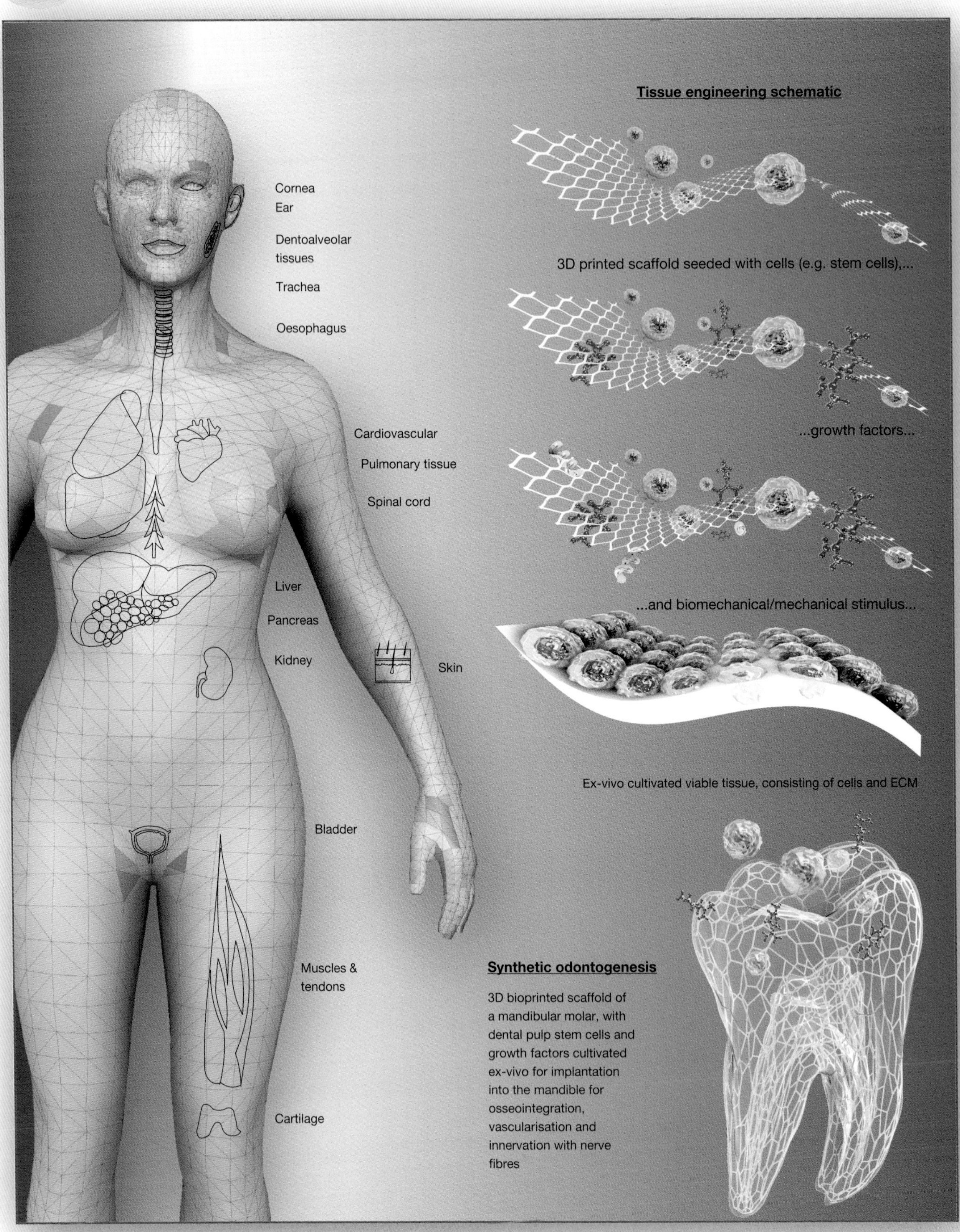

Prosthodontics at a Glance, Second Edition. Irfan Ahmad.

This chapter of the **Regenerative Medicine (RM)** section discusses **tissue engineering (TE)**, while the next chapter concentrates on **stem cells**.

Ambiguous TERM

TE is a narrow branch of RM, a type of **translation medicine** that delivers laboratory research to clinical practice for the benefit of patients. The **end goals of TE and RM are identical**, i.e. repair, restore [function] or improve damaged tissues or organs, but the methods used to achieved these objectives are different. **RM is a broader field incorporating cell-based therapy (e.g. stem cells), cellular gene therapy, pharmacology and immunomodulation *in vivo* or *ex vivo*,** while **TE is reliant on biomaterials, and limited to bioengineering artificial tissues or whole organs on a scaffold *ex vivo*.** However, there is considerable ambiguity and overlap of the terms TE and RM, and the concepts are often interchangeable and inseparable. For example, some authorities opine that **RM incorporates the concept of 'self-healing', i.e. maximising the body's innate ability to regenerate itself**, while the modus operandi of **TE is to create *de novo* tissues**. Conversely, with RM, the tissues are endogenously formed using various technologies. Therefore, TE and RM may either be considered as distinct fields, or combined as a single entity, represented by the acronym **TERM**.

Historical perspective

Although the term **'tissue engineering' was coined in 1987** following the seminal Harvard Mouse experiment, tissues-based therapies, predominately **skin grafts, can be traced back to India in 300 BCE.** In the 1930s, Alexis Carrel proposed **bioengineering organs *ex vivo*.** At the time, research was **cytocentric**, i.e. cells were regarded as the protagonist for TE, but later the paradigm shifted to emphasise that the **extracellular matrix (ECM)** plays an equally import role. The first TE skin allografts were introduced in the late 1970s/early 1980s, followed by **synthetic biodegradable polymers** in late 1980s. With the discovery of **stem cells** at the turn of this century, the term 'regenerative medicine' was born, and a bioartificial bladder and trachea engineered in 2006 and 2008, respectively.

Principles of TE

In nature, cells secrete an **ECM to form scaffolds** that organise cells into a tissue and eventually build organs. **For TE, the starting point is a scaffold** (mimicking the ECM) that is **infused with cells, growth factors and biomechanically stimulated to create a viable tissue.** The latter is then transplanted to **repair damaged tissues/organs**, synthetic **extracorporeal life-supporting units** (kidney dialysis or liver function) or **test new drugs and medical devices**.

Materials for **scaffolds are autologous, allogeneic, xenogeneic or synthetic. Scaffolds based on natural materials are the gold standard**, including collagen, fibrin and polysaccharide-based (e.g. hyaluronic acid). Also, autologous decellularised tissue avoids immunogenicity concerns. **Synthetic biomaterials** include resorbable collagen-based polylactic, polyglycolic (e.g. Poly(lactic-Co-Glycolic) Acid [PLGA]) or polycaprolactone (e.g. polyether ether ketone [PEEK], high-strength poly[*N*-acryloyl glycinamide] hydrogels), but the degradation process releases toxic acid that are harmful to cells. Another material is small **oligopeptides** that assemble into **nanofibres**, similar to natural ECM. **Methods of fabricating scaffolds include electrospinning, microfluidic, molecular self-assembly, thermally induced phase separation (TIPS) and 3D printing. 3D bioprinting** uses a bioink, consisting of polymers (e.g. nanocomposite hydrogel), cells and growth factors or decellularised ECM, to print scaffolds by a variety of 3D printing technologies such as stereolithographic, inkjet and microextrusion. The major **drawbacks are viability of the cells, and adequate vascularisation.** To overcome these issues, **stem cells are preferred since they can withstand the bioprinting process better than organs specific cells**, and **incorporating angiogenic growth factors** (VEGF, bFGF, PDGF) and endothelial cells generate a vascular network. The **organ-on-a-chip** is yet another ingenious method of combining 'smart hydrogels' and cells to 3D bioprint micro-organs for transplantation. The cells' source for TE is varied. Stem cells (SC) offer the advantage of high proliferation and differentiation into other types of cell lineage, e.g. **pluripotent embryo SC, induced pluripotent SC (iPSCs) from adults or multipotent mesenchymal SC (MSCs).** The **biochemical stimulus** for the scaffold/cell complex is from growth factors, e.g. bone morphogenetic proteins (BMPs), basic fibroblast growth factor (bFGF or FGF-2), transforming growth factor-β (TGF-β), plus chemokines and cytokines. Examples of **mechanical stimuli** are magnetic, electrical, cyclic loading, osmotic pressure, mechanosensitive ion channels, photobiomodulation or mechanosensors. Finally, to confer **antimicrobial, antioxidant and anti-inflammatory properties**, pharmacological agents are added, e.g. medicinal plant extracts (Curcumin longa L. and Mucuna gigantea), resveratrol, ethanol and dichloromethane, L-DOPA.

Challenges and opportunities

Without doubt, there is a tangible need for tissues and organ substitutes, and while **TE can potentially synthesise any tissue** of the body, it is in its infancy with many challenges. Although **academics and researches are enamoured by the TE vernacularism,** the reality is different. The initial promising success with relatively simple, avascular tissues cannot be translated to more complex ones, and incorporating these therapies in clinical practice has been slow. In addition, research funding has evaporated, as sponsors perceive this technology as complex, expensive and with a long gestation period before becoming commercially viable. Furthermore, clinical applications face legal, ethical and regulatory obstacles. However, there is renewed interest due to emerging microtechnologies such as **3D nanolithographic printing** (fabricating intricate scaffolds with a 0.1 μm micro-precision), and stem cells. Also, **precise regulation and sustained release of growth factors at crucial stages** to enhance cell differentiation and maturation, **immunomodulation by MSCs**, improving safety issues with cell transplantation, **altering the recipient microenvironment** for favourable acceptance by pre-vascularising the donor site and understanding the role **microbiome** plays in grafting integration.

The **future applications of TE in dentistry are cell sheet technology** (delivering stem cells without a scaffold) for **regenerating the periodontal ligament**, using IOS and CBCT scans for **bioprinting customised scaffolds for guided bone regeneration (GBR)** and **guided tissue regeneration (GTR)**, and perhaps **synthetic odontogenesis (biotooth engineering).**

Key points

- TE and RM achieve the same objective of regeneration but by difference means.
- The term TE was coined in the 1980s, but the concept dates back to BCE.
- Building blocks of TE are a scaffold, cells and bioactive stimuli.
- TE is used for transplants, life-supporting devices and drug development.
- Currently, 'off-the-shelf' organs and teeth are elusive and fanciful.

75 Stem cells

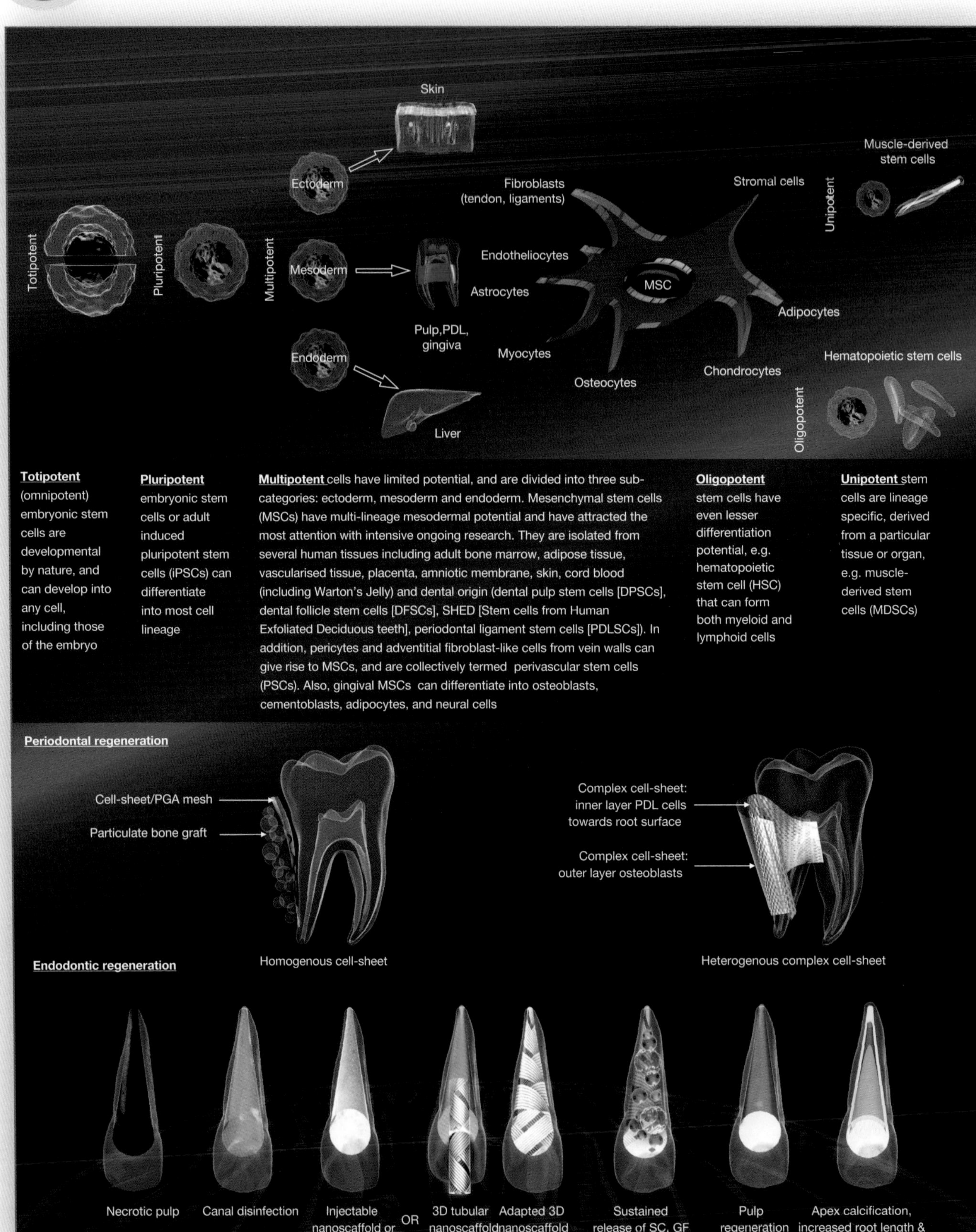

Stem cells are a key component of **tissue engineering (TE)** and **regenerative medicine (RM)**. Although in nascency, stem cell technology is perceived as the augury of personalised medicine and **personalised dentistry**. Stem cells are defined as **progenitor cells** with the **capability to differentiate into other cell lineage**. The nomenclature of stem cells varies, and is named after the donor animal, the source of tissue or organ or more commonly according to the differentiation potential.

Mesenchymal stem cells (MSCs)

Mesodermal differentiation cells were termed **'mesenchymal stem cells' (MSCs)** by Arnold Caplan in the 1990s and have several backronyms. But in light of recent research regarding the importance of the **secretome containing bioactive agents** (cytokine/growth factors) for creating a microenvironment termed **trophic activity**, Caplan has suggested **a revised appellation, 'medicinal signalling cells'**, respecting the original MSCs acronym. The first application of MSCs in RM was in 2004. MSCs are **multipotent cells** with the ability to differentiate into a particular mesenchymal tissue. Besides their differentiation ability, **human MSCs (hMSCs)** possess unique properties of **immunomodulation (both immunosuppression and immunostimulation)**, anti-inflammation, antimicrobial, angiogenesis, antifibrosis, antiscarring and anti-apoptosis (by mitochondrial transfer). This allows **allogenic MSCs to be administered via blood transfusions or TE for treating a variety of diseases** such as myocardial infarct ischaemia, graft-versus-host disease (GVHD), Crohn's Disease, rheumatoid arthritis, tendinitis, cartilage and meniscus repair, stroke, anticarcinogenic therapy, spinal cord injuries and **periodontitis**. Furthermore, it was previously assumed MSCs needed to be placed at the site of the damaged or injured tissues to initiate regeneration, but the current thinking is that the signals or **'commands' from the secretome macromolecules trigger regeneration.** However, identifying which bioactive factor in the secretome is therapeutic for a specific disease is still unclear.

Stem cells of dental origin

DPSCs are considered a type of MSCs but with a **higher clonogenic and proliferative potential** compared to those derived from the bone marrow. The popularity of dental stem cells for research and clinical applications is attractive since harvesting is cost-effective and relatively simple from extracted teeth (e.g. wisdom teeth, following trauma or for orthodontic reasons). Also, **autologous and allogenic dental stem cells** are available from many cell banks around the world. **DPSCs have the innate differentiation ability** for **neurogenesis, adipogenesis, osteogenesis, chondrogenesis, angiogenesis, dentinogenesis and calcification.** These mechanisms are governed by growth factors released from DPSCs, e.g. basic fibroblast growth factor b (bFGF), transforming growth factor-β (TGF-β3), nerve growth factor (NGF), platelet-derived growth factor (PDGF) and insulin-like growth factors (IGF) I and II to name a few.

Regenerative dentistry

Although **currently no specific dental treatment modality exists using stem cells**, research in this field has increased exponentially in the last decade, primarily **concentrating on periodontal and endodontic regeneration.** The aim of **periodontal regeneration is to regenerate the periodontal ligament (PDL), cementum and alveolar bone. Cytotherapy represents a novel cell-sheet** approach by combining stem cells with a modified **TE technology without a scaffold**. The benefits of a scaffold-free cell-sheet are that no artificial materials are used, thus **avoiding the toxic byproducts of synthetic biodegradable polymers**. Also, both **odontogenic (PDLSCs and DPSCs) and non-odontogenic (iPSCs or bone marrow MSCs)** can be utilised. Autologous PDLSCs are obtained from extracted teeth, or allogeneic MSCs or PDLSCs from a stem cell bank. The cells are cultured with growth factors (e.g. 4-(4-methoxyphenyl)pyrido[40,30:4,5]thieno[2,3-*b*]pyridine-2-carboxamide [TH]) and umbilical vein endothelial cells (for angiogenesis) at reduced temperature to form cell-sheets that are immersed in a collagen gel carrier ready for transplantation by conventional open flap surgery. The **cell-sheets can be homogenous,** using exclusively PDL or bone cells, and the regeneration limited to a specific type of tissue. Conversely, a **heterogeneous complex cell-sheet**, consisting of several layers of PDL and bone cells, simultaneously **regenerates both PDL-like and bone-like tissue** in three dimensions. Moreover, a **complex cell-sheet** is thicker and allows contouring to the desired anatomical form, whereas single cell-sheets require particulate bone-grafting materials, which are prone to dislodge and stray from the defect. The main issue with this technique is stem cell stabilisation and sufficient quantity, plus the fabrication process is costly and protracted.

The methods for **regenerating the pulp-dentine complex are tissue engineering (TE) using a nanofibrous scaffold** fabricated by electrospinning, molecular self-assembly, thermally induced phase separation (TIPS) and 3D bioprinting, or injecting a cocktail of stem cells ladened with growth factors without using a scaffold. The **nanoscaffolds** are biocompatible, biodegradable, mimics the ECM, support and promote stem cells proliferation and differentiation, maintain cell phenotype and allow sustained physical and chemical stimuli from antibiotics and antigenic factors.

Rejuvenation

Ageing is genetically determined, manifested by decreased reparative and regenerative capacity due to depletion and dysfunction of stem cells. The **theories of chronological ageing** are **cumulative DNA damage** or the **epigenectic model**. The former suggests escalating degradation of DNA as the cause of ageing, but **fails to explain resetting of the clock to zero at conception.** The epigenectic mode is gaining popularity, stating that **ageing is reversible** and modulated by progressive changes in chromatin regulation due to DNA methylation. **If adult somatic cells are reprogrammed to an embryonic-like state,** using genes such as NANOG and LIN28, **the induced pluripotent stem cells' (iPSCs) epigenetic age is reset to zero**, and can then be used as **anti-senescence therapy** for rejuvenating tissues, organs and possibly the entire body, turning back the clock and **having a second chance!**

Key points

- Stem cells are capable of differentiating into another cell lineage.
- Stem cells are classified according to their differentiation potential.
- Sources of stem cells include embryonic and adult tissues.
- Stem cells are used for TE and RM.
- MSCs are the subject of intense research due to their unique therapeutic properties.
- Regenerative dentistry includes endodontic and periodontal regeneration.
- Stem cells are forerunners of personalised medicine/dentistry and rejuvenation therapies.

Index

Note: Bold page numbers denote images/illustration pages

C

D

E

F

G

H

P